SITE-SPECIFIC CANCER SERIES

Central Nervous System Cancers

Edited by
Deborah Hutchinson Allen, RN, MSN, CNS, FNP-BC, AOCNP®,
and Laurie L. Rice, RN, MSN, ANP-BC

Oncology Nursing Society
Pittsburgh, Pennsylvania

ONS Publications Department
Publisher: Leonard Mafrica, MBA, CAE
Director of Publications: Barbara Sigler, RN, MNEd
Managing Editor: Lisa M. George, BA
Technical Content Editor: Angela D. Klimaszewski, RN, MSN
Staff Editor II: Amy Nicoletti, BA
Copy Editor: Laura Pinchot, BA
Graphic Designer: Dany Sjoen

Library of Congress Cataloging-in-Publication Data
Central nervous system cancers / edited by Deborah Hutchinson Allen and Laurie L. Rice.
    p. ; cm. -- (Site-specific cancer series)
  Includes bibliographical references.
  ISBN 978-1-890504-98-4 (alk. paper)
  1. Central nervous system--Cancer. 2. Central nervous system--Cancer--Nursing. I. Allen, Deborah Hutchinson. II. Rice, Laurie L. III. Oncology Nursing Society. IV. Series: Site-specific cancer series.
  [DNLM: 1. Central Nervous System Neoplasms--nursing. WY 156]
  RC280.N43C457 2010
  616.99'481--dc22

                                                                                      2010030814

Publisher's Note
This book is published by the Oncology Nursing Society (ONS). ONS neither represents nor guarantees that the practices described herein will, if followed, ensure safe and effective patient care. The recommendations contained in this book reflect ONS's judgment regarding the state of general knowledge and practice in the field as of the date of publication. The recommendations may not be appropriate for use in all circumstances. Those who use this book should make their own determinations regarding specific safe and appropriate patient-care practices, taking into account the personnel, equipment, and practices available at the hospital or other facility at which they are located. The editors and publisher cannot be held responsible for any liability incurred as a consequence from the use or application of any of the contents of this book. Figures and tables are used as examples only. They are not meant to be all-inclusive, nor do they represent endorsement of any particular institution by ONS. Mention of specific products and opinions related to those products do not indicate or imply endorsement by ONS. Web sites mentioned are provided for information only; the hosts are responsible for their own content and availability. Unless otherwise indicated, dollar amounts reflect U.S. dollars.

ONS publications are originally published in English. Publishers wishing to translate ONS publications must contact the ONS Publishing Division about licensing arrangements. ONS publications cannot be translated without obtaining written permission from ONS. (Individual tables and figures that are reprinted or adapted require additional permission from the original source.) Because translations from English may not always be accurate or precise, ONS disclaims any responsibility for inaccuracies in words or meaning that may occur as a result of the translation. Readers relying on precise information should check the original English version.

Printed in the United States of America

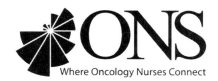

Oncology Nursing Society
Integrity • Innovation • Stewardship • Advocacy • Excellence • Inclusiveness

Contributors

Editors

Deborah Hutchinson Allen, RN, MSN, CNS, FNP-BC, AOCNP®
Clinical Nurse Specialist, Inpatient Oncology
Duke University Medical Center
Durham, North Carolina
Chapter 4. Pathology, Histology, and Molecular Markers of Primary Brain Tumors

Laurie L. Rice, RN, MSN, ANP-BC
Clinical Nurse Practitioner, Neuro-Oncology Brain Tumor Institute
Northwestern Medical Faculty Foundation
Chicago, Illinois
Chapter 1. Introduction

Authors

Jean M. Arzbaecher, RN, MS, APN, CNRN
Clinical Nurse Specialist
University of Chicago Brain Tumor Center
Chicago, Illinois
Chapter 2. Anatomy and Physiology of the Brain and Spine

Mary Beth Baer, BS
Research Associate
University of Pittsburgh School of Nursing
Pittsburgh, Pennsylvania
Chapter 11. Symptom Management and Psychological Issues

Rosemary Cashman, RN, MA, MSc(A), ACNP
Nurse Practitioner
BC Cancer Agency, Vancouver Centre
Vancouver, British Columbia, Canada
Chapter 5. Adult Cancers of the Brain and Spinal Cord

Sharon S. Cush, RN, OCN®
Neuro-Oncology Nurse Coordinator
Department of Neurosurgery
University of North Carolina
Chapel Hill, North Carolina
Chapter 7. Treatment Modalities: Surgical Treatments

Maureen Daniels, BScN, RN
Coordinator
The Gerry & Nancy Pencer Brain Tumor Centre
Princess Margaret Hospital, University Health Network
Toronto, Ontario, Canada
Chapter 9. Treatment Modalities: Radiotherapy

Annick Desjardins, MD, FRCPC
Assistant Professor of Medicine
Duke University Medical Center
Durham, North Carolina
Chapter 4. Pathology, Histology, and Molecular Markers of Primary Brain Tumors

Corrine Hoeppner, MSN, ARNP
Neuro-Oncology Nurse Practitioner
Seattle Children's Hospital
Seattle, Washington
Chapter 10. Special Considerations: Pediatric Therapeutic Modalities

Eva Lu T. Lee, MSN, RN, ANP-BC
Supervisor, Mid-Level Provider, Advanced Practice Nurse
University of Texas MD Anderson Cancer Center
Houston, Texas
Chapter 3. Patient Assessment

Maurene A. McQuestion, RN, BScN, MSc, CON(C)
Clinical Nurse Specialist, Advanced Practice Nurse
Princess Margaret Hospital, University Health Network
Toronto, Ontario, Canada
Chapter 9. Treatment Modalities: Radiotherapy

Kara Penne, RN, MSN, ANP, AOCNP®
Adult Nurse Practitioner—Senior
Duke Medical Center
Durham, North Carolina
Chapter 7. Treatment Modalities: Surgical Treatments

Paula R. Sherwood, RN, PhD, CNRN
Associate Professor
University of Pittsburgh
Pittsburgh, Pennsylvania
Chapter 11. Symptom Management and Psychological Issues

Alixis Van Horn, RN, CHPN
Clinical Coordinator, Brain Tumor Center
Tufts Medical Center
Boston, Massachusetts
Chapter 8. Treatment Modalities: Chemotherapy

Nancy E. Villanueva, PhD, CRNP, BC, CNRN
Neurosurgery Nurse Practitioner-Researcher
Penn State Milton S. Hershey Medical Center
Hershey, Pennsylvania
Chapter 12. Evidence-Based Practice: Where We Are Now

Melody Ann Watral, MSN, RN, CPNP-PC, CPON®
Certified Pediatric Nurse Practitioner (Pediatric Neuro-Oncology)
Department of Surgery, Division of Neurosurgery (Pediatrics)
Duke University Health Systems
Durham, North Carolina
Chapter 6. Pediatric Cancers of the Brain and Spinal Cord

Laurel J. Westcarth, MSN, RN, ANP-BC
Advanced Practice Nurse, Neuro-Oncology
University of Texas MD Anderson Cancer Center
Houston, Texas
Chapter 3. Patient Assessment

Disclosure

Editors and authors of books and guidelines provided by the Oncology Nursing Society are expected to disclose to the readers any significant financial interest or other relationships with the manufacturer(s) of any commercial products.

A vested interest may be considered to exist if a contributor is affiliated with or has a financial interest in commercial organizations that may have a direct or indirect interest in the subject matter. A "financial interest" may include, but is not limited to, being a shareholder in the organization; being an employee of the commercial organization; serving on an organization's speakers bureau; or receiving research from the organization. An "affiliation" may be holding a position on an advisory board or some other role of benefit to the commercial organization. Vested interest statements appear in the front matter for each publication.

Contributors are expected to disclose any unlabeled or investigational use of products discussed in their content. This information is acknowledged solely for the information of the readers.

The contributors provided the following disclosure and vested interest information:
Annick Desjardins, MD, FRCPC: AstraZeneca Pharmaceuticals, consultant; UCB Pharma, honorarium
Laurie L. Rice, RN, MSN, ANP-BC: Clinical Care Options, consultant, other remuneration
Alixis Van Horn, RN, CHPN: Sigma Tau Pharmaceuticals, consultant, honorarium

Contents

CHAPTER 1

Introduction

Laurie L. Rice, RN, MSN, ANP-BC

Introduction

Cancers of the central nervous system (CNS) are considered to be among the most devastating of all cancers. The brain and spinal cord are complex organs that control the CNS, the peripheral nervous system, and many of the voluntary and involuntary systems of the body. The effects can be devastating for the patient and the family when cancer attacks the CNS. It has been found that 20%–40% of all cancers metastasize to the brain (Cairncross, Kim, & Posner, 1980; Gavrilovic & Posner, 2005; Nathoo, Chahlavi, Barnett, & Toms, 2005; Posner, 1992).

Many families have experienced the effects of a CNS cancer. The diagnosis and death of Senator Edward Kennedy in 2009 brought public awareness to this disease state. All patients will have some change in personality, memory, motor skills, or executive functioning during the illness trajectory that compromises their quality of life. Care of those living with a brain and spinal tumor requires a broad knowledge base in neuro-oncology and a sensitive and realistic approach that optimizes quality of life and permits a sense of hopefulness to prevail. Care of informal caregivers also is an area of ongoing study.

Historical Perspective

The brain being the domicile for all the mysteries of the body has been suspected for ages. Dating back to the middle Stone Age period, archeologists found skulls with holes bored into them, a procedure called trepanation. The healed holes reveal that the surgeries had been successful and the patients had survived. Trepanation was carried out until the beginning of the 20th century. This treatment was believed to permit evil spirits to be removed and to treat seizures, headaches, and blindness. The first experiential physiologists, Galen, Vesalius, and Willis, whose work dated back to 130–200 AD, described on parchment paper the anatomy of the brain. Galen's view

of human anatomy dominated European medicine for 1,500 years (Kaye & Laws, 1995).

Modern brain surgery was first reported by Rickman Godlee in 1884. He operated on a 25-year-old Scottish farmer who suffered from epilepsy and progressive hemiparesis. He was found to have an oligodendroglioma and subsequently died from an infection (Kaye & Laws, 1995). The discoveries in the 19th century of asepsis, anesthesia, and neurologic localization of the brain tumor allowed modern brain surgery to flourish. The 20th century found a surge of technologic advances mostly focused on diagnostic and surgical techniques. Treatment choices have remained few with no grand slams, but the discovery of temozolomide provided hope.

The 21st century has just begun to reveal advances. Personalized treatments based on tumor typing may be on the horizon. MGMT (chemically known as O-6-methylguanine DNA methyltransferase) status of the tumor was found to differentiate those patients who may be more receptive to temozolomide (Hegi et al., 2005) (see Chapters 5 and 8 for discussions regarding MGMT). Scientists are working to find the genomic makeup of tumors and to work on effective treatments to possibly cure them. Thus far, CNS cancer death rates have not declined. Oncology nurses are also more sensitive to the overall psychosocial needs of patients and family caregivers.

Epidemiology

Low-grade (grade 2) tumors, including low-grade oligodendrogliomas, astrocytomas, and mixed oligoastrocytomas, have been found over time to progress to grade 3 or 4 tumors. The time may vary depending on the genetic makeup of the tumor, which can only be determined if a surgical pathology specimen is obtained and analyzed (Whittle, 2004). Despite the surgical and oncologic advances in technology, the prognosis remains poor for high-grade tumors. The diagnosis of

CNS cancer, with the daunting statistics on median survival of patients with high-grade tumors being less than 12 months, leaves little hope for the patient. Current knowledge reveals that most low-grade tumors will progress to high-grade tumors (van den Bent et al., 2005).

The National Cancer Institute (NCI, n.d.) estimated that 22,070 new cases of brain and other CNS cancers would be diagnosed in the United States in 2009. The American Brain Tumor Association (ABTA, 2010) clarifies this statistic further by estimating that 62,930 new cases of primary brain tumors would be diagnosed in 2010. Of this total, 23,720 are malignant and 39,210 are nonmalignant (ABTA, 2010). The death toll from cancers of the CNS is estimated to reach approximately 13,000 (NCI, n.d.).

An estimated 12,920 deaths were attributed to primary CNS cancers in 2009 (Central Brain Tumor Registry of the United States, 2010). The incidence of CNS tumors is highest in developed, industrialized countries where approximately 6–11 new cases are diagnosed annually per 100,000 population; mortality rates for all types of primary CNS tumors are 3–7 per 100,000 (Feraly, Bray, Pisani, & Parkin, 2000; Parkin, Whelan, Feraly, Teppo, & Thomas, 2002). Gliomas comprise 70% of all brain tumors with the most common type, glioblastoma multiforme, also being the most lethal (Ohgaki, 2009). From 2003 to 2007, the median age of patients at the time of a brain cancer diagnosis was 56 years old (NCI Surveillance, Epidemiology, and End Results, 2009).

Some controversy exists regarding a possible increase in the incidence of brain tumors, particularly in older adults. This may be due to improvements in neuroimaging access and technology (Christensen, Kosteljanetz, & Johansen, 2003; Legler et al., 1999). Population-based incidence data from the Netherlands Cancer Registry showed a stable incidence of adult and childhood gliomas (Houben et al., 2006). In this study, an increase in incidence of high-grade astrocytomas in adults was balanced by a decrease in low-grade astrocytomas.

Although the exact incidence of metastatic brain tumors is unknown, estimates range from double to 10 times the number of primary brain tumors, with at least 20%–40% of patients with cancer developing brain metastases at some point in their disease (Cairncross et al., 1980; Gavrilovic & Posner, 2005; Nathoo et al., 2004; Posner, 1992).

Risk Factors

Little consensus exists regarding the risk factors for developing primary brain tumors. The general principles of tumorigenesis implicate an accumulation of inherited and acquired genetic alterations that allow cells to evade normal regulatory mechanisms and divide abnormally. The relationship between chromosome instability and cancer susceptibility is well established, as is the association of defective DNA repair mechanisms in individuals harboring chromosomal alterations (Busch, 1994; Wei et al., 1996). Heritable factors are implicated in a few rare autosomal dominant tumor syndromes (only one mutant gene is required to express the disease), including Li-Fraumeni syndrome, neurofibromatosis types 1 and 2, and Turcot syndrome (Ohgaki, 2009).

Environmental factors associated with this malignant transformation have been difficult to positively identify. Exposure to ionizing radiation has been established as a risk factor for CNS tumors through studies on atomic bomb survivors, as well as children treated with radiation for tinea capitis (ringworm of the scalp) (Hodges, Smith, Garrett, & Tate, 1992; Preston et al., 2002; Socié et al., 2000).

The observation that brain tumor incidence is increased in certain occupations, including firefighters, physicians, farmers, embalmers, and pathologists, has prompted studies of the effects of industrial and occupational chemical exposure, but no definitive causative agent has been found (Mazumdar et al., 2008). Studies on diet, alcohol consumption, tobacco, electromagnetic fields, and cell phone use have similarly resulted in conflicting and inconclusive findings about risk factors (Parascandola, 2001). Some viruses have been implicated in brain tumor development in animal models, but only HIV has been causally linked to brain cancer in humans (Brittain, 2002; McLaughlin-Drubin & Munger, 2008).

Clinical Practice Implications

The brain tumor diagnosis continues to provoke fear and anxiety in patients. Because of the brief median overall survival of less than 12 months for patients with glioblastoma multiforme, specialists in neuro-oncology have systematically researched the natural history of brain tumors. Through the tireless effort of those committed to improve outcomes, advances have been made in the initial surgical management of brain tumors, with a reduction in the morbidity while achieving the surgical objectives. For decades, radiation therapy has been shown to be an effective postsurgical adjuvant therapy, and the current fractionated regimen maximizes the efficacy while minimizing the toxicity of this therapy. Only recently have definitive results shown a benefit from chemotherapy drugs, particularly alkylating agents (Hegi et al., 2005).

With these therapeutic advances, the median survival today has increased several months compared to earlier last century. This is thought to be a result of both the aggressive and resistant biology of brain tumors and the difficulty with which promising agents can be delivered to the brain. To circumvent these barriers, innovations in the form of surgical bed polymer-based therapeutics delivery and positive-pressure interstitial therapy delivery have been tested in the surgical arena. Although the polymer-based therapeutics delivery methods, such as chemotherapy-impregnated wafers, have shown modest activity (Lassman & Holland, 2005), trials investigating the utility of positive-pressure interstitial therapy delivery used to deliver chemotherapeutic agents directly into the tumor have not yet yielded positive results (Debinski, 2002).

Scientists have embraced the challenge of advancing care by dissecting the molecular biologic basis of brain tumor formation and the molecular signatures that dictate tumors' behavior. By identifying unique molecules that appear to play important roles in brain tumor biology, the field of neuro-oncology has moved forward with a tailored approach to targeting and modifying treatment. Through these efforts, the U.S. Food and Drug Administration has approved promising new agents for use against brain tumors, with the most recent approval for bevacizumab, which targets the activity of vascular endothelial growth factor. Interestingly, as the fight against these tumors advances, the use of newer agents has rewritten what is known about the radiographic changes that occur when treating brain tumors, necessitating reevaluation of previous knowledge.

Summary

Today, tools and methods to analyze tumors and their behavior are becoming more prevalent. Clearly, efforts over the past century have yielded real advances; however, we have also come to realize that gains in survival must be balanced with the maintenance of quality of life. Recognizing that what is more important to patients is the length of their good quality of life, more and more researchers have incorporated measures into clinical trials that follow quality of life. Although we have yet to cure brain tumors, clear steps forward have been taken toward reaching this ultimate goal. Each advance injects hope to the team of caregivers and, more importantly, to those who live with this diagnosis.

This book will explore the current treatment for cancers of the CNS. Nurses are trying to make a difference in the outcomes of our patients in survival and quality of life. Our future endeavors will focus on not only basic science questions but also on quality of life for patients, caregivers, and families.

The author wishes to acknowledge Kenji Muro, MD, and Rosemary Cashman, RN, MA, MSc(A), ACNP, for their contributions to this chapter.

References

American Brain Tumor Association. (2010). *Facts and statistics, 2010.* Retrieved from http://www.abta.org/sitefiles/pdflibrary/ABTA-FactsandStatistics2010.pdf

Brittain, D. (2002). Management of cancer in patients with HIV. *Southern African Journal of HIV Medicine, 3,* 24–28. Retrieved from http://ajol.info/index.php/sajhivm/article/viewFile/44742/28241

Busch, D. (1994). Genetic susceptibility to radiation and chemotherapy injury: Diagnosis and management. *International Journal of Radiation Oncology, Biology, Physics, 30,* 997–1002.

Cairncross, J.G., Kim, J.H., & Posner, J.B. (1980). Radiotherapy for brain metastases. *Annals of Neurology, 7,* 529–541. doi:10.1002/ana.410070606

Central Brain Tumor Registry of the United States. (2010). *CBTRUS statistical report: Primary brain and central nervous system tumors diagnosed in the United States in 2004–2006.* Retrieved from http://www.cbtrus.org/2010-NPCR-SEER/CBTRUS-WEBREPORT-Final-3-2-10.pdf

Christensen, H.C., Kosteljanetz, M., & Johansen, C. (2003). Incidences of gliomas and meningiomas in Denmark, 1943 to 1997. *Neurosurgery, 52,* 1327–1333. doi:10.1227/01.NEU.0000064802.46759.53

Debinski, W. (2002). Local treatment of brain tumours with targeted chimera cytotoxic proteins. *Cancer Investigation, 20,* 801–809.

Feraly, J., Bray, F., Pisani, P., & Parkin, D.M. (2000). *Globocan 2000: Cancer incidence, mortality and prevalence worldwide.* Lyon, France: International Agency for Research on Cancer.

Gavrilovic, I.T., & Posner, J.B. (2005). Brain metastases: Epidemiology and pathophysiology. *Journal of Neuro-Oncology, 75,* 5–14. doi:10.1007/s11060-004-8093-6

Hegi, M.E., Diserens, A.C., Gorlia, T., Hamou, M.F., de Tribolet, N., Weller, M., … Stupp, R. (2005). MGMT silencing and benefit from temozolomide in glioblastoma. *New England Journal of Medicine, 352,* 997–1003. doi:10.1056/NEJMoa043331

Hodges, L.C., Smith, J.L., Garrett, A., & Tate, S. (1992). Prevalence of glioblastoma multiforme in subjects with prior therapeutic radiation. *Journal of Neuroscience Nursing, 24,* 79–83.

Houben, M.P., Aben, K.K., Teepen, J.L., Schouten-Van Meeteren, A.Y., Tijsen, C.C., Van Dujin, C.M., & Coebergh, J.W. (2006). Stable incidence of childhood and adult glioma in the Netherlands, 1989–2003. *Acta Oncologica, 45,* 272–279. doi:10.1080/02841860500543190

Kaye, A.H., & Laws, E.R. (1995). Historical perspective. In A.H. Kaye & E.R. Laws (Eds.), *Brain tumors: An encyclopedic approach* (pp. 3–8). New York, NY: Churchill Livingstone.

Lassman, A., & Holland, E. (2005, October). Glioblastoma multiforme—past, present and future. *US Neurology Review,* pp. 1–6. Retrieved from http://www.touchneurology.com/files/article_pdfs/neuro_1887

Legler, J.M., Ries, L.A.G., Smith, M.A., Warren, J.L., Heineman, E.F., Kaplan, R.S., & Linet, M.S. (1999). Brain and other central nervous system cancers: Recent trends in incidence and mortality. *Journal of the National Cancer Institute, 91,* 1382–1390. doi:10.1093/jnci/91.16.1382

Mazumdar, M., Liu, C.-Y., Wang, S.-F., Pan, P.-C., Wu, M.-T., Christiani, D.C., & Kaohsiung Brain Tumor Research Group. (2008). No association between parental or subject occupation and brain tumor risk. *Cancer Epidemiology, Biomarkers and Prevention, 17,* 1835–1837. doi:10.1158/1055-9965.EPI-08-0035

McLaughlin-Drubin, M.E., & Munger, K. (2008). Viruses associated with human cancer. *Biochimica et Biophysica Acta, 1782,* 127–150. doi:10.1016/j.bbadis.2007.12.005

Nathoo, N., Chahlavi, A., Barnett, G.H., & Toms, S.A. (2005). Pathobiology of brain metastases. *Journal of Clinical Pathology, 58,* 237–242. doi:10.1136/jcp.2003.013623

National Cancer Institute. (n.d.). Brain tumor. Retrieved from http://www.cancer.gov/cancertopics/types/brain

National Cancer Institute Surveillance, Epidemiology, and End Results. (2009, November). SEER stat fact sheets: Brain and other nervous system. Retrieved from http://seer.cancer.gov/statfacts/html/brain.html

Ohgaki, H. (2009). Epidemiology of brain tumors. *Methods in Molecular Biology, 472,* 323–342. doi:10.1007/978-1-60327-492-0_14

Parascandola, M. (2001, January). Cell phones, aluminum, Agent Orange: No? Yes? Maybe? Retrieved from http://www.dana.org/news/cerebrum/detail.aspx?id=3034

Parkin, D.M., Whelan, S.L., Feraly, J., Teppo, L., & Thomas, D.B. (Eds.). (2002). *Cancer incidence in five continents* (Vol. VIII). Lyon, France: International Agency for Research on Cancer.

Posner, J.B. (1992). Management of brain metastases. *Revue Neurologique, 148,* 477–487.

Preston, D.L., Ron, E., Yonehara, S., Toshihiro, K., Hideharu, F., Kishikawa, M., ... Mabuchi, K. (2002). Tumors of the nervous system and pituitary gland associated with atomic bomb radiation exposure. *Journal of the National Cancer Institute, 94,* 1555–1563.

Socié, G., Curtis, R.E., Deeg, H.J., Sobocinski, K.A., Filipovich, A.H., Travis, L.B., ... Horowitz, M.M. (2000). New malignant diseases after allogeneic marrow transplantation for childhood acute leukemia. *Journal of Clinical Oncology, 18,* 348–357.

van den Bent, M.J., Afra, D., de Witte, O., Ben Hassel, M., Schraub, S., Hoang-Huan, K., ... UK Medical Research Council. (2005). Long-term efficacy of early versus delayed radiotherapy for low-grade astrocytoma and oligodendroglioma in adults: The EORTC 22845 randomised trial. *Lancet, 366,* 985–990. doi:10.1016/S0140-6736(05)67070-5

Wei, Q., Spitz, M.R., Gu, J., Cheng, L., Xu, X., Strom, S.S., ... Hsu, T.C. (1996). DNA repair capacity correlates with mutagen sensitivity in lymphoblastoid cell lines. *Cancer Epidemiology, Biomarkers and Prevention, 5,* 199–204. Retrieved from http://cebp.aacrjournals.org/content/5/3/199.full.pdf

Whittle, I.R. (2004). The dilemma of low grade glioma. *Journal of Neurology, Neurosurgery and Psychiatry With Practical Neurology, 75,* 31–36. doi:10.1136/jnnp.2004.040501

CHAPTER 2

Anatomy and Physiology of the Brain and Spine

Jean M. Arzbaecher, RN, MS, APN, CNRN

Introduction

This chapter offers an overview of basic neuroanatomy and neurophysiology. Basic cellular and anatomic structures, cerebrospinal fluid (CSF), circulation, and general functions of structures will be reviewed as they relate to the care of patients with central nervous system (CNS) cancers. An understanding of the cells and structures of the brain and spinal cord will give the nurse insight into the complex needs and problems that these patients encounter.

Cells of the Central Nervous System

The human brain is composed of billions of cells (Hickey, 2003b; Martin, 1989). Primary brain tumors resemble specific native cellular structures. The two predominant types of cells in the CNS are neurons and neuroglial cells (Martin, 1989). Neurons are the primary functional unit in the nervous system. They are membrane-excitable cells that are capable of conducting electrical impulses. They respond to stimuli, conduct impulses, and release specific chemical regulators. The word *glia* comes from the Greek word for "glue." Neuroglial or glial cells provide structural support, nutrition, and protection of the neurons, as well as modulation of their activity. The four different types of neuroglial cells are astrocytes, oligodendrocytes, ependymal cells, and microglia (Hickey, 2003b).

Astrocytes (*astro* is Greek for "star") are the most abundant type of glial cells and have a star-like appearance from the multiple processes that extend from the cell body (Hickey, 2003b) (see Figure 2-1). Their functions include providing nutrition for neurons, reinforcing the structural network that provides support for neurons, removing cellular debris, and regulating neurotransmitters. They may form "foot processes" or "astrocytic feet," which are extensions that extend to capillaries and control the movement of molecules from blood to the brain, thus providing a building block for the blood-brain

Figure 2-1. Astrocytes Lie Within Brain Tissues

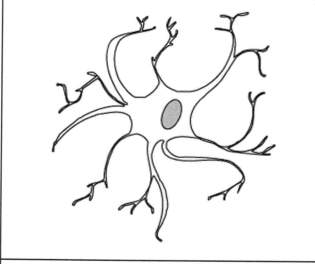

Note. From *A Primer of Brain Tumors: A Patient's Reference Manual* (8th ed., p. 28), by the American Brain Tumor Association, 2004. Retrieved from http://www.abta.org/siteFiles/SitePages/E2E7B6E1D9BBEAD2103 BCB9F2C80D588.pdf. Copyright 2004 by the American Brain Tumor Association. Reprinted with permission.

barrier (Zuccarelli, 2004), which will be discussed later in this chapter.

Oligodendrocytes have few branching processes. They line themselves along neurons and form the myelin sheath of the axon, which provides insulation and protection, allowing more efficient signal transmission to and from the brain and along the spinal cord (Hickey, 2003b; Martin, 1989).

Ependymal cells are epidermal cells, which line the ventricles of the brain and the central canal of the spinal cord (see Figure 2-2). They produce and secrete CSF and have a protective role in regulating the movement of substances from the bloodstream to the brain (Zuccarelli, 2004). Cilia on ependymal cells help to circulate the CSF.

Figure 2-2. Ependymal Cells Line the Ventricles

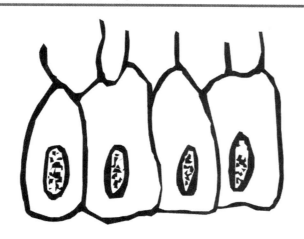

Note. From *A Primer of Brain Tumors: A Patient's Reference Manual* (8th ed., p. 35), by the American Brain Tumor Association, 2004. Retrieved from http://www.abta.org/siteFiles/SitePages/E2E7B6E1D9BBEAD2103 BCB9F2C80D588.pdf. Copyright 2004 by the American Brain Tumor Association. Reprinted with permission.

Microglia are neuroglial cells that are the resident macrophages of the brain and spinal cord. These cells act as the first and main form of active immune defense in the CNS, responding to infection or damage (Martin, 1989). They remove and disintegrate the waste products of neurons.

Transformation of glial or neuronal cells into primary brain tumors is a complex process that still is not completely understood. It is hypothesized that primary brain tumors arise from neural precursor cells (Gilbertson & Rich, 2007). This will be discussed in a later chapter.

Overview of the Brain

The brain, upon gross inspection, is gray in color and slightly smaller than the skull that encases it. The brain constitutes approximately 2% of body weight. The average weight of the brain of a young adult male is 1,400 g (Hickey, 2003b). Brain tissue including cell bodies and neuronal projections is gray in color and commonly referred to as *gray matter*. Regions that contain axons appear white and are commonly referred to as *white matter* (Martin, 1989).

The meninges are membranous layers of connective tissue that surround the brain and the spinal cord (see Figure 2-3). These layers or coverings line the brain and include the dura mater, arachnoid, and pia mater (Martin, 1989).

The four interconnected ventricles within the brain are filled with CSF (see Figure 2-4). The two lateral ventricles are on either side of the midline in the lower and inner portion of each cerebral hemisphere. The third ventricle is a single structure located in the midline with the thalamus surrounding it on both sides. It connects to the fourth ventricle via the aqueduct of Sylvius. The fourth ventricle forms the roof of the pons and the medulla in the brain stem. The central canal of the spinal cord is continuous with the fourth ventricle (Martin, 1989). The walls of each ventricle contain a cauliflower-like structure called the *choroid plexus*, which secretes most of the CSF (Littlejohns, 2004; Martin, 1989).

The tentorium cerebelli or cerebellar tentorium is an extension of the dura mater that separates the cerebellum from the inferior portion of the occipital lobes, as shown in Figure 2-4. The supratentorial space contains the cerebral hemispheres and the diencephalon. The diencephalon is a division of the cerebrum and is composed of the thalamus, hypothalamus, subthalamus, and epithalamus. These are many of the more "primitive" or evolutionarily conserved subcortical supratentorial structures. The corpus callosum is a thick area of nerve fibers in the midline that connects the left and right cerebral hemispheres. Every lobe of one hemisphere is connected with the corresponding lobe of the opposite hemisphere. The supratentorial part of the brain is further identified by lobes: the frontal lobe, parietal lobe, temporal lobe, and occipital lobe (see Figure 2-5).

The infratentorial space (also called the *posterior fossa*) contains the cerebellum and the brain stem. The cerebellum (Latin for "little brain") is the large, bilaterally symmetrical structure in the posterior fossa. The brain stem is composed of the midbrain, pons, and medulla (see Figure 2-6).

These structures will be referred to throughout this chapter and the remainder of the text. It is incumbent upon the nurse to use the figures to imprint the locations of specific components of the brain.

Blood-Brain Barrier

The brain and spinal cord are considered "immunologically privileged sites" (Nicholas & Lukas, 2010, p. 169) in that they are separated from the rest of the body by the blood-brain barrier. The blood-brain barrier is composed of a tightly bound network of tight junctions of endothelial cells and astrocytic foot processes (Hickey, 2003b; Littlejohns, 2004). Before molecules in the blood can enter the CNS, they must go through the blood-brain barrier, which restricts passage of substances to a greater extent than endothelial cells in the rest of the body. This protects the brain from blood-borne substances, toxins, and pathogens, thus maintaining a stable environment for neural tissue (Zuccarelli, 2004). One clinical consequence of the blood-brain barrier is that many chemotherapeutic agents do not have access to the CNS and, in turn, to brain tumor cells. The blood-brain barrier is deemed to be less robust in the setting of brain tumors (Posner, 1995); however, it still effectively prevents the delivery of the majority of chemotherapeutic agents at effective doses to CNS tumor cells (Hickey, 2003a).

Figure 2-3. Structure of the Meninges

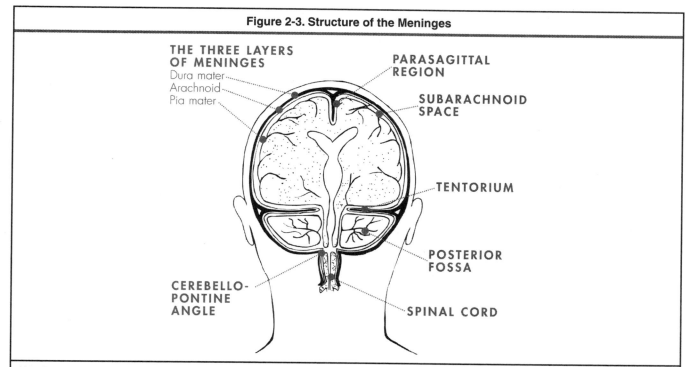

Note. From *A Primer of Brain Tumors: A Patient's Reference Manual* (8th ed., p. 44), by the American Brain Tumor Association, 2004. Retrieved from http://www.abta.org/siteFiles/SitePages/E2E7B6E1D9BBEAD2103BCB9F2C80D588.pdf. Copyright 2004 by the American Brain Tumor Association. Reprinted with permission.

Figure 2-4. The Tentorium Displaying Supratentorial and Infratentorial Structures

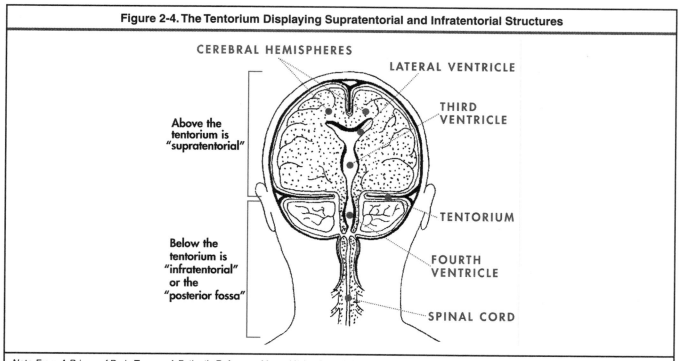

Note. From *A Primer of Brain Tumors: A Patient's Reference Manual* (8th ed., p. 6), by the American Brain Tumor Association, 2004. Retrieved from http://www.abta.org/siteFiles/SitePages/E2E7B6E1D9BBEAD2103BCB9F2C80D588.pdf. Copyright 2004 by the American Brain Tumor Association. Reprinted with permission.

Figure 2-5. Lobes of the Brain

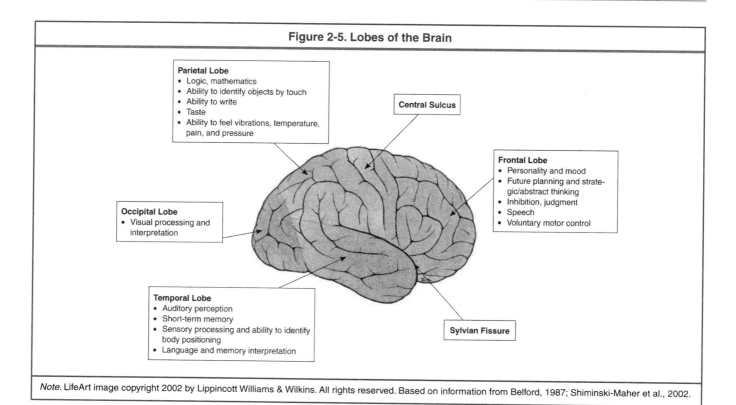

Parietal Lobe
- Logic, mathematics
- Ability to identify objects by touch
- Ability to write
- Taste
- Ability to feel vibrations, temperature, pain, and pressure

Central Sulcus

Frontal Lobe
- Personality and mood
- Future planning and strate-gic/abstract thinking
- Inhibition, judgment
- Speech
- Voluntary motor control

Occipital Lobe
- Visual processing and interpretation

Temporal Lobe
- Auditory perception
- Short-term memory
- Sensory processing and ability to identify body positioning
- Language and memory interpretation

Sylvian Fissure

Note. LifeArt image copyright 2002 by Lippincott Williams & Wilkins. All rights reserved. Based on information from Belford, 1987; Shiminski-Maher et al., 2002.

Figure 2-6. Major Structures of the Brain, Sagittal View

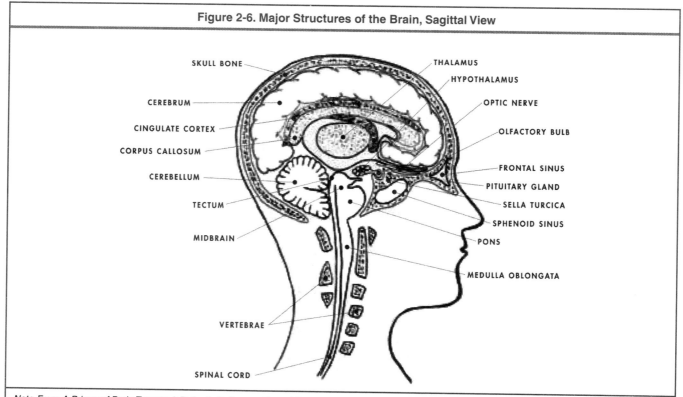

SKULL BONE

CEREBRUM

CINGULATE CORTEX

CORPUS CALLOSUM

CEREBELLUM

TECTUM

MIDBRAIN

VERTEBRAE

SPINAL CORD

THALAMUS

HYPOTHALAMUS

OPTIC NERVE

OLFACTORY BULB

FRONTAL SINUS

PITUITARY GLAND

SELLA TURCICA

SPHENOID SINUS

PONS

MEDULLA OBLONGATA

Note. From *A Primer of Brain Tumors: A Patient's Reference Manual* (8th ed., p. 7), by the American Brain Tumor Association, 2004. Retrieved from http://www.abta.org/siteFiles/SitePages/E2E7B6E1D9BBEAD2103BCB9F2C80D588.pdf. Copyright 2004 by the American Brain Tumor Association. Reprinted with permission.

Meninges

The meninges are membranous layers of connective tissue that surround the brain and the spinal cord (see Figure 2-3). The three layers from the outermost layer inward are the dura mater, arachnoid, and pia mater (Martin, 1989). The term *leptomeninges*, or "thin meninges," is used to refer to the two innermost layers, the pia mater and the arachnoid mater (Littlejohns, 2004). Leptomeningeal metastasis, also known as carcinomatosis meningitis, is the spread of cancer via the leptomeninges and will be discussed further in Chapter 5.

Cerebrospinal Fluid and the Ventricular System

CSF is a clear, odorless solution that fills the ventricles of the brain and the subarachnoid space of the brain and spinal cord (Adams, 2008). Its purpose is to provide buoyancy and act as a shock absorber, cushioning the brain and spinal cord against injury caused by movement.

CSF flows in a closed system from the lateral ventricles into the third ventricle and then the fourth. From there, it passes into the subarachnoid space. The CSF can flow all the way down to the end of the spinal cord around the cauda equina, where lumbar punctures are performed, and then back up (Hickey, 2003b). This flow of the CSF explains the potential spread of cancer cells leading to leptomeningeal metastasis and causing leptomeningeal disease, which is discussed in further detail in a later chapter.

Most of the CSF produced daily is reabsorbed into the arachnoid villi, which are projections from the subarachnoid space into the venous sinus of the brain. Arachnoid villi are very permeable and allow CSF to exit easily from the subarachnoid space into the venous sinuses (Hickey, 2003b). Figure 2-7 illustrates the ventricular system and flow of CSF.

CSF is produced at a rate of 500 ml per day (Hickey, 2003b). The average volume in the CNS is 150 ml, with 25 ml in each lateral ventricle (one-third of the total fluid) and the remaining fluid in the other ventricles and over the surface and base of the brain and spinal cord (Littlejohns, 2004). Much more CSF is produced each day than the CNS can hold, and CSF in the normal brain is cycled three to four times per day. In turn, it is important that the arachnoid granulations continue to filter CSF. When they are unable to, communicating hydrocephalus develops. Tumors that grow within or near the ventricle may become of sufficient size to obstruct the flow of CSF. When flow between the ventricles in the brain is blocked, noncommunicating hydrocephalus can develop (Hickey, 2003a).

Intracranial pressure (ICP) is the pressure normally exerted by CSF that circulates around the brain and spinal cord and within the cerebral ventricles. The normal range of ICP when monitored in a clinical setting is generally 0–15 mm Hg (Hickey, 2003a) or 50–200 mm H_2O (Adams, 2008). ICP monitoring is generally reserved for the intensive care setting. However, the majority of patients with a CNS cancer are

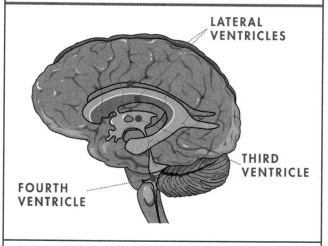

Figure 2-7. Flow of Cerebrospinal Fluid Through the Brain Lining and Ventricular Spaces

LATERAL VENTRICLES

THIRD VENTRICLE

FOURTH VENTRICLE

Note. From *A Primer of Brain Tumors: A Patient's Reference Manual* (8th ed., p. 4), by the American Brain Tumor Association, 2004. Retrieved from http://www.abta.org/siteFiles/SitePages/E2E7B6E1D9 BBEAD2103BCB9 F2C80D588.pdf. Copyright 2004 by the American Brain Tumor Association. Reprinted with permission.

treated as an outpatient and not hospitalized in an intensive care unit, thus the homecare or outpatient treatment team must determine whether the patient has signs and symptoms of increased ICP. Signs and symptoms of increased ICP include headache, nausea and vomiting, decreased level of consciousness, papilledema, and neurologic worsening.

An understanding of the pathophysiologic effects of brain tumors requires an understanding of the Monroe-Kellie hypothesis and increased ICP. Its premise is that the skull, a rigid compartment, is filled to capacity with essentially incompressible contents: brain tissue (80%), blood (10%), and CSF (10%). If the volume of any one component increases, another component must decrease reciprocally for the overall volume to remain constant or ICP will rise (Littlejohns, 2004). Depending on the rate of tumor growth, there is little time for the intracranial compartment to accommodate the lesion, and signs and symptoms of increased ICP may be noted in a shorter time frame.

As noted previously, if a tumor blocks the flow of CSF between the ventricles, noncommunicating hydrocephalus occurs, with symptoms of rapidly increased ICP within hours. In most patients with brain tumors, vasogenic edema develops in the surrounding tissue as a result of compression, and increased ICP may occur within days to weeks, but not as rapidly as with CSF obstruction (Hickey, 2003a).

Circulation

The brain receives its blood supply predominantly from two pairs of arteries: the internal carotid arteries and the vertebral arteries. The internal carotid arteries are termed the *anterior circulation*, and the vertebral arteries are termed the *posterior circulation*. The cerebral hemispheres receive blood from both anterior and posterior circulation, whereas the brain stem receives its blood supply only from the posterior circulation (Martin, 1989).

The internal carotid arteries have several branches, which include (Hickey, 2003b)
- Ophthalmic arteries to supply the retina and other structures in the orbit
- Posterior communicating artery, which connects the anterior circulation with the posterior circulation
- Anterior choroidal artery, which supplies the optic tract, choroid plexus, and portions of the internal capsule and basal ganglia
- Anterior cerebral artery, which supplies medial surfaces of the frontal and parietal lobes
- Middle cerebral artery, which forms the largest branches, which in turn supply parts of the basal ganglia, internal capsule, and the entire lateral cortical surface of the brain.

The vertebrobasilar system supplies the posterior circulation to the brain. The two vertebral arteries join each other at the level of the brain stem near the junction of the pons and medulla to form the single basilar artery. The basilar artery ends at the junction of the midbrain and pons where it divides into two posterior cerebral arteries, which supply the inferior part of the temporal lobe and the occipital lobe. It also gives rise to anterior inferior and superior cerebellar arteries, which supply blood to the cerebellum (Martin, 1989).

The circle of Willis, located at the base of the skull, is a circle of connected arteries that supply blood to the brain. It is significant in that it allows communication of blood from the anterior to the posterior areas of the brain, as well as between the right and the left cerebral hemispheres. If one of the arteries supplying the circle is blocked or narrowed, blood flow from the other vessels can often preserve the perfusion of the brain (Brazis, Masdeu, & Biller, 2001; Martin, 1989).

The components of the circle of Willis are the anterior cerebral arteries; the anterior communicating arteries, which connect the two anterior cerebral arteries; the internal carotid arteries; the posterior cerebral arteries; and the posterior communicating arteries, which connect the anterior and posterior circulation. The basilar artery and middle cerebral arteries are not considered part of the circle (Goldberg, 2003; Martin, 1989).

The venous drainage of the brain and dura includes the veins of the brain itself, the dural venous sinuses, the dura's meningeal veins, and the diploic veins between the tables of the skull. Communication exists among most of these channels. Cerebral veins, unlike systemic veins, are thin walled, have no valves, and seldom accompany the corresponding cerebral arteries. Cerebral veins empty into the dural sinuses, a collection of large channels between the layers of the dura, which function as low-pressure channels for venous flow.

They, in turn, empty into the jugular veins, which return the blood to the systemic circulation (Martin, 1989).

General Functions According to Lobes

When discussing brain tumors, it is important to differentiate whether the lesions are supratentorial (above the tentorium) or infratentorial (below the tentorium) (see Figure 2-4). The location of the tumor can aid in determining the type of tumor, as different tumors occur with different frequencies at each location. Additionally, most childhood tumors are infratentorial, whereas most adult tumors are supratentorial. The supratentorial structures receive approximately 80% of the cerebral blood volume, so the majority of hematogenous metastases also develop there (Gavrilovic & Posner, 2005).

The location of a tumor in the brain plays an important role in the overall neurologic picture of the patient. A small, slow-growing tumor in a critical area of the brain (for example, the brain stem) can cause a devastating neurologic picture, whereas a large, fast-growing tumor in another area (for example, the right frontal lobe) can cause minimal deficits. For this reason, the terms *benign* and *malignant* are often not emphasized in discussions with patients about brain tumors. A benign tumor that is surgically unresectable or does not respond to conventional therapy may continue to grow and result in loss of significant neurologic function and ultimately life. In other words, a patient may have a benign tumor in a "malignant" location and vice versa.

Location of tumor will often give rise to focal (pertaining to that area of the brain) signs and symptoms. The brain is organized so that lesions in the supratentorial structures have an effect on the opposite (contralateral) side of the body with the exception of the cerebellum, where effects are on the same (ipsilateral) side (Brazis et al., 2001). A basic understanding of the lobes of the brain and their functions and common focal signs and symptoms will assist the nurse in explaining and perhaps predicting outcomes in patients with a tumor in these areas. Figure 2-5 illustrates the lobes of the brain and their functions.

Supratentorial Structures

Frontal Lobe

The frontal lobe is located at the front of each cerebral hemisphere and positioned anterior to the parietal lobe and above and anterior to the temporal lobes. It is separated from the parietal lobe by the central sulcus. Just anterior to the central sulcus is the primary motor cortex.

The major functions of the frontal lobes are cognition, higher-level executive functions (abstract thinking and reasoning), regulation of personality, and memory (Hickey, 2003b; Littlejohns, 2004). The motor control of speech is located in the dominant hemisphere of the frontal lobe in an area called the Broca area. Nearly all right-handed individuals have their dominant hemisphere on the left side of the brain. It is interesting to note, however, that a large majority of left-handed individuals also have their dominant hemisphere on the left. It may be important to determine the cerebral dominance in a left-handed individual in planning for a surgical resection of a tumor in the frontal lobe near the Broca area. Neurodiagnostic methods of determining cerebral dominance, such as functional magnetic resonance imaging, will be discussed in Chapter 3.

The motor cortex is located in the posterior aspect of the frontal lobe and separates the frontal lobe from the parietal lobe. It is responsible for the planning, control, and execution of voluntary movements of specific body parts.

Focal signs commonly seen in patients with frontal lobe tumors include difficulties in higher-level functioning; personality, behavior, and mood changes; fluent speech deficits; and unilateral (opposite the tumor) weakness (Hickey, 2003a; Lupica, 2004).

Parietal Lobe

The parietal lobe is located above the occipital and temporal lobe and behind the frontal lobe. The primary sensory cortex is located in the parietal lobe. The main function of the parietal lobe is the integration of sensory information, allowing interpretation of pain, temperature, light touch, vibration, spatial orientation, and position sense. In addition, awareness of the parts of one's body is controlled by the parietal lobe.

Focal signs commonly seen in patients with parietal lobe tumors include sensory deficits; inability to recognize objects; inability to distinguish left from right; and neglect syndrome, which is manifested by lack of awareness of one side (opposite the tumor) of the body or visual field (Hickey, 2003a; Lupica, 2004). Patients and families frequently mistake neglect for weakness. When testing for neurologic strength in a patient with parietal lobe dysfunction, it is important to ask the patient to focus on the affected side for more accurate assessment.

Temporal Lobe

The temporal lobe is directly below the frontal and parietal lobes. The primary auditory cortex is located in the temporal lobe, and its main functions are hearing and processing of spoken language. The auditory association area located in the dominant hemisphere of the temporal lobe is an area called Wernicke area (Hickey, 2003b; Littlejohns, 2004).

The temporal lobe is also associated with memory skills. An area called the interpretive area is located in the temporal lobe at the junction where the temporal, parietal, and occipital lobes meet and provides an integration of the somatic, auditory, and visual association areas (Hickey, 2003b).

Focal signs commonly seen with temporal lobe tumors are weakness, visual field deficits, memory deficits, and when the dominant lobe is involved, speech and language deficits (difficulty understanding the spoken word). Seizures arising from the temporal lobe are common and may include visual, auditory, or olfactory hallucinations; automatism; and amnesia for events. They may be preceded by an aura, which is part of the actual seizure. This can be an unusual emotion or peculiar sensation of the abdomen, epigastrium, or thorax or an abnormal smell. They are characteristic and repetitive in nature (Hickey, 2003a; Lupica, 2004).

Occipital Lobe

The occipital lobe is the smallest of the four lobes, located in the most posterior aspect of the cerebral hemispheres. The primary visual cortex is located in the occipital lobe. The major function of the occipital lobe is visual perception.

Focal signs commonly seen in occipital lobe lesions are associated with vision. These symptoms may include loss of vision in one half of the visual field (homonymous hemianopia) or one quarter of the visual field (homonymous quadrantanopia), visual hallucinations, and failure to recognize familiar objects (Hickey, 2003a; Lupica, 2004).

Diencephalon

The diencephalon is the portion of the brain that contains the thalamus and the hypothalamus. The thalamus surrounds the third ventricle. Its function includes relaying sensation, special sense, and motor signals to the cerebral cortex along with the regulation of consciousness, sleep, and alertness. The thalamus plays a role in conscious pain awareness, and damage to this area frequently causes a significant hypersensitivity to pain syndrome that usually only includes one half of the body (Brazis et al., 2001). The hypothalamus is directly below the thalamus and forms part of the walls of the third ventricle. One of the functions of the hypothalamus is to connect the nervous system with the endocrine system via the pituitary gland. The hypothalamus controls body temperature, hunger, thirst, sexual drive, and sleep-wake cycles (Hickey, 2003b).

Pituitary Gland

The hypophysis or pituitary gland is an endocrine gland located at the bottom of the hypothalamus (see Figure 2-6). It sits in a bony saddle called the *sella turcica*. Directly above the pituitary gland is the optic chiasma. The optic nerves, which are responsible for vision, leave the eyeballs and travel back to the optic chiasma where they partially cross before continuing to the back of the brain where vision is processed (Martin, 1989).

The pituitary gland modulates functions throughout the body by secreting hormones that control the other endocrine glands. The secretion of the pituitary gland is controlled by the hypothalamus. When pituitary lesions are detected, it is important to determine which hormones are oversecreted in order to identify treatment options.

Common symptoms resulting from tumors in the pituitary gland and hypothalamus are visual deficit caused by optic nerve involvement; specifically, compression of the optic chiasma can cause loss of the peripheral vision bilaterally (bitemporal hemianopia) (Brazis et al., 2001). Other symptoms include headache and endocrine dysfunction (Hickey, 2003a).

Infratentorial Structures

Brain Stem

The brain stem is in the lower part of the brain, which is continuous with the spinal cord. It is responsible for controlling our most vegetative functions. The three major divisions of the brain stem are (from superior to inferior) the midbrain, pons, and medulla (see Figure 2-6). Though small, this is an extremely important part of the brain, as the nerve connections of the motor and sensory systems from the main part of the brain to the rest of the body pass through the brain stem. The brain stem also plays a crucial role in the regulation of cardiac and respiratory function (Hickey, 2003b; Littlejohns, 2004; Martin, 1989). Cranial nerves 2–12 are found in the brain stem. Chapter 3 reviews each cranial nerve and its assessment in detail. Figure 2-8 illustrates the location of each of the cranial nerves in the brain as well as their basic function.

A lesion in the brain stem can cause devastating neurologic deficits. These may include lower cranial nerve deficits (swallowing, articulation, and gag reflex), motor and sensory deficits, vertigo, hiccups, ataxic gait, incoordination, nystagmus, and nausea and vomiting. Sudden death can occur from damage to vital respiratory and cardiac centers (Hickey, 2003a; Lupica, 2004). Obstructive hydrocephalus and rapidly increased ICP may develop from tumor encroachment on the ventricles.

Cerebellum

The cerebellum (see Figure 2-4) plays an important role in the integration of sensory perception, coordination, and motor control. All sensory modalities are circuited through the cerebellum, which provides input about muscle activity through feedback loops. The cerebellum controls fine movement, coordinates muscle groups, and maintains balance through these feedback loops (Hickey, 2003b; Littlejohns, 2004; Martin, 1989).

Movements are not lost when the cerebellum is damaged; however, the movements that were once automatic and precise become uncoordinated and erratic (Martin, 1989). Focal signs seen in cerebellar tumors include ataxic gait, incoordination, nystagmus, vertigo, and nausea. Obstruction of CSF and increased ICP are also common. A phenomenon called *cerebellar mutism* is common in children with posterior fossa tumors. It is a symptom complex including decreased or absent speech followed by dysarthria or slurred speech. It is thought to be a result of a transient decrease in

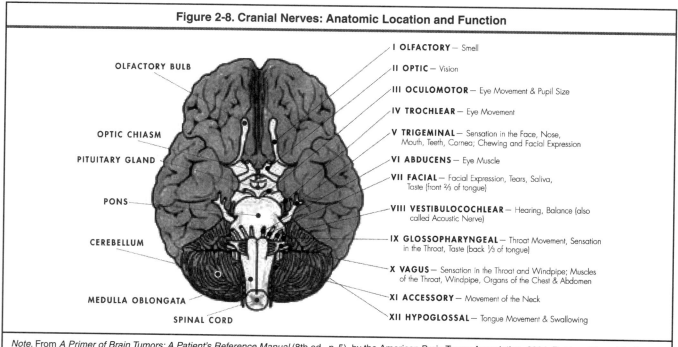

Figure 2-8. Cranial Nerves: Anatomic Location and Function

OLFACTORY BULB
OPTIC CHIASM
PITUITARY GLAND
PONS
CEREBELLUM
MEDULLA OBLONGATA
SPINAL CORD

I OLFACTORY — Smell
II OPTIC — Vision
III OCULOMOTOR — Eye Movement & Pupil Size
IV TROCHLEAR — Eye Movement
V TRIGEMINAL — Sensation in the Face, Nose, Mouth, Teeth, Cornea; Chewing and Facial Expression
VI ABDUCENS — Eye Muscle
VII FACIAL — Facial Expression, Tears, Saliva, Taste (front ⅔ of tongue)
VIII VESTIBULOCOCHLEAR — Hearing, Balance (also called Acoustic Nerve)
IX GLOSSOPHARYNGEAL — Throat Movement, Sensation in the Throat, Taste (back ⅓ of tongue)
X VAGUS — Sensation in the Throat and Windpipe; Muscles of the Throat, Windpipe, Organs of the Chest & Abdomen
XI ACCESSORY — Movement of the Neck
XII HYPOGLOSSAL — Tongue Movement & Swallowing

blood flow to the cerebellum (Charalambides, Dinopoulos, & Sgouros, 2009).

The Spinal Cord

The spine is a flexible column formed by a series of 33 bones called vertebrae, which are stacked on top of each other to support the head and trunk and protect the spinal cord. This vertebral column is composed of 33 vertebrae: 7 cervical, 12 thoracic, 5 lumbar, 5 sacral (fused into one), and 4 coccygeal (fused into one) (Hickey, 2003b; Littlejohns, 2004). Figure 2-9 shows the vertebral column details.

Each vertebra consists of an anterior solid segment known as the vertebral body and a posterior segment known as the arch. The vertebrae become larger as they descend in the vertebral column.

The spinal cord is a cylindrical structure within the vertebral column. It is an elongated mass of nerve tissue and support cells that starts from the base of the medulla. The spinal cord is the main pathway for information connecting the brain and the rest of the body. It extends from the first cervical vertebra to the lower border of the first lumbar vertebra. As the cord reaches the lower two levels of the thoracic region, it becomes tapered and is called the *conus medullaris*. The spinal cord may vary on where it forms the conus medullaris but approximately is at the level of the L1 or L2 vertebra. The range is from one vertebra higher to one vertebra lower: T12 to L3 (Reimann & Anson, 1944). The lumbar puncture is done at this level because the risk of cord injury is minimal when the patient is positioned properly (Adams, 2008). A non-neural filament, the filum terminale, continues until it attaches to the second segment of the fused coccyx (Hickey, 2003b; Littlejohns, 2004).

Spinal Cord Meninges

The spinal cord coverings that surround and protect it are the same as the brain: the dura, arachnoid, and pia. The spinal dura is a continuation of the inner layer of the cerebral dura. The spinal dura encases the spinal roots, spinal ganglia, and spinal nerves. The spinal dural sac terminates at the second or third sacral level. The arachnoid layer of the spinal meninges is a continuation of the cerebral arachnoid. The innermost layer, the pia, in the spinal cord is thicker, firmer, and less vascular than that found in the brain (Hickey, 2003b; Littlejohns, 2004; Martin, 1989).

When discussing spinal cord lesions, it is important to identify the lesion's location in relationship to the meninges. The lesion can be identified as extramedullary, which means outside of the spinal cord. This includes extradural, which is outside of the spinal dura within the epidural space, or intradural, which is within the spinal dura but not within the spinal cord. The lesion may also be identified as intramedullary, which is within the substance of the spinal cord (Schellinger, Propp, Villano, & McCarthy, 2008). Spinal cord tumors will

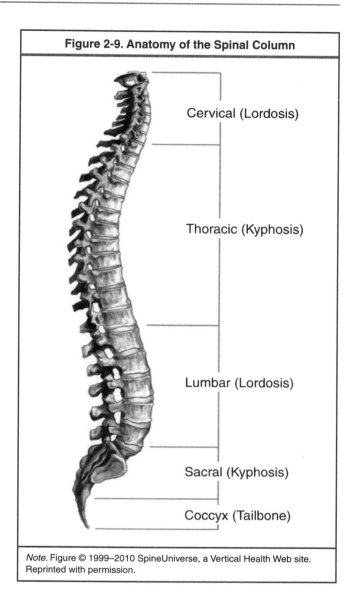

Figure 2-9. Anatomy of the Spinal Column

Cervical (Lordosis)

Thoracic (Kyphosis)

Lumbar (Lordosis)

Sacral (Kyphosis)

Coccyx (Tailbone)

Note. Figure © 1999–2010 SpineUniverse, a Vertical Health Web site. Reprinted with permission.

be discussed in Chapter 5 for adult tumors and Chapter 6 for pediatric tumors.

Spinal Circulation

The upper cervical cord receives its arterial blood supply from branches of the vertebral arteries. Below this, the spinal cord receives its arterial blood supply, for the most part, from the anterior spinal artery and two posterior spinal arteries. The venous system of the spine includes an intradural and extradural system (Hickey, 2003b; Littlejohns, 2004; Martin, 1989).

Cross Section of the Spinal Cord

When viewed in cross section, the spinal cord is an "H" or butterfly-shaped area of gray matter surrounded by white matter. Cross sections of the cord at various levels have differences in the shape and extent of gray and white matter. The gray matter consists of cell bodies and neuronal projections. This central region surrounds the central canal (an anatomic extension of the ventricles in the brain) and contains CSF. The white matter includes longitudinally running fiber tracts containing both sensory and motor neurons.

The white matter is composed of three columns: posterior, lateral, and anterior. Functional spinal cord tracts are located in the columns. Ascending tracts provide a pathway from the environment to the CNS and are mostly for sensory perception. Descending tracts provide a pathway from the CNS to the environment and are mostly for motor function. The name of the tract often gives an indication of whether it is an ascending or descending tract; the first structure in the name indicates where the tract originates. The location of the tumor on cross section will help to determine functional loss (Goldberg, 2003; Hickey, 2003b; Lupica, 2004).

- The posterior columns convey pressure, deep pain, position, and vibration sensations. They include the fasciculus gracilis, which carries impulses from the lower extremities, and fasciculus cuneatus, which carries impulses from the upper extremities.
- The lateral columns include the lateral spinothalamic tracts, which ascend from the cord to terminate in the thalamus and convey pain and temperature sensations, and the anterior and posterior spinocerebellar tracts, which convey information regarding touch and pressure from the muscles to regulate precise movement.
- The anterior columns include the anterior spinothalamic tract, which conveys light touch.
- The descending tracts are the anterior and lateral corticospinal tracts, which control all voluntary muscle activity from the cerebral cortex.

Spinal Nerves

Spinal nerves are a part of the peripheral nervous system. The 31 pairs of spinal nerves each have a right and left nerve that exit from the spinal cord below the corresponding vertebra. These include 8 cervical, 12 thoracic, 5 lumbar, 5 sacral, and 1 coccygeal nerve pairs. Afferent impulses conduct signals from the periphery to the CNS. Efferent impulses conduct signals from the CNS to the periphery. Each spinal nerve has a posterior (dorsal) root by which afferent impulses enter the cord and a ventral root by which efferent impulses leave (Hickey, 2003b; Littlejohns, 2004).

Dermatomes and Myotomes

The afferent fibers conduct impulses from a particular region on the surface of the skin, called a dermatome, to the spinal canal. The efferent fibers conduct impulses from a single segment on the spinal cord to a group of muscles they innervate, called myotomes. Although slight variations exist, dermatome and myotome patterns of distribution are relatively consistent from person to person. Locating a tumor as precisely as possible helps to correlate the dermatome and myotome with specific functional assessment for that level (Hickey, 2003c). See Figure 2-10 for specific landmarks of dermatomes and myotomes.

The lumbar and sacral nerves develop long roots, which dangle from the end of the spinal cord and are collectively referred to as the cauda equina (Latin for "horse's tail") (Littlejohns, 2004), a bundle-like structure of nerve fibers that extends caudally from the end of the spinal cord and gradually declines in number further down as individual pairs leave the spinal column (Hickey, 2003b; Littlejohns, 2004). It is bathed in CSF and is where lumbar punctures are performed.

A specific syndrome known as cauda equina syndrome is a serious neurologic condition in which the patient experiences complete loss of function of the nerve roots below the termination of the spinal cord. Specific deficits include saddle anesthesia, absent anal reflex, lower motor neuron weakness, and flaccid bladder (Adams, 2008). The signs and symptoms of cauda equina syndrome are low back pain, radicular pain, numbness in the groin, bowel and bladder incontinence, lower extremity muscle weakness (especially foot dorsiflexion), and reduced or absent lower extremity reflexes. It is considered a neurologic emergency, and immediate intervention may prevent permanent neurologic damage (Hickey, 2003c; Prendergast, 2004).

Reflexes

A reflex is an involuntary and nearly instantaneous movement in response to a stimulus. The deep tendon reflexes provide information on the integrity of the central and peripheral nervous system. The following are common sites for testing reflexes, the name of the reflex, and the location in the spinal cord that maintains the integrity of that reflex (Adams, 2008; Hickey, 2003b; Littlejohns, 2004).

- Biceps (biceps)—C5–C6
- Triceps (triceps)—C7
- Brachioradialis (brachioradialis)—C5–C6
- Patellar (quadriceps)—L3–L4
- Achilles (gastrocnemius soleus)—S1–S2

Regardless of the type or location of a spinal tumor, the associated pathophysiologic changes can lead to spinal cord dysfunction and neurologic deficits. These changes result from direct cord compression, ischemia secondary to arterial or venous obstruction, or, in the case of intramedullary tumors, direct invasion.

Cord compression alters the normal physiology involved in providing an adequate blood supply, maintaining stable cellular membranes, and facilitating afferent and efferent impulses for specific sensory, motor, and reflex functions of the spinal cord and related spinal nerves. Signs and symp-

---

Figure 2-10. Landmarks of Dermatomes and Myotomes

Dermatome Landmarks
- C2—Occiput
- C4—Neck, upper shoulder
- C6—Thumb, radial aspect of arm, index finger
- C7—Middle finger, middle palm, back of hand
- C8—Ring and little finger, ulnar aspect of arm
- T4—Nipple line
- T10—Umbilicus
- T12–L1—Groin region
- L3–L4—Anterior knee and lower leg
- L5—Outer aspect of lower leg, dorsum of foot, great toe
- S4–S5—Genitals and saddle area

Myotome Landmarks
- C1–C4—Neck
- C3–C5—Diaphragm
- C5–C6—Shoulder movement, elbow flexion
- C6–C8—Extension of forearm, wrist
- C7–T1—Wrist flexion
- T1–T12—Thoracic, abdominal, back muscles
- L1–L3—Hip flexion
- L2–L4—Extension of leg, adduction of thigh
- L4–L5—Dorsiflexion of foot
- L4–S2—Abduction of thigh, flexion of lower leg
- L5–S2—Plantar flexion of foot
- S2–S4—Perineal area and sphincters

C—cervical; L—lumbar; S—sacral; T—thoracic

Note. Based on information from Adams, 2008; Hickey, 2003b.

---

toms of spinal cord compression are sudden and progressive motor and sensory impairment. Interventions for spinal cord compression will be discussed in a later chapter.

Summary

Understanding the normal function of the brain and spine will assist the nurse in anticipating issues that patients may have or appreciate why they have deficits. It will improve the nurse's ability to support and educate the family as they go through the journey of cancer of the CNS.

References

Adams, A.C. (2008). *Mayo Clinic essential neurology.* Rochester, MN: Mayo Foundation for Medical Education and Research.

Belford, K. (1987). Central nervous system cancers. In S.L. Groenwald, M.H. Frogge, M. Goodman, & C.H. Yarbro (Eds.), *Cancer nursing: Principles and practice* (4th ed., pp. 980–1035). Sudbury, MA: Jones and Bartlett.

Brazis, P.W., Masdeu, J.C., & Biller, J. (2001). *Localization in clinical neurology* (4th ed.). Philadelphia, PA: Lippincott Williams & Wilkins.

Charalambides, C., Dinopoulos, A., & Sgouros, S. (2009). Neurological sequelae and quality of life following treatment of posterior fossa ependymomas in children. *Child's Nervous System, 25,* 1313–1320. doi:10.1007/s00381-009-0927-2

Gavrilovic, I.T., & Posner, J.B. (2005). Brain metastasis: Epidemiology and pathophysiology. *Journal of Neuro-Oncology, 75,* 5–14. doi:10.1007/s11060-004-8093-6

Gilbertson, R.J., & Rich, J.N. (2007). Making a tumour's bed: Glioblastoma stem cells and the vascular niche. *Nature Reviews Cancer, 7,* 733–736. doi:10.1038/nrc2246

Goldberg, S. (2003). *Clinical neuroanatomy made ridiculously simple* (3rd ed.). Miami, FL: MedMaster.

Hickey, J.V. (2003a). Brain tumors. In J.V. Hickey (Ed.), *The clinical practice of neurological and neurosurgical nursing* (5th ed., pp. 483–508). Philadelphia, PA: Lippincott Williams & Wilkins.

Hickey, J.V. (2003b). Overview of neuroanatomy and neurophysiology. In J.V. Hickey (Ed.), *The clinical practice of neurological and neurosurgical nursing* (5th ed., pp. 45–92). Philadelphia, PA: Lippincott Williams & Wilkins.

Hickey, J.V. (2003c). Spinal cord tumors. In J.V. Hickey (Ed.), *The clinical practice of neurological and neurosurgical nursing* (5th ed., pp. 509–520). Philadelphia, PA: Lippincott Williams & Wilkins.

Littlejohns, L.R. (2004). Anatomy of the nervous system. In M.K. Bader & L.R. Littlejohns (Eds.), *AANN core curriculum for neuroscience nursing* (4th ed., pp. 30–86). St. Louis, MO: Saunders.

Lupica, K. (2004). Nervous system tumors. In M.K. Bader & L.R. Littlejohns (Eds.), *AANN core curriculum for neuroscience nursing* (4th ed., pp. 511–535). St. Louis, MO: Saunders.

Martin, J.H. (1989). *Neuroanatomy: Text and atlas.* New York, NY: Elsevier.

Nicholas, M.K., & Lukas, R. (2010). Immunologic privilege and the brain. In I. Berczi & B.G.W. Arnason (Eds.), *NeuroImmune Biology: The brain and host defense* (Vol. 9, pp. 169–181). New York, NY: Elsevier.

Posner, J.B. (1995). Foreword. In R.G. Wiley (Ed.), *Neurological complications of cancer* (pp. v–vi). New York, NY: Marcel Dekker.

Prendergast, V. (2004). Spine disorders. In M.K. Bader & L.R. Littlejohns (Eds.), *AANN core curriculum for neuroscience nursing* (4th ed., pp. 511–535). St. Louis, MO: Saunders.

Reimann, A.F., & Anson, B.J. (1944). Vertebral level of termination of the spinal cord with report of a case of sacral cord. *Anatomical Record, 88,* 127–138. doi:10.1002/ar.1090880108

Schellinger, K.A., Propp, J.M., Villano, J.L., & McCarthy, B.J. (2008). Descriptive epidemiology of primary spinal cord tumors. *Journal of Neuro-Oncology, 87,* 173–179. doi:10.1007/s11060-007-9507-z

Shiminski-Maher, T., Cullen, P.M., & Sansalone, M. (2002). *Childhood brain and spinal cord tumors: A guide for family, friends and caregivers.* Sebastopol, CA: O'Reilly.

Zuccarelli, L. (2004). Cellular physiology of the nervous system. In M.K. Bader & L.R. Littlejohns (Eds.), *AANN core curriculum for neuroscience nursing* (4th ed., pp. 511–535). St. Louis, MO: Saunders.

CHAPTER 3

Patient Assessment

Eva Lu T. Lee, MSN, RN, ANP-BC, and Laurel J. Westcarth, MSN, RN, ANP-BC

Introduction

Although cancers of the central nervous system (CNS) account for a small percentage of all cancers and cancer-related deaths (Bondy, El-Zein, & Scheurer, 2007), the neurologic sequelae of both the disease and treatment have a devastating impact on quality of life. Clinical manifestations develop from either regional parenchymal or diffuse intracranial effects from brain neoplasms (Yung, Aaron, & Aldape, 2005). The clinical symptoms of a brain neoplasm depend on its anatomic location in the brain (Drevelegas, Chourmouzi, & Papanicolaou, 2008). Patients most commonly present with headaches, seizures, nausea, vomiting, altered mental status, or focal deficits (Hickey, 2003a). The nature of focal deficits varies by tumor location and aids the clinician in localizing the tumor (Hickey, 2003a). A comprehensive patient health history, thorough neurologic assessment, and advanced diagnostic technology tests are essential in the early assessment of patients with CNS tumors. In addition to detecting neurologic deficits on examination, it is important to recognize symptoms associated with CNS tumors because some patients may have a normal or near normal neurologic examination (McAllister, Ward, Schulman, & De Angelis, 2002).

Spinal cord tumors are rare and constitute approximately 15% of all CNS neoplasms (Belford, 2005). Similar to brain tumors, slower-growing spinal tumors have minimal or no neurologic sequelae, whereas rapidly growing tumors such as high-grade gliomas can produce significant neurologic consequences on presentation (Rosenberg & Theodosopoulos, 2002). Patients with spinal cord tumors can present with complaints of pain, weakness, sensory loss, or alterations in bladder and bowel control (Kornblith, Walker, & Cassady, 1987).

Neuroimaging plays a vital role in the management of patients with CNS neoplasm. The roles of neuroimaging include refinement of the preoperative differential diagnosis, preoperative planning, assessment of treatment response, and diagnosis of tumor progression or therapy-related effects (Henson & Gonzalez, 2005). The most commonly employed neuroradiologic tools that provide valuable diagnostic information are magnetic resonance imaging (MRI) and computed tomography (CT). However, MRI is the imaging tool of choice because it is more sensitive in differentiating between tumor and normal brain tissue (Keles, Tihan, Burton, Prados, & Berger, 2005; Yamada & Sorensen, 2008). MRI, in comparison to CT, has the ability to visualize brain anatomy and detect pathology; however, CT is more sensitive for identifying bone abnormalities such as abnormal calcifications and lytic lesions. Additionally, CT scans are faster and may be particularly useful in diagnosing acute conditions such as intracranial hemorrhage or hydrocephalus (Yung et al., 2005).

Examination

The evaluation of a patient with a possible brain tumor starts with a history and physical; the neurologic examination being an integral component of both. While the history defines the clinical problem (what), the physical examination is performed to localize the lesion (where). A thorough and complete neurologic history requires a good knowledge base of the basic principles of neurologic functions and potential disorders. The neurologic examination is usually performed and documented in a uniform and chronologic manner but can be modified according to the clinical problem and condition of the patient (Oommen, 2009). The American Association of Neuroscience Nurses (AANN) has a clinical practice guideline series for nurses available online. Information pertaining to a neurologic examination of the older adult is concisely presented at www.aann.org/pdf/cpg/aannneuroassessmentolderadult.pdf.

History

Clinical history is an important part of the neurologic examination. It tells the story and, if possible, should be obtained in the patient's own words. The history begins by identifying the chief complaint. If the patient is unable to answer the questions because of comprehension or insight failure or the illness, information should be obtained from the accompanying family member. The focal point of the history is the chief complaint, which is also the key to subsequent analysis of the information leading to a differential diagnosis (Gilroy, 2000). Once the chief complaint is identified, the next step is to record the history of the present illness. The history should be documented in chronologic order; hence, the examiner must learn to encourage the flow of information while minimizing the interpolation of insignificant statements made by the patient or family. Control of the interview must be maintained, and the interviewer should remain polite, firm, and tactful, which will assist in keeping the interview on track so that the maximum amount of information is obtained. The interviewing process is a time to observe the patient's expression, demeanor, affect, eye movement, asymmetry of movement, and the family dynamics (Gilroy, 2000).

The neurologic review is the next step of the history and will supply additional information regarding the presence of common neurologic symptoms. This includes headache; visual symptoms; hearing, speech, memory, writing, reading, walking, or sphincter problems; weakness, numbness, loss of consciousness; or change in sleep patterns. The nurse should question the patient regarding new symptoms or a change in the pattern of an old symptom. Additionally, the nurse must discover whether the pattern is gradual or of sudden onset, what makes it better or worse, or if it is associated with other neurologic symptoms (Gilroy, 2000).

The next section of the history should record the past medical history, family history, and social history. The past medical history should question whether the patient has a prior history of cancer because the neurologic complaints may be due to metastatic disease from a primary cancer causing symptoms consistent with brain or spinal cord disorder. This information is critical in prioritizing the subsequent evaluation. For example, metastatic disease to the brain and spine is more common in malignant melanoma and lung, breast, prostate, and thyroid cancers (Westcarth & Armstrong, 2007), and a history of one of these cancers would increase the likelihood that neurologic abnormalities are the result of either tumor spread (metastases) or the remote effects of the cancer (paraneoplastic syndromes). Similarly, a history of a prior cancer may provide a crucial clue in ascertaining a diagnosis of spinal neoplasm (Huff, 2009). One of the earliest signs that patients usually report with spinal neoplasm is back pain. In this situation, determining exacerbating factors, whether the pain is getting better or worse, or if it is accompanied by sensory or motor symptoms are crucial components of the history. "Emergence of leg weakness, paresthesias in the lower extremities, and/or bowel or bladder dysfunction in patients with a history of cancer should evoke immediate concern for cord compression" (Huff, 2009, Clinical, History, bullet 7). However, many patients with impending spinal cord compres-

sion present with pain, and prompt assessment may prevent neurologic dysfunction by permitting early intervention. A complete history should also include inquiry about unusual childhood diseases and a history of systemic disease such as hypertension, diabetes, or heart disease (Gilroy, 2000).

The family history will provide essential inherited information such as migraine, metabolic, muscle, nerve, and neurodegenerative disorders. On the other hand, unusual infections and exposure to toxins and parasites can be obtained by information provided in the social, occupational, and travel history (Beers, Porter, Jones, Kaplan, & Berkwits, 2006). In the social history, include questions regarding smoking, alcohol consumption, illicit drug use, occupation, and exposure to unusual chemicals or toxins. Finally, prior to proceeding to the physical examination, obtain a list of all current medications and note if they are prescribed or over the counter, including herbal remedies and other alternative medical treatments (Gilroy, 2000).

Physical Examination

The physical assessment includes evaluation of general health in addition to the neurologic examination. The general physical examination includes evaluation of vital signs, HEENT (head, ears, eyes, nose, and throat), cardiovascular, respiratory, gastrointestinal, genitourinary, skin, and musculoskeletal systems (Westcarth & Armstrong, 2007). The neurologic examination is part of the general health examination and should be interpreted in the context of the general physical examination. The neurologic examination begins with watchful observation from the time the patient enters the room. Note the patient's speech, speed of response, gait, posture, demeanor, mood, and coordination. Deficits can be evident during history taking and while moving to the examination table (Beers et al., 2006). The following tools are used in a neurologic examination: stethoscope, ophthalmoscope, reflex hammer, tuning fork, and other supplies including gloves, tongue depressor, and cotton swabs.

The comprehensive neurologic examination is typically performed in a stepwise fashion and includes evaluation of mental status, cranial nerves, motor system, sensory examination, reflexes, coordination, cerebellar examination, and gait testing (Gelb, 2005).

Mental Status

The mental status evaluation assesses level of consciousness, speech, language, and communication. Voice, speech, language, and cognition (mentation) are four forms of verbal communication that consist of complex neurophysiologic processes. A voice disorder is known as *dysphonia*, speech and voice disorder is known as *dysarthria*, and loss or deficiency in the understanding and production of language is called *dysphasia* or *aphasia*. Several types of dysarthria and dysphasia exist; therefore, an accurate assessment of verbal communication, cognition, and swallowing will aid in the early identification and management of these patients. Difficulty in articulation, or dysarthria, is commonly caused by paralysis, paresis, or a lack of coordination between physical voice production and actual speech (Gilroy, 2000). Disorder of language, or dysphasia, is clearly distinguished from dysarthria, and deficits may affect some or all components of language. Language function and dysfunction is complex, but deficiency occurs when there is a lesion in the dominant hemisphere. Most deficits are related to the loss of receptive function (receptive or Wernicke aphasia) or loss of expressive function (expressive or Broca aphasia). Some of the common language symptom terminology includes "anomia (naming and word finding problem), auditory agnosia (word recognition problem), dysgraphia (writing difficulty), dyslexia (reading difficulty), paraphasia (word substitution), and agrammatism (grammatical errors)" (Gilroy, 2000, p. 7).

Patients with lesions in the nondominant hemisphere will present with a unique pattern of dysfunction called *nondominant hemisphere dysfunction*. This dysfunction includes impairment in judgment and reasoning, memory problems with extinction or neglect of stimuli on the opposite side of the body, loss of visual perception, lack of insight, attention deficits, and poor organizational and task initiation skills. Nondominant hemisphere dysfunctions also involve impairments of dysarthria and dysphasia (Gilroy, 2000).

Assessing orientation to date, time, and place will identify if the patient is in correlation with his or her surrounding and time. Therefore, ask the patient about current events (e.g., "Who is the president of the United States?"), and this information will provide insight into orientation and recent memory (Gilroy, 2000). Attention is assessed by spelling the word WORLD forward and backward, and calculation is assessed by serial 7 subtraction, counting backwards by 3s or 7s, or naming the months backward (Goldberg, 1999). If the patient fails to calculate in a serial fashion, he or she should be asked to do simple addition instead. The term used to describe difficulty performing simple arithmetic function is *dyscalculia*, whereas failure to perform mathematical calculation is *acalculia* (Gilroy, 2000). Memory function is complex and involves the ability to form, imprint, and retain information. Bedside testing of short-term memory can be performed by asking the patient to recall three objects over a period of three to five minutes. The loss of recent memory with retention of remote memory is common in progressive disease involving the medial temporal lobe (Gilroy, 2000).

Cranial Nerves

Cranial nerves are responsible for providing motor and sensory innervations for the head and neck. Cranial nerves are tested to localize a lesion in the CNS. Cranial nerves (CN) I–XII are tested in the following order (see Figure 3-1).

Cranial Nerve I (Olfactory)

In clinical practice, CN I is rarely tested unless the patient has a specific complaint. Use a distinct odor such as coffee or a nonirritant material such as peppermint, soap, orange, vanilla, or cloves. Avoid a noxious trigger such as ammonia that can stimulate the pain fibers of the trigeminal nerve (Bickley & Szilagyi, 2007). Each nostril is tested separately with eyes closed (Lindsay & Bone, 2004).

Cranial Nerve II (Optic)

To assess the integrity of the visual pathways, check the visual acuity, visual fields, pupils, and the optic fundus. Use a Snellen chart to test each eye for visual acuity. Test the visual fields by confrontation. Have the patient cover one eye and focus on the examiner's nose. Show one to three fingers in each of the four visual quadrants of each uncovered eye, and ask the patient to state the number of fingers visualized (Martin, Lee, & Langston, 2001). Visual field defect is described as homonymous if the same side or quadrant of the visual field is affected on both eyes (Fuller, 2004). Check for pupillary size, equality, and reaction to light and accommodation, and perform a funduscopic examination of each eye. Ask the patient to focus on a distant object away from the light. To view the macula, ask the patient to focus on the light. Note the width of blood vessels, and look for arteriovenous nipping. Look for hemorrhages or white patches of exudates, and note the clarity of the disc margins (Lindsay & Bone, 2004).

Cranial Nerves III (Oculomotor), IV (Trochlear), and VI (Abducens)

These three cranial nerves are responsible for eye movement; therefore, they are evaluated together. CN IV controls the superior oblique muscle, which allows each eye to look down and medially. CN VI controls the lateral rectus muscle, which allows each eye to move laterally. An easy way to remember the functions of these CNs is the mnemonic "SO 4 LR 6 All the Rest 3": **s**uperior **o**blique CN **4**, **l**ateral **r**ectus CN **6**, **all the rest** of the muscles are innervated by CN **3** (Goldberg, 2008).

Cranial Nerve V (Trigeminal)

The sensory component of CN V is composed of three branches: V1 ophthalmic, V2 maxillary, and V3 mandibular. Test sensation of the trigeminal nerve from V1 to V3 distribution (Russell & Triola, 2006). The motor component of CN V innervates the temporalis and masseter muscles. Palpate the temporalis and ask the patient to clench his or her jaw, and do the same examination with the masseter muscles (Goldberg, 2008; Russell & Triola, 2006).

Cranial Nerve VII (Facial)

The facial nerve innervates all the muscles of facial expression. Test the muscle of facial expression by asking the patient to smile, raise the eyebrows, squeeze the eyes

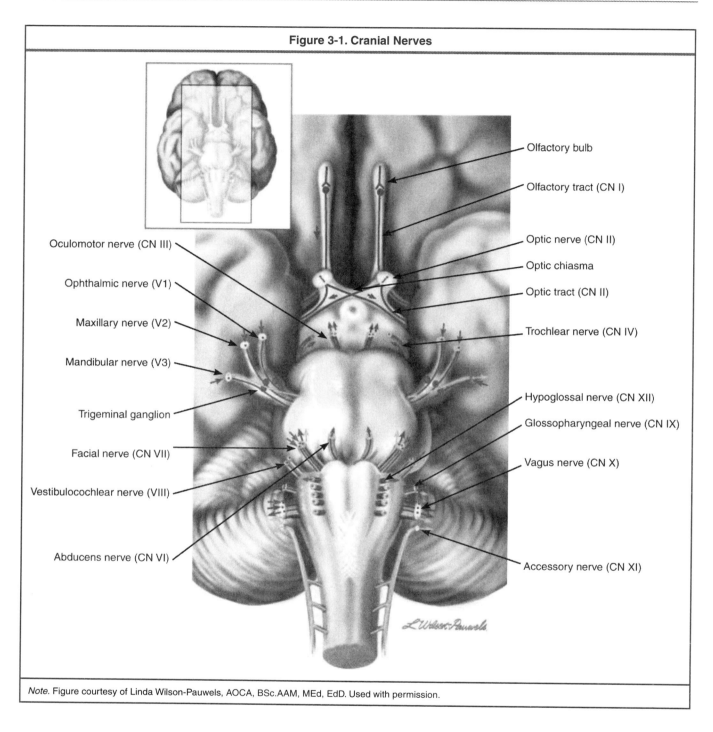

Figure 3-1. Cranial Nerves

Olfactory bulb

Olfactory tract (CN I)

Optic nerve (CN II)

Optic chiasma

Optic tract (CN II)

Trochlear nerve (CN IV)

Hypoglossal nerve (CN XII)

Glossopharyngeal nerve (CN IX)

Vagus nerve (CN X)

Accessory nerve (CN XI)

Oculomotor nerve (CN III)

Ophthalmic nerve (V1)

Maxillary nerve (V2)

Mandibular nerve (V3)

Trigeminal ganglion

Facial nerve (CN VII)

Vestibulocochlear nerve (VIII)

Abducens nerve (CN VI)

Note. Figure courtesy of Linda Wilson-Pauwels, AOCA, BSc.AAM, MEd, EdD. Used with permission.

shut tightly, and puff the cheeks while you observe for asymmetry. Facial weakness may result from either upper or lower motor neuron palsy. Upper motor palsy can result from a lesion contralateral to the side of the facial palsy disrupting the face motor fibers from the primary motor cortex to the facial nucleus within the pons. Lower motor neuron palsy can result from a lesion involving the facial nerve at the nucleus in the pons or along the course of the

facial nerve ipsilateral to the side of the facial weakness (Martin et al., 2001).

Cranial Nerve VIII (Acoustic or Vestibulocochlear)

The acoustic nerve is composed of the cochlear and the vestibular nerves. The cochlear nerve is responsible for hearing, and the vestibular for balance (Martin et al., 2001). Each ear is tested separately. First, test the hearing by rubbing your fingers approximately six inches away from each ear. If findings are abnormal, perform the Weber and Rinne tests. Using a 512 Hz tuning fork, perform the Weber test by tapping the fork and placing it on the vertex of the head, assessing which ear hears the sound louder, the good ear or the deaf ear (Fuller, 2004). Normal hearing allows sound to be heard equally in both ears. With conductive hearing loss, the sound is louder on the deaf ear because bone conduction is greater than air conduction. Conversely, in sensorineural loss, the sound is louder on the good ear because normally air conduction is greater than bone conduction (Lindsay & Bone, 2004). The Rinne test is performed by tapping the fork and placing it at the mastoid process. The patient is instructed to signal when the sound is no longer audible. The tuning fork is then transferred immediately in front of the external auditory canal. A patient with normal hearing will continue to hear the sound by air conduction. In conductive hearing loss, the patient will not be able to hear the sound as soon as it is transferred in front of the deaf ear because, in this case, bone conduction is greater than air conduction (Oomen, 2009; Russell & Triola, 2006). However, sensorineural loss will result in decreased bone and air conduction (Lindsay & Bone, 2004; Oommen, 2009). The vestibular function is not normally tested unless the patient has a specific complaint such as vertigo.

Cranial Nerves IX (Glossopharyngeal) and X (Vagus)

These nerves are examined together, and their actions are seldom separately impaired because they both contribute to the same functions such as soft palate elevation and gag reflex. Ask the patient to open the mouth and say "ahh," and observe for symmetrical elevation of the soft palate while the uvula remains at midline. The gag reflex is an important component of the examination if brain stem pathology is suspected or a complaint of dysarthria or dysphagia is present in the history or examination (Goldberg, 2008; Russell & Triola, 2006). The sensory component of CN IX is responsible for taste in the posterior one-third of the tongue but is not routinely tested, as this is rarely a clinically important problem and is impractical. Listen to the patient's voice, and note for vocal cord palsy characterized by a high-pitched voice (Lindsay & Bone, 2004).

Cranial Nerve XI (Spinal Accessory)

Ask the patient to push head from side to side against resistance to assess the strength of the sternocleidomastoid muscle. To test the trapezius, ask the patient to shrug the shoulders and to hold them against resistance (Lindsay & Bone, 2004).

Cranial Nerve XII (Hypoglossal)

The hypoglossal nerve is responsible for tongue movement. Ask the patient to open the mouth, and inspect for atrophy or fasciculations (involuntary muscle twitching). Then ask the patient to protrude the tongue, and note for any deviation. To check for subtle weakness, have the patient push the tongue against the wall of the cheek while providing counter pressure

from the outer cheek (Goldberg, 2008; Lindsay & Bone, 2004; Martin et al., 2001).

Motor System

Evaluate body position, movement, muscle (bulk, strength, and tone), coordination, gait, and stance. Muscles tested are C5 (elbow flexion), C6 (wrist extension), C7 (elbow extension), C8 (finger flexion), T1 (finger abduction), L2 (hip flexion), L3 (knee extension), L4 (ankle dorsiflexion), L5 (toe extension), and S1 (ankle plantar flexion). Muscle strength is graded on a six-point scale developed by the Medical Research Council and ranges from 0 to 5: 0 (absent muscular contraction), 1 (trace), 2 (active movement with gravity eliminated resistance), 3 (active movement against gravity), 4 (active movement against gravity with some resistance), and 5 (normal strength) (Adams, 2008; Bickley & Szilagyi, 2007).

Sensory System

Primary modalities of sensation that are tested include light touch, vibration, pain, temperature, and position sense. Assess pain and temperature, position, vibration, and discriminative sensations (stereognosis, number identification, and two-point discrimination). Evaluation of sensory dermatomes is important if there are concerns about peripheral nerve root involvement in the disease process (Adams, 2008; Bickley & Szilagyi, 2007).

Deep Tendon Reflexes

The neurologic examination includes evaluation of biceps, triceps, brachioradialis, patella, and Achilles tendon reflexes. Reflexes are graded on a scale from 0 to 4+: 0 (absent reflexes), 0.5 (present with reinforcement using the Jendrassik maneuver [the fingers of both hands are locked together and pulled against each other while the tendon is tapped to elicit the reflex]), 1+ (present but diminished), 2+ (average/normal), 3+ (brisker than average or increased reflex), and 4+ (hyperactive, very brisk with clonus) (Bickley & Szilagyi, 2007; Fuller, 2004). If reflexes are hyperactive, evaluate for ankle clonus (sustained contractions after reflex testing) (Goldberg, 1999).

Coordination and Cerebellar Testing

Test for rapid alternating movements, finger-nose test, heel-shin test, and feet tapping; assess for tremor, nystagmus with eye movements, and truncal ataxia.

Gait

Gait is assessed by observing the patient's stance, posture, stability, and rate and speed of walking. Adams (2008) recommended that practitioners "watch the patient walk" (p. 1) as they assess the patient's equilibrium and locomotion. Practitioners should observe how the patient sits, stands, and initiates walking, without the patient becoming aware of being watched, if possible (Adams, 2008). The patient should be asked to walk across the room and observe for any gait abnormality, then next to do the tandem walk (one foot in front of the other), then to walk on the heels, and, last, on the toes.

The information received from the history and physical examination should answer the questions "What?" (clinical problems) and "Where?" (lesion location within the brain or spine). It will shed light on the patient's mental intactness and motor or sensory deficit and provide a clue or insight as to the location of the lesion. The history and physical examination will guide the healthcare provider to the diagnostic testing process required and aid in the establishment of a diagnosis and plan.

Neurologic Examination of Patients With Spinal Cord Tumors

A complete neurologic assessment of the patient with a suspected spinal cord tumor involves a detailed history taking and a complete neurologic examination. This should include an assessment of pain in the history with specifics as to the level of pain, onset, location, and aggravating and relieving factors. Also assess for bladder, bowel, and sexual dysfunction. Perform a sensory examination, and carefully note the deficits, particularly if they are at a particular sensory level. The sensory examination can point out which ascending fibers of the spinal cord are affected. When posterior columns are affected, the patient will manifest impairments of light touch, vibration, and joint position sense. Conversely, when the spinothalamic tract is affected, pain and temperature impairment will be noted. The motor examination involves evaluation for muscle weakness, wasting, and spasticity, as well as an evaluation of tendon reflexes and Babinski sign (the big toe raises and other toes flex or spread with plantar stimulation) (Fuller, 2004).

Signs and Symptoms

General Signs and Symptoms

An intracranial mass or spinal tumor is often diagnosed because patients present with symptoms. Presenting symptoms are typically characterized as either general or localized. The general symptoms of an intracranial mass are headaches, seizures, altered mental status, nausea, and vomiting. Headaches are a common symptom in patients with brain tumors, although the diagnosis of a brain tumor accounts for only a small percentage of patients presenting

with headaches (Cavaliere, 2008) (see Table 3-1 and Figure 3-2). Headaches associated with brain tumors usually awaken the patient at night or occur upon waking in the morning (Adams, 2008). Frontal lesions may cause frontal headache, and occipital or posterior fossa lesions may cause occipital or posterior cervical pain. However, many patients will present with a diffuse headache of a vertex location (upper-most surface or top of the head) (Kornblith et al., 1987). The acute-onset headache may occur with intratumoral bleeding or increased intracranial pressure (ICP) (Cavaliere, 2008). It is important to note that headaches caused by an increase in ICP from a brain tumor can be affected by and worsen with coughing, exercise, or position change (Adams, 2008). Headaches are a result of stimulation of the pain-sensitive structures on the head.

Similarly, seizures are typically not localizing but are a common presenting sign of intracranial tumors. Seizures may develop because of direct extension of the tumor into the brain or meninges, metabolic imbalance from cancer therapy or the tumor, or the neurotoxicity of cancer treatment (Gilbert & Armstrong, 1995). Interestingly, intracranial tumors that cause seizures generally have a slow

Table 3-1. Headache Characteristics in Brain Tumors (Including Low- and High-Grade Tumors)

Characteristic	Description
Description	"Tension-type," "dull ache," "pressure-like," and "sinus-like headache" in 77% of patients "Migrainous" in 9%–26% of cases
Timing	Intermittent, develops and resolves over several hours Worse with cough, Valsalva maneuver, and bending in 23% Interferes with sleep in 32%
Duration	Less than 1 month: 29% 1–6 months: 26% Greater than 6 months: 45%
Location	72% bilateral and 25% unilateral Frontal in 68%
Intensity	May be mild, moderate, or severe Mean intensity of 8.5/10 when associated with increased intracranial pressure and 6.5/10 if no evidence of increased intracranial pressure
Associated symptoms	Nausea and vomiting (38%) Visual disturbance (40%) Seizures (50%)

Note. From "Headache" (p. 58), by R. Cavaliere in D. Schiff, S. Kesari, and P.Y. Wen (Eds.), *Cancer Neurology in Clinical Practice: Neurologic Complications of Cancer and Its Treatment* (2nd ed.), 2008, Totowa, NJ: Humana Press. Copyright 2008 by Humana Press. Reprinted with permission.

Figure 3-2. Clinical Factors That Suggest a Structural Cause for Headache

- Any change in preexisting headache pattern
- Headaches unresponsive to previously effective therapies
- Any focal symptom or sign
- Papilledema
- Change in behavior, personality, or mentation
- Vomiting
- Awake patient from sleep or worse upon awakening in the morning
- Worse with bending over, coughing, sneezing, or Valsalva

Note. From "Headache" (p. 59), by R. Cavaliere in D. Schiff, S. Kesari, and P.Y. Wen (Eds.), *Cancer Neurology in Clinical Practice: Neurologic Complications of Cancer and Its Treatment* (2nd ed.), 2008, Totowa, NJ: Humana Press. Copyright 2008 by Humana Press. Reprinted with permission.

growth rate, and tumors with a faster growth rate produce fewer seizures (Adams, 2008). Patients with status epilepticus and seizures that occur frequently require emergency management to prevent permanent neurologic sequelae (Gilbert & Armstrong, 1995). A diagnostic evaluation is required to determine the etiology of all cases of seizures (see Figure 3-3).

Alteration in mental status is another common complication of CNS tumors. It can result from a multitude of etiologies, including metabolic disorders, toxic encephalopathies, treatment side effects, tumor, increased ICP, infection, vascular disease, seizures, or psychiatric disorder. Changes in mental status can present in various forms from a subtle cognitive dysfunction to overt disorientation, hallucinations, or lethargy (Kraker & Blakeley, 2009). Projectile vomiting is a manifestation of a posterior fossa lesion, which is more common in children than adults. Nausea without accompanying neurologic signs can be seen with tumors of the floor of the fourth ventricle or of the insula (Batchelor & Byrne, 2008). Some tumors, such as those that are located in the frontal poles of the brain, do not cause symptoms to develop until they reach a substantial size, whereas small tumors that are located on eloquent areas of the brain, such as the language regions in the dominant cerebral hemisphere, may cause the patient to become symptomatic. Tumors that are slow growing may not produce symptoms because they allow the brain to adapt to infiltration and distortion (Schold et al., 1997).

Increased ICP is a common complication in patients with brain tumors because the mass, lesion, or associated edema caused by irritation of the cortex around the lesion adds to the volume of tissue in the brain. The majority of the symptoms associated with increased ICP arise from secondary effects mediated by pressure gradients, compartmental shifts, brain herniation, and vascular changes. The most common symptoms of increased ICP are headache, nausea, and vomiting (Lee & Armstrong, 2008).

Focal Signs and Symptoms

Focal symptoms include contralateral weakness, contralateral sensory loss, visual field deficits, speech disturbance, behavioral change, and partial seizures (McAllister et al., 2002). The location of the brain neoplasm will dictate the symptoms that the patient experiences. When cranial nerves are involved, the patient may manifest symptoms such as loss of smell, vision changes, eye movement problems, ptosis, diplopia, unilateral facial numbness, one-sided facial paralysis, hearing loss, or swallowing problems.

Anatomic Correlates

Frontal Lobe

The frontal lobe controls higher mental functions, motor function, behavior, contralateral head and gaze preference, cortical inhibition of bowel and bladder, and speech. Patients with frontal lobe lesions may manifest lack of motivation, inattention, irritability, lack of initiative, poor judgment, or depression. These mood disturbances have a slow and progressive course and may initially be diagnosed as a psychiatric disorder. Involvement of the motor cortex may cause contralateral weakness. The Broca area is located in the inferior part of the dominant frontal lobe; a lesion affecting the Broca area results in expressive aphasia. The patient with Broca aphasia or nonfluent aphasia may have normal language comprehension but will have hesitant speech with articles and conjunctions omitted (Lindsay & Bone, 2004).

Temporal Lobe

Lesions affecting the temporal lobe may cause memory problems, partial complex seizures, auditory problems, visual field deficits, emotion and behavior changes, and prosopagnosia (the inability to recognize faces). The dominant hemisphere is important in the understanding of language, and the nondominant hemisphere in the hearing of sounds, rhythm, and music (Lindsay & Bone, 2004).

Parietal Lobe

Tumors of the parietal lobe of either the dominant or nondominant sensory cortex (postcentral gyrus) will manifest in contralateral sensory disturbance affecting joint position sense, localization of light touch, two-point discrimination, stereognosis (difficulty distinguishing objects placed in hand), graphesthesia (difficulty distinguishing numbers or letters written in palm of hands), or sensory inattention to double simultaneous stimulation with contralateral body or limb neglect (Kaye & Edward, 2001; Lindsay & Bone, 2004). Damage to the dominant parietal lobe at the supramarginal and angular gyri is associated with Wernicke aphasia (receptive or fluent aphasia). The patient with this disorder will have comprehension difficulty, problems with fluent but nonsensical speech, making nonexistent words (neologisms) or saying half-correct

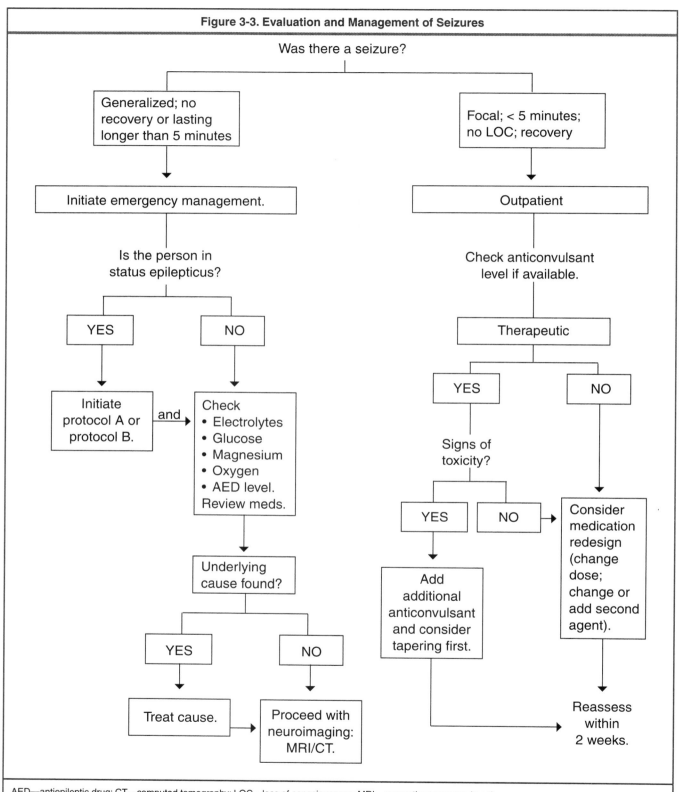

Figure 3-3. Evaluation and Management of Seizures

Was there a seizure?

Generalized; no recovery or lasting longer than 5 minutes

Focal; < 5 minutes; no LOC; recovery

Initiate emergency management.

Outpatient

Is the person in status epilepticus?

Check anticonvulsant level if available.

YES

NO

Therapeutic

Initiate protocol A or protocol B.

and

Check
• Electrolytes
• Glucose
• Magnesium
• Oxygen
• AED level.
Review meds.

YES

NO

Signs of toxicity?

YES

NO

Consider medication redesign (change dose; change or add second agent).

Underlying cause found?

YES

NO

Add additional anticonvulsant and consider tapering first.

Treat cause.

Proceed with neuroimaging: MRI/CT.

Reassess within 2 weeks.

AED—antiepileptic drug; CT—computed tomography; LOC—loss of consciousness; MRI—magnetic resonance imaging

Note. From "Seizures" (p. 971), by T.S. Armstrong, K.E. Baumgartner, and S.J. Min in D. Camp-Sorrell and R.A. Hawkins (Eds.), *Clinical Manual for the Oncology Advanced Practice Nurse* (2nd ed.), 2006, Pittsburgh, PA: Oncology Nursing Society. Copyright 2006 by the Oncology Nursing Society. Reprinted with permission.

words (paraphasia), and poor handwriting (Lindsay & Bone, 2004). Lesions in the nondominant parietal lobe, however, are associated with dressing apraxia (difficulty in dressing), geographic agnosia (disturbance of geographic memory), constructional apraxia (difficulty copying geometric patterns), or anosognosia (patient denies weakness of affected limb) (Lindsay & Bone, 2004). A constellation of symptoms known as the Gerstmann syndrome is associated with tumors of the dominant parietal lobe. These symptoms include acalculia (reduced ability or inability to perform simple mathematical calculation), agraphia (disturbance of writing), finger agnosia (difficulty distinguishing fingers of hands), and right-left confusion. Homonymous visual field defect and sensory seizures are also possible symptoms with parietal lobe tumors (Hickey, 2003a).

Occipital Lobe

The occipital lobe constitutes a small area in relation to the entire cerebral cortex, which explains the infrequent occurrence of tumors in this area (Fortuna, 2002). It contains the primary visual cortex responsible for perception of vision. Impairment of the occipital lobe function by a brain neoplasm results in homonymous hemianopsia (partial blindness that causes vision loss in the same visual field of both eyes). Other symptoms associated with occipital lobe lesions are visual hallucinations, visual illusions (objects may appear smaller or larger than reality), prosopagnosia, and color agnosia (impaired recognition of colors).

Cerebellum

The cerebellum is located in the posterior fossa separated from the cerebrum by the tentorium cerebelli. Tumors that grow in the cerebellum produce symptoms involving equilibrium, fine motor movements, tremors, ataxia, wide-based gait, nystagmus, or dysarthria.

Brain Stem

The brain stem is located in the posterior fossa and comprises the midbrain, pons, and medulla. Cranial nerves, with the exception of CNs I and II, emerge from the brain stem; therefore, patients with tumors in the brain stem manifest lower cranial nerve deficits, vision changes, eye movement problems, ptosis, diplopia, unilateral facial numbness or paralysis, nausea and vomiting, hearing loss, hiccups, or swallowing problems. Rapid evolution of symptoms is one of the hallmarks of diffuse brain stem tumors (Kan & Kestle, 2008).

Fourth Ventricle

The location of the fourth ventricle is critical because tumors located in this area can obstruct the flow of cerebrospinal fluid (CSF), causing hydrocephalus and subsequently causing increased ICP. Symptoms associated with hydrocephalus are headache, gait imbalance, and urinary incontinence. Tumors of the fourth ventricle cause vertigo on head movements and change in voice (Fortuna, 2002).

Spinal Cord Tumors

Spinal cord tumors may be grouped by location to include extradural, extramedullary (meningiomas and neurofibromas), and intramedullary (ependymomas, astrocytomas, oligodendrogliomas, hemangioblastomas), as well as metastatic tumors (Adams, 2008). Signs and symptoms associated with spinal cord tumors are usually associated with spinal cord compression (Belford, 2005). Patients with suspected spinal cord lesions should be evaluated emergently to rule out neurologic compromise such as spinal cord compression (McAllister et al., 2002). Signs and symptoms and sensory deficits depend on the location of the lesion in the spinal cord (Belford, 2005). A combination of motor and sensory deficits known as the Brown-Séquard syndrome may be present, manifesting as spinothalamic symptoms (alteration in pain and temperature) on the contralateral side of the tumor and loss of motor function, light touch, vibration, and position sense on the ipsilateral side (Hickey, 2003c). Spinal cord tumors cause symptoms characteristic of vertebral, radicular, or spinal cord pain followed by motor weakness, sensory deficit (paresthesia or hypoesthesia), bowel or bladder dysfunction, sexual dysfunction, neurogenic intermittent claudication (pain in the buttock, thigh, or leg), and subarachnoid hemorrhage (Fortuna, 2002). Pain is the most common presenting symptom with epidural spinal cord compression, often but not always localized to the region of the tumor and worse when the patient is supine (Schold et al., 1997). Pain usually precedes signs of spinal cord compression by weeks or months and is progressive once cord compression occurs (Hickey, 2003c).

Spinal cord tumor pain is characterized as progressive and unrelenting in nature. Patients describe the pain as band-like and following a dermatomal distribution (Belford, 2005). Pain is much less commonly associated with intramedullary tumor. When present, this pain is typically axial, aching, dull, of gradual onset, and not easily explained by pathologic changes of sensory pathways (Ogden & McCormick, 2008). Ascending and descending pathways are interrupted, causing decreased sensation distal to the lesion (Martin et al., 2001). Patients with spinal tumors may not always present with neurologic symptoms; however, neurologic symptoms are rather common in those who have aggressive or malignant tumors (Whitehead & Illner, 2006).

Neoplastic Meningitis

Neoplastic meningitis (NM) or leptomeningeal disease is the product of multifocal seeding of the subarachnoid space with tumor cells (Adams, 2008) and affects the entire neural axis, making clinical signs and symptoms variable (Blaney & Poplack, 2005). Signs and symptoms are assigned or grouped to the sites of CNS involvement: cerebral, cranial nerve, and spinal (Groves, 2004). Patients present with facial weakness, gait difficulty, difficulty swallowing, headache, confusion, nausea and vomiting, loss of consciousness, and dizziness (Kraker & Blakeley, 2009; Omar & Mason, 2008). Cranial nerve deficit is one of the most common symptoms of leptomeningeal spread (Kraker & Blakeley, 2009). Headache and diplopia (CN VI) are the most common signs and symptoms in patients with hematologic cancer, whereas cerebral or spinal/radicular symptoms are present with solid tumor malignancies (Blaney & Poplack, 2005). Headache can result from inflammation of the pain-sensitive dura, whereas symptoms associated with cranial nerves and lumbosacral roots can result from frequent accumulation of malignant cells around the skull base and lumbosacral regions (Groves, 2004). It is also common for patients with leptomeningeal involvement to present with isolated syndromes such as symptoms of increased ICP, cauda equina syndrome, or cranial neuropathy (Chamberlain, 2008). Refer to Chapter 5 for additional discussion of leptomeningeal disease.

Metastatic Disease

Metastatic tumor is the most common cause of brain cancer, surpassing the incidence rate of all other types of primary brain tumors combined (Armstrong & Gilbert, 2000). Although the CNS is partially protected by the blood-brain barrier and does not have a lymphatic system, it is still a common site for metastasis, typically at the gray-white matter junction (Ribalta & Fuller, 2004). Metastatic tumors to the brain can present with symptoms similar to that of any intracranial mass lesions. Brain metastases should be suspected in patients with a known history of primary cancer who develop new neurologic symptoms (American College of Surgical Oncology [ACSO] CNS Working Group, 2005). Signs and symptoms of brain metastases can be divided into two categories: general symptoms and focal symptoms. General symptoms are typically associated with cerebral edema or increased ICP such as headaches, nausea and vomiting, and cognitive deficits. Focal symptoms result from localized compression or destruction of brain tissue and most often manifest as focal weakness, numbness, speech problems, and seizures (ACSO CNS Working Group, 2005).

Diagnostic Tests

Neuroimaging plays a critical role in formulating the diagnosis, evaluating therapeutic effects, detecting early recurrence, and planning therapy for brain or spinal cord tumors. The diagnosis of a brain or spinal cord tumor is typically based on history and findings on neurologic examination; however, neuroimaging improves the accuracy of the diagnosis and is needed for presurgical planning (Yamada & Sorensen, 2008).

Imaging studies refine preoperative differential diagnosis, locate anatomic landmarks for operative planning, and identify treatment-related side effects. The need for noninvasive diagnostic studies paved the way to the widespread use of neuroimaging in the field of neuro-oncology (Nabors, 2005).

Computed Tomography

CT was invented in the early 1970s and revolutionized clinical neuroscience because never before was a machine able to noninvasively image a living person's whole brain (Bryan, 2005). The CT scan gives more detailed information on bony structures such as the skull. It can also diagnose disease in the soft tissue and blood vessels although not as detailed as MRI. The CT scan allows physicians to diagnose a wide array of conditions in the brain and spine. A spine CT test is most commonly used to diagnose a herniated disk or spinal stenosis. The CT is a valuable diagnostic tool in emergency centers to provide rapid information in the management of trauma and is widely used because of its cost-effectiveness. It is indicated when a patient is not able to undergo MRI or has metal implants or fragments in the body (Barker & Chao, 2002; Henson & Gonzalez, 2005).

The CT scan is obtained by a rotating x-ray beam that passes through the patient's head. The extent of its absorption is measured by a diametrically opposed detector (Lindsay & Bone, 2004). The patient receives an IV iodine contrast medium when the scan without contrast reveals some abnormality or dye study is clinically indicated. Cross-sectional, axial, and coronal images of the brain and spine are produced (Barker & Chao, 2002). Blood and calcification (arteriovenous malformation, hamartoma) will show as high-density lesions. Lesions that appear as low density on CT are infarction, tumor, abscess, edema, encephalitis, or resolving hematoma (Lindsay & Bone, 2004). Although MRI is known to be more sensitive than CT, some tumors have a specific radiologic feature on CT scans (Wen, Teoh, & McLaren, 2002). Tumors such as low-grade astrocytoma usually show as a hypodense area (Armstrong, Cohen, Weinberg, & Gilbert, 2004). On postcontrast CT, astrocytoma will reveal as a nonenhancing lesion (Henson & Gonzalez, 2005). Glioblastomas may show on precontrast CT as centrally hypodense lesions representing necrosis (Drevelegas et al., 2008). When MRI is not available, CT with myelography, which was originally the imaging of choice for intramedullary tumor, is still considered a useful diagnostic tool (Marmor & Gokaslan, 2002).

Magnetic Resonance Imaging

MRI was introduced in the mid-1980s and has evolved into the premier neuroimaging of choice (Jolesz et al., 2008). MRI is able to produce multiplanar imaging without the use of ionizing radiation. It is the most sensitive test for detecting leptomeningeal enhancement seen in metastatic disease (Groves,

2007). The contrast used in MRI is gadolinium. Although MRI has replaced CT in CNS imaging, CT is important and can be used as an adjunct to planning in vertebral neoplasms. MRI has replaced CT because of its sensitivity to pathologic alterations in brain tissues, advanced anatomic resolution, and ability to distinguish between the different forms of tissue in lesions within the tumors. The ability of MRI to obtain multiplanar images and its higher contrast resolution make it the imaging of choice in the diagnosis of brain neoplasms (Drevelegas et al., 2008). MRI uses radiofrequency waves and a powerful magnetic field to produce images.

The principles of physics involved in the production of MRI images are complex (Armstrong et al., 2004). When a patient is placed in a magnetic field, hydrogen nuclei referred to as *spins* align themselves within the field (Armstrong et al., 2004; Lindsay & Bone, 2004; Yamada & Sorensen, 2008). A radiofrequency pulse is then introduced at a specific frequency, which causes the hydrogen protons to move out of alignment (Armstrong et al., 2004; Lindsay & Bone, 2004). When the radiofrequency pulse is stopped, the protons realign themselves with the magnetic field, producing radiofrequency energy, which is a signal that is localized by the rapid turning on and off of the partially varied magnetic field (Armstrong et al., 2004; Wen et al., 2002). The MRI machine contains radio antennae or coils that generate the image. The T1 component (or spin-lattice relaxation) is dependent on time taken for realignment of protons within the magnetic field and represents how these protons interact with the lattice of surrounding molecules and their return to thermal equilibrium (Lindsay & Bone, 2004). The T2 component (spin-spin relaxation) reflects the time taken for the protons to recover to the out-of-phase or original state and is dependent on the locally energized protons' return to electromagnetic equilibrium (Lindsay & Bone, 2004). The image pixel or intensity of volume element depends on the concentration of hydrogen atoms that are variable between types of tissues. Therefore, it is easy to detect any irregularity such as tumors, vascular abnormality, necrotic tissue, and other injuries because of the variation in intensity between tissues (Nabors, 2005). Two MRI techniques used for control of tissue contrast are repetition time (TR), which is the time between successive applications of radiofrequency pulse sequence, and the echo time (TE), which is time between the 90° pulse and the echo (Armstrong et al., 2004; Yamada & Sorensen, 2008).

Primary glial tumors have typical but not diagnostic imaging features. In low-grade astrocytoma, MRI typically demonstrates T2-weighted signal hyperintensity within the white matter and a cerebral cortex with ill-defined margins and varying degrees of mass effect. Linear enhancement along the periphery may be visible with little or no vasogenic edema. Oligodendroglioma, an uncommon glial tumor, has an imaging hallmark of intratumoral calcification (Cha, 2005). Other MRI features include well-defined margins surrounded by normal brain, hypointense on T1-weighted and hyperintense on T2-weighted imaging, as seen in Figure 3-4. Tumor-

associated cysts may be seen along with areas of contrast enhancement. The latter is the result of leaky vasculature in the poorly formed blood-tumor barrier and disruption of the blood-brain barrier (Henson & Gonzalez, 2005). Table 3-2 provides a differential diagnosis of brain tumors based on neuroimaging characteristics.

Figure 3-4. Magnetic Resonance Imaging Showing an Oligodendroglioma

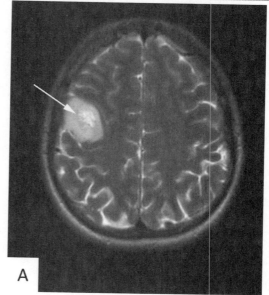

A

Right frontal hyperintense signal on T2-weighted imaging

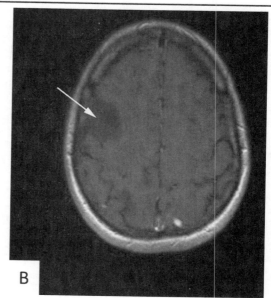

B

Right frontal hypointense signal on T1-weighted postcontrast imaging

Note. Photos courtesy of MD Anderson Cancer Center. Used with permission.

Table 3-2. Differential Diagnosis of Brain Tumors Based on Imaging Characteristics

Imaging Characteristic	Appearance	Tumor Type
Contrast enhancement pattern	Homogeneous	Juvenile pilocytic astrocytoma Glioblastoma Metastases
	Heterogeneous, irregular	Glioblastoma Anaplastic astrocytoma Oligodendroglioma Metastases
	Focal nodular	Oligodendroglioma Ganglioglioma
	Absent	Low-grade fibrillary astrocytoma Gliomatosis cerebri
T2 signal	Low to isointense to gray matter	Meningioma Primary cerebral lymphoma Ependymoma Medulloblastoma Pineoblastoma Metastases (mucinous variant)
	Hyperintense to gray matter	Glial tumor
Cyst		Juvenile pilocytic astrocytoma Ganglioglioma Oligodendroglioma Hemangioblastoma Pleomorphic xanthoastrocytoma
Hemorrhage		Glioblastoma Anaplastic astrocytoma Ependymoma Oligodendroglioma
Calcification		Oligodendroglioma Ependymoma
Necrosis		Glioblastoma Metastases

Note. From "Diagnostic Imaging" (p. 21), by S. Cha in M.S. Berger and M.D. Prados (Eds.), *Textbook of Neuro-Oncology*, 2005, Philadelphia, PA: Elsevier Saunders. Copyright 2005 by Elsevier Saunders. Reprinted with permission.

Mixed tumors with oligodendroglial and glial features are known as *anaplastic oligodendrogliomas*. These tumors have low-grade oligodendroglioma characteristics but with additional features such as necrosis and contrast enhancement common to anaplastic cells. Cystic features and calcification are also common. These tumors are unique among the gliomas

because of their oligodendroglioma characteristics. These lesions are more common in the temporal and frontal lobes. MRI will reveal a hypointense mass lesion on T1-weighted imaging, and a well-circumscribed hyperintense mass lesion expanding the cortex with white matter involvement on T2-weighted imaging (Henson & Gonzalez, 2005). Anaplastic astrocytomas, World Health Organization (WHO) grade 3, and glioblastoma multiforme, WHO grade 4, are high-grade diffuse fibrillary astrocytomas. Anaplastic gliomas have ill-defined borders on T2-weighted images and are heterogeneous hyperintense with either absent, focal, or patchy contrast enhancement. A glioblastoma mass lesion is typically irregular with a thick wall, ring-like enhancement on post-contrast T1-weighted images, prominent mass effect, and peritumoral edema (Tanaka, 2006) (see Figure 3-5).

Figure 3-5. Magnetic Resonance Imaging of the Brain Showing Glioblastoma

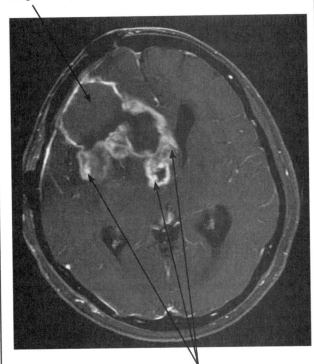

Surgical cavity

Multinodular residual/ recurrent neoplasm

This magnetic resonance image shows right frontal craniotomy with multinodular residual recurrent neoplasm that is periventricular subependymal and involves the septum pellucidum and fornix. There is an associated mass effect, midline shift, and entrapment of the right lateral ventricle.

Note. Photo courtesy of MD Anderson Cancer Center. Used with permission.

Brain tumors are not only classified by tumor type but also by tumor location. They can be located either intra-axial (within the brain parenchyma) or extra-axial (outside the brain parenchyma (Cha, 2005). Table 3-3 provides the differential diagnosis of brain tumors based on location.

Intracranial metastasis constitutes approximately 50% of all supratentorial brain tumors. Metastatic disease spreads into the CNS through a hematogenous route and induces neovascularization as the metastatic lesions spread and enlarge. On imaging, vasogenic edema is common and is associated with neurologic symptoms. These tumors are multiple and well circumscribed and are more common in the gray-white matter junction. Metastatic tumors to the spine are more common than primary spinal cord tumors (Boriani & Weinstein, 2006).

Although T1, T2, and postcontrast sequences provide information in the evaluation of brain tumors, they fail to discriminate tumor cells from peritumoral edema and to accurately determine tumor margins (Drevelegas et al., 2008). The fluid-attenuated inversion recovery sequence (also known as FLAIR) is useful in detecting nonenhancing lesions. The CSF signal is nullified, allowing pathology close to the CSF to be viewed more clearly (Wen et al., 2002). Other advanced neuroimaging techniques that clinicians use to evaluate brain neoplasms and other intracranial abnormalities are diffusion-weighted imaging (DWI) and perfusion-weighted imaging (PWI). Additionally, these techniques are used for treatment planning and evaluation of treatment response.

Diffusion-Weighted Imaging

The basic principle in DWI is derived from the physical phenomenon called *Brownian motion of water molecules* (Nabors, 2005). The random motion of all molecules driven by thermal energy is called *diffusion*. The diffusion of water molecules in human tissue can be sampled using MRI techniques (Yamada & Sorensen, 2008). DWI provides an additional MRI modality to examine the structure of tissue and diagnose diseases (Nabors, 2005). In clinical practice, DWI has been used to delineate and grade tumor, as well as to evaluate tumor extent and invasion (Nabors, 2005). In acute ischemia, diffusion is restrained by cytotoxic edema. The degree of restricted diffusion is measured using a parameter termed as the *apparent diffusion coefficient* (ADC) (Lindsay & Bone, 2004). Lower ADCs usually point to malignant glioma, whereas higher ADCs signify low-grade gliomas (Drevelegas et al., 2008). DWI is now regarded as the standard imaging technique in the timely diagnosis of cerebral ischemia (Cha, 2008). It is also valuable in the precise interpretation of new abnormal enhancement that may develop shortly after surgical resection (Cha, 2008).

Perfusion-Weighted Imaging

PWI provides hemodynamic information complementing the anatomic imaging data from a conventional MRI (Cha, 2008). This technique combines quick imaging with timed contrast injection. Neuroimaging data show quantitative estimates of cerebral blood volume reflecting the underlying microvasculature and angiogenesis. Tumors that are more

Table 3-3. Differential Diagnosis of Brain Tumors Based on Tumor Location

Intra-Axial	Extra-Axial	Intraventricular Supratentorial
Glial, Astrocytic Low-grade fibrillary astrocytoma Anaplastic astrocytoma Glioblastoma multiforme	**Dural** Meningioma Hemangiopericytoma Metastases	Choroid plexus tumor Neurocytoma Meningioma Metastases
Glial, Nonastrocytic Oligodendroglioma Ganglioglioma Dysembryoplastic neuroepithelial tumor	**Pituitary** Adenoma	
Nonglial Primary cerebral lymphoma Metastases	**Pineal** Pineocytoma Germ cell tumor Pineoblastoma	
	Suprasellar Craniopharyngioma Germ cell tumor Lymphoma Metastases Juvenile pilocytic astrocytoma	
	Skull Base Chordoma Plasmacytoma Metastases Chondroid tumor	
Infratentorial		
Glial, Astrocytic Juvenile pilocytic astrocytoma Astrocytoma (low-grade, anaplastic, glioblastoma)	**Dural** Meningioma Hemangiopericytoma Metastases	Ependymoma/ subependymoma Choroid plexus tumor
Nonglial Medulloblastoma Hemangioblastoma Metastases	**Cerebellopontine Angle** Meningioma Schwannoma Epidermoid	

Note. From "Diagnostic Imaging" (p. 20), by S. Cha in M.S. Berger and M.D. Prados (Eds.), *Textbook of Neuro-Oncology*, 2005, Philadelphia, PA: Elsevier Saunders. Copyright 2005 by Elsevier Saunders. Reprinted with permission.

malignant have been associated with increased vascularity as a result of increased angiogenesis (Armstrong et al., 2004). Hence, this imaging technique is useful in characterizing glial neoplasms (Wen et al., 2002).

Spinal cord tumors are classified as either benign or malignant based on the results of pathologic evaluation. These tumors are further categorized by location: extramedullary (outside the parenchyma) or intramedullary (within the cord parenchyma) (see Figure 3-6). Gliomas (ependymomas, low-grade astrocytomas) are the most common intramedullary tumors. Hemangioblastomas, which are associated with Hippel-Lindau syndrome, are the third most common intramedullary tumors (Marmor & Gokaslan, 2002). Intramedullary tumors are also found in metastatic disease from primary sites such as the lung, breast, prostate, kidney, thyroid, or lymph nodes. Infiltration and destruction of cord parenchyma and extension over multiple spinal cord segments are common to intramedullary tumors, whereas extramedullary tumors cause neurologic damage by compressing the spinal cord or nerve roots. They first destroy bone prior to compressing the spinal cord. Diagnosis is typically made initially using imaging studies such as MRI that focus on the anatomic area based on the patient's complaint. MRI is advantageous over CT not only for analyzing brain lesions but also for analyzing

spinal lesions because it provides sagittal views of the spine, separates tumors from nontumorous conditions, and is able to categorize tumors by location (e.g., intramedullary, intradural extramedullary, extradural) (Marmor & Gokaslan, 2002). Spinal x-ray may also reveal bone destruction, widening of the vertebral pedicles, or paraspinal tissue distortion especially with metastatic disease (Beers et al., 2006). Intramedullary ependymoma is isointense on T1-weighted images and hyperintense on T2-weighted images. They are enhanced after the contrast is administered. Cervical ependymoma often has hemosiderin at the periphery. Astrocytoma will reveal diffuse cord enlargement on T1-weighted images, and contrast is usually heterogeneous with irregular borders. Hemangioblastoma and ependymoma are often associated with syrinx formation (a fluid-filled cavity within the spinal cord). This occurs less frequently with astrocytomas of the spinal cord. Hemangioblastomas are less hyperintense on T1-weighted images but are commonly isointense, enhanced on contrast with edema, and usually associated with a cyst or a syrinx (Marmor & Gokaslan, 2002).

Magnetic Resonance Spectroscopy

Magnetic resonance spectroscopy (MRS) is used to measure metabolic activity in the brain to differentiate tumor from

---

Figure 3-6. Magnetic Resonance Imaging of the Spine Showing Intramedullary Lesion

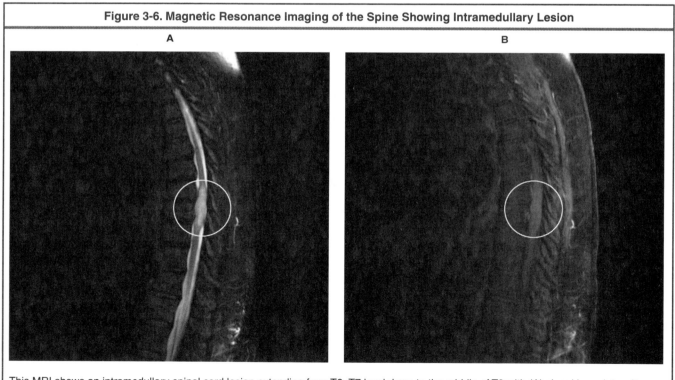

This MRI shows an intramedullary spinal cord lesion extending from T6–T7 level down to the middle of T9 with (A) signal hyperintensity on T2-weighted imaging and (B) abnormal signal intensity on postcontrast T1-weighted imaging.

Note. Photo courtesy of MD Anderson Cancer Center. Used with permission.

radiation necrosis by characteristic spectral patterns (Beers et al., 2006). MRS details the relative concentration of choline, which is the marker of membrane turnover; N-acetyl aspartate (NAA), marker for neuronal health; creatine, component of energy pool; and lactate, marker of anaerobic metabolism (Weingart, McGirt, & Brem, 2006). In brain tumors, choline peaks tend to be high because actively dividing cells require membrane turnover, and NAA peaks tend to be low because neurons are destroyed (Cha, 2008). A rise in the choline along with a low NAA peak is evidence of tumor recurrence. MRS is also used to distinguish between abscess, infarction, and demyelinating disease.

Functional Magnetic Resonance Imaging

Functional magnetic resonance imaging (fMRI) is used to locate the eloquent cortex in the brain (i.e., the bilateral precentral gyrus, left frontal operculum and angular gyrus, and superior temporal gyrus—areas that control motor skills and speech [Ali, Fadel, & Abouldahab, 2009]) before surgical resection or for radiation therapy planning (Cha, 2005). The most common fMRI studies are used to localize the primary motor cortex and somatosensory cortex, typically performed by stimulation of the hand or repetitive movement of the finger during imaging (Piepmeier & Baehring, 2008).

Positron-Emission Tomography

Positron-emission tomography (PET) provides physiologic and biochemical information in terms of tumor metabolism, rate of tumor proliferation, and tumor invasiveness and information related to essential functional tissue (Kracht, Jacobs, & Heiss, 2008). The PET scan uses positron-emitting isotopes (radionuclides) administered intravenously. The isotope's positrons combine with the electrons that release two photons, thus creating a signal detected by the positron detectors (Nabors, 2005). MRI is the imaging of choice for diagnosing and staging brain tumors; however, PET may be valuable in diagnosing nonenhancing, low-grade gliomas that are undergoing malignant transformation (Podoloff et al., 2009). PET may also be useful for differentiating radiation effect from tumor recurrence and guiding biopsy to the site of maximum uptake (Podoloff et al., 2009). This imaging technology is also emerging as a tool for radiation planning and dose confirmation (Podoloff et al., 2009).

Lumbar Puncture

The lumbar puncture (LP), also known as spinal tap, is commonly indicated to evaluate ICP and the extent of leptomeningeal disease, to administer chemotherapy or a radiopaque agent, and for CSF analysis. This procedure involves the introduction of a hollow spinal needle with a stylet into the lumbar subarachnoid space of the spinal canal using aseptic technique (Hickey, 2003c). Once the indication

for LP is established, the necessary preprocedure tests are obtained, and an informed consent is signed, the LP can be performed. The patient is positioned in a lateral decubitus position (knees drawn up to abdomen or fetal position). The landmark is identified between L3 and L4 or L4 and L5 interspace in adults. The alternative position for LP is sitting up and bent over a table if CSF pressure is not indicated or when a difficult LP is performed. This position makes the landmark easier to locate. The site is then prepped and draped in a sterile fashion, and local anesthesia with 1% lidocaine is administered. The spinal needle is advanced into the subarachnoid space, keeping the needle parallel to the spine with the tip pointed toward the umbilicus. Possible complications after LP include CSF leak, headache, bleeding from venous plexus, nerve root damage, risk for infection, or herniation (Gilroy, 2000; Remmel, Bunyan, Brumback, Gascon, & Olson, 2002). The nurse's role in patient care before, during and after the procedure involves patient assessment, patient education, preparation of procedure equipment, assisting the proceduralist with positioning, facilitation of CSF specimen transport to the laboratory, monitoring of vital signs, and documentation.

Electroencephalography

Electroencephalography (EEG) is a painless, noninvasive diagnostic test that uses electrodes distributed over the scalp to capture the electrical activity of the brain. It is commonly used for the diagnosis of seizure disorder, metabolic encephalopathies, herpes simplex encephalitis, structural pathology, and sleep disorders. Continuous EEG monitoring is also helpful in patients with subclinical seizures (without physical manifestation) or in comatose patients with undiagnosed seizures that may affect altered consciousness (Hickey, 2003b).

EEG brain waves are classified according to the number of cycles per second into four frequency bands known as alpha, beta, theta, and delta rhythms. Alpha rhythms are most prominent in the occipital lobes and will disappear or "block" with eye opening (Lindsay & Bone, 2004). Beta waves are present in the frontal and central areas of the brain and are prominent on patients who are on barbiturates and benzodiazepines. Theta rhythms are common in patients who are older than 60 and primarily originate from the temporal lobes, whereas delta rhythms are normally present in sleep (Hickey, 2003b; Lindsay & Bone, 2004).

In patients with a brain tumor, the following EEG abnormalities are described.
- Focal abnormality related to the location of the tumor. For example, right parietal tumor can cause focal right parietal EEG abnormalities.
- Epileptiform discharges, which are interictal phenomena and suggest propensity for having seizures. These abnormal discharges can be focal or generalized. For example, left frontal tumor can result in left frontal epileptiform dis-

charges. This could result in focal seizures arising from the left frontal region. However, focal-onset seizure can secondarily generalize. Patients with generalized epileptiform discharges on EEG can develop generalized seizures.

- EEG background can become slow when the patient develops encephalopathy from metabolic etiology (infections, hepatic and renal dysfunction, respiratory acidosis) or toxins including medications (excessive antiepileptics). Neoplastic meningitis or gliomatosis cerebri (diffusely infiltrating glial tumor of the cerebral cortex) can result in generalized background slowing.
- Patients with cancer are at increased risk for nonconvulsive status epilepticus (seizures with primary manifestation as altered sensorium without clear motor manifestation). EEG remains the standard bedside test to diagnose this condition.
- Patients with cancer are at increased risk for herpetic infections and autoimmune inflammatory disease like limbic encephalitis. EEG in these conditions can show focal temporal lobe abnormalities (Aminoff, 2007; Ropper & Brown, 2005).

Summary

The diagnosis of nervous system tumors involves a detailed and accurate history coupled with a neurologic examination. Patient assessment is a key component in the diagnosis and management of brain and spine neoplasms because it can localize the lesion and provide crucial information about the nervous system. The neurologic examination, when practiced and mastered, becomes second nature to the clinician.

Neuroimaging plays a vital role in the planning and management of patients with brain and spine neoplasms. Besides the CT scan and MRI, newer imaging techniques and studies have proved useful to aid in tumor diagnosis and characterization. The clinician is faced with many challenges, as symptoms can drastically affect the patient's quality of life. Thus, symptom management plays a paramount role in the management of this patient population. Early diagnosis and intervention of brain and spine tumors can potentially increase patient survival and maintain quality of life.

References

Adams, A.C. (2008). *Mayo clinic essential neurology.* Rochester, NY: Informa Healthcare.

Ali, M.Z., Fadel, N.A., & Abouldahab, H.A. (2009). Awake craniotomy versus general anesthesia for managing eloquent cortex low-grade gliomas. *Neurosciences, 14,* 263–272. Retrieved from http://www.neurosciencesjournal.org/PDFFiles/Jul09/Awake.pdf

American College of Surgical Oncology CNS Working Group. (2005). The management of brain metastases. In D. Schiff & B.P. O'Neill (Eds.), *Principles of neuro-oncology* (pp. 553–579). New York, NY: McGraw-Hill.

Aminoff, M.J. (2007). Electrophysiology. In C. Goetz (Ed.), *Textbook of clinical neurology* (3rd ed., pp. 477–497). Philadelphia, PA: Elsevier Saunders.

Armstrong, T.S., Cohen, M.Z., Weinberg, J., & Gilbert, M.R. (2004). Imaging techniques in neuro-oncology. *Seminars in Oncology Nursing, 20,* 231–239. doi:10.1016/S0749-2081(04)00087-7

Armstrong, T.S., & Gilbert, M.R. (2000). Metastatic brain tumors: Diagnosis, treatment, and nursing interventions. *Clinical Journal of Oncology Nursing, 4,* 217–225.

Barker, E.M., & Chao, P.W. (2002). Neurodiagnostic and laboratory studies. In E. Barker (Ed.), *Neuroscience nursing: A spectrum of care* (2nd ed., pp. 99–128). St. Louis, MO: Mosby.

Batchelor, T.T., & Byrne, T.N. (2008). Neurologic complications of primary brain tumors. In D. Schiff, S. Kesari, & P.Y. Wen (Eds.), *Cancer neurology in clinical practice: Neurologic complications of cancer and its treatment* (2nd ed., pp. 381–396). Totowa, NJ: Humana Press.

Beers, M.P., Porter, R.S., Jones, T.V., Kaplan, J.L., & Berkwits, M. (2006). Approach to the neurologic patient. In M.P. Beers, R.S. Porter, T.V. Jones, J.L. Kaplan, & M. Berkwits (Eds.), *The Merck manual of diagnosis and therapy* (18th ed., pp. 1748–1757). Whitehouse Station, NJ: Merck Research Laboratories.

Belford, K. (2005). Central nervous system cancers. In C.H. Yarbro, M.H. Frogge, & M. Goodman (Eds.), *Cancer nursing: Principles and practice* (6th ed., pp. 1089–1136). Sudbury, MA: Jones and Bartlett.

Bickley, L.S., & Szilagyi, P.G. (2007). *Bates' guide to physical examination and history taking* (9th ed.). Philadelphia, PA: Lippincott Williams & Wilkins.

Blaney, S.M., & Poplack, D.G. (2005). Leptomeningeal metastases and dural/skull metastases. In D. Schiff & B.P. O'Neill (Eds.), *Principles of neuro-oncology* (pp. 607–628). New York, NY: McGraw-Hill.

Bondy, M.L., El-Zein, R., & Scheurer, M.E. (2007). Epidemiology of brain tumors. In F. De Monte, M.R. Gilbert, A. Mahajan, & I.E. McCutcheon (Eds.), *M.D. Anderson cancer series: Tumors of the brain and spine* (pp. 1–22). New York, NY: Springer.

Boriani, S., & Weinstein, J.N. (2006). Oncologic classification of vertebral neoplasm. In C.F. Dickman, M.G. Fehlings, & Z.L. Gokaslan (Eds.), *Spinal cord and spinal column tumors: Principles and practice* (pp. 24–37). New York, NY: Thieme.

Bryan, N.R. (2005). Introduction. In J. Gillard, A. Walman, & P. Barker (Eds.), *Clinical MR neuroimaging: Diffusion, perfusion and spectroscopy* (pp. 1–4). Cambridge, United Kingdom: Cambridge University Press.

Cavaliere, R. (2008). Headache. In D. Schiff, S. Kesari, & P.Y. Wen (Eds.), *Cancer neurology in clinical practice* (2nd ed., pp. 57–63). Totowa, NJ: Humana Press.

Cha, S. (2005). Diagnostic imaging. In M.S. Berger & M.D. Prados (Eds.), *Textbook of neuro-oncology* (pp. 19–27). Philadelphia, PA: Elsevier Saunders.

Cha, S. (2008). Physiological imaging. In M. Bernstein & M.S. Berger (Eds.), *Neuro-oncology: The essentials* (2nd ed., pp. 79–90). New York, NY: Thieme.

Chamberlain, M.C. (2008). Neoplastic meningitis. In H.B. Newton & F.A. Jolesz (Eds.), *Handbook of neuro-oncology neuroimaging* (pp. 58–67). New York, NY: Elsevier.

Drevelegas, A., Chourmouzi, D., & Papanicolaou, N. (2008). Malignant astrocytomas. In H.B. Newton & F.A. Jolesz (Eds.), *Handbook of neuro-oncology neuroimaging* (pp. 325–340). New York, NY: Academic Press.

Fortuna, A. (2002). *Early diagnosis in neuro-oncology.* Milan, Italy: Springer.

Fuller, G. (2004). *Neurological examination made easy* (3rd ed.). Edinburg, United Kingdom: Elsevier Churchill Livingstone.

Gelb, D.J. (2005). The neurologic examination. In D.J. Gelb (Ed.), *Introduction to clinical neurology* (3rd ed., pp. 43–54). Philadelphia, PA: Elsevier Butterworth-Heinemann.

Gilbert, M.R., & Armstrong, T.S. (1995). Management of seizures in the adult patient with cancer. *Cancer Practice, 3,* 143–149.

Gilroy, J. (2000). The neurological evaluation. *Basic neurology* (3rd ed., pp. 1–60). New York, NY: McGraw-Hill.

Goldberg, C. (2008). A practical guide to clinical medicine: The neurological examination. Retrieved from http://meded.ucsd.edu/clinicalmed/neuro2.htm

Goldberg, S. (1999). *The four-minute neurologic exam.* Miami, FL: MedMaster.

Groves, M.D. (2007). Neoplastic meningitis. In F. De Monte, M.R. Gilbert, A. Mahajan, & I.E. McCutcheon (Eds.), *M.D. Anderson cancer series: Tumors of the brain and spine* (pp. 245–262). New York, NY: Springer.

Groves, M.D., Jr. (2004). Leptomeningeal carcinomatosis: Diagnosis and management. In R. Sawaya (Ed.), *Intracranial metastases: Current management strategies* (pp. 309–330). Malden, MA: Blackwell Futura.

Henson, J.W., & Gonzalez, R.G. (2005). Imaging in central nervous system tumors. In P.M. Black & J.S. Loeffler (Eds.), *Cancer of the nervous system* (2nd ed., pp. 53–88). Philadelphia, PA: Lippincott Williams & Wilkins.

Hickey, J.V. (2003a). Brain tumors. In J.V. Hickey (Ed.), *The clinical practice of neurological and neurosurgical nursing* (5th ed., pp. 483–508). Philadelphia, PA: Lippincott Williams & Wilkins.

Hickey, J.V. (2003b). Seizures and epilepsy. In J.V. Hickey (Ed.), *The clinical practice of neurological and neurosurgical nursing* (5th ed., pp. 619–640). Philadelphia, PA: Lippincott Williams & Wilkins.

Hickey, J.V. (2003c). Spinal cord tumors. In J.V. Hickey (Ed.), *The clinical practice of neurological and neurosurgical nursing* (5th ed., pp. 509–520). Philadelphia, PA: Lippincott Williams & Wilkins.

Huff, J.S. (2009, July). Neoplasms, spinal cord. Retrieved from http://emedicine.medscape.com/article/779872-overview

Jolesz, F.A., Talos, I.F., Warfield, S.K., Kacher, D., Hata, N., Foroglou, N., & Black, P.M. (2008). Magnetic resonance image guided neurosurgery. In H.B. Newton & F.A. Jolesz (Eds.), *Handbook of neuro-oncology neuroimaging* (pp. 171–180). New York, NY: Academic Press.

Kan, P., & Kestle, J.R.W. (2008). Brainstem tumors. In M. Bernstein & M.S. Berger (Eds.), *Neuro-oncology: The essentials* (2nd ed., pp. 277–286). New York, NY: Thieme.

Kaye, A.H., & Edward, R.J.L. (2001). Historical perspective. In A.H. Kaye & R.J.L. Edward (Eds.), *Brain tumors: An encyclopedic approach* (2nd ed., pp. 3–8). London, United Kingdom: Churchill Livingstone.

Keles, E.G., Tihan, T., Burton, E.C., Prados, M.D., & Berger, M.S. (2005). Diffuse astrocytoma. In M.S. Berger & M.D. Prados (Eds.), *Textbook of neuro-oncology* (pp. 111–121). Philadelphia, PA: Elsevier Saunders.

Kornblith, P.L., Walker, M.D., & Cassady, R.J. (1987). *Neurologic oncology* (pp. 55–65). London, United Kingdom: Lippincott.

Kracht, L.W., Jacobs, A.H., & Heiss, W.-D. (2008). Metabolic imaging. In M. Bernstein & M.S. Berger (Eds.), *Neuro-oncology: The essentials* (2nd ed., pp. 70–78). New York, NY: Thieme.

Kraker, J., & Blakeley, J. (2009). Neurologic manifestations of brain metastases. In L.R. Kleinberg (Ed.), *Brain metastasis: A multidisciplinary approach* (pp. 1–26). New York, NY: Demos Medical.

Lee, E.L.T., & Armstrong, T.S. (2008). Increased intracranial pressure. *Clinical Journal of Oncology Nursing, 12,* 37–41. doi:10.1188/08.CJON.37-41

Lindsay, K.W., & Bone, I. (2004). *Neurology and neurosurgery illustrated* (4th ed.). New York, NY: Churchill Livingstone.

Marmor, E., & Gokaslan, Z.L. (2002). Primary spinal cord tumors. In V. Levin (Ed.), *Cancer in the nervous system* (2nd ed., pp. 149–157). New York, NY: Oxford University Press.

Martin, R.A., Lee, E.K., & Langston, E.L. (2001). The neurologic examination. In R.A. Martin (Ed.), *Family practice curriculum in neurology* [Online version of the CD-ROM]. Retrieved from http://www.aan.com/familypractice/html/menu.htm

McAllister, L.D., Ward, J.H., Schulman, S.F., & De Angelis, L.M. (2002). *Practical neuro-oncology: A guide to patient care.* Boston, MA: Butterworth-Heinemann.

Nabors, L.B. (2005). Neuroimaging. In D. Schiff & B.P. O'Neill (Eds.), *Principles of neuro-oncology* (pp. 53–80). New York, NY: McGraw-Hill.

Ogden, A.T., & McCormick, P.C. (2008). Intradural spinal tumors. In M. Berstein & M.S. Berger (Eds.), *Neuro-oncology: The essentials* (2nd ed., pp. 379–390). New York, NY: Thieme.

Omar, A.I., & Mason, W.P. (2008). Leptomeningeal metastases. In D. Schiff, S. Kesari, & P.Y. Wen (Eds.), *Cancer neurology in clinical practice: Neurologic complications of cancer and its treatment* (2nd ed., pp. 181–201). Totowa, NJ: Humana Press.

Oommen, K.J. (2009, November 25). Neurological history and physical examination. Retrieved from http://emedicine.medscape.com/article/1147993-overview

Piepmeier, J.M., & Baehring, J.M. (2008). Perioperative management. In M. Bernstein & M.S. Berger (Eds.), *Neuro-oncology: The essentials* (2nd ed., pp. 103–111). New York, NY: Thieme.

Podoloff, D.A., Ball, D.W., Ben-Josef, E., Benson, A.B., III, Cohen, S.J., Coleman, R.E., ... Wong, R.J. (2009). NCCN Task Force: Clinical utility of PET in a variety of tumor types. *Journal of the National Comprehensive Cancer Network, 7*(Suppl. 2), S1–S23.

Remmel, K.S., Bunyan, R., Brumback, R.A., Gascon, G.G., & Olson, W.H. (2002). Neurodiagnostic procedures. In *Handbook of symptom-oriented neurology* (3rd ed., pp. 12–29). St. Louis, MO: Mosby.

Ribalta, T., & Fuller, G.N. (2004). Brain metastases: Histopathological evaluation and diagnostic pitfalls. In R. Sawaya (Ed.), *Intracranial metastases: Current management strategies* (pp. 55–70). Malden, MA: Blackwell Futura.

Ropper, A.H., & Brown, R.H. (2005). Special techniques for neurologic diagnosis. In A.H. Ropper & R.H. Brown (Eds.), *Adams and Victor's principles of neurology* (8th ed., pp. 11–34). New York, NY: McGraw-Hill.

Rosenberg, W.S., & Theodosopoulos, P.V. (2002). Spinal tumors. In M.D. Prados (Ed.), *American Cancer Society atlas of clinical oncology series: Brain cancer* (pp. 365–374). Hamilton, Ontario, Canada: Decker Inc.

Russell, S., & Triola, M. (2006). The precise neurological exam. Retrieved from http://cloud.med.nyu.edu/modules/pub/neurosurgery

Schold, S.C.J., Burger, P., Mendelsohn, D.B., Glatstein, E.J., Mickey, B.E., & Minna, J.D. (1997). *Primary tumors of the brain and spinal cord.* Boston, MA: Butterworth-Heinemann.

Tanaka, A. (2006). Imaging diagnosis and fundamental knowledge of common brain tumors in adults. *Radiation Medicine, 24,* 482–492. doi:10.1007/s11604-006-0051-0

Weingart, J.D., McGirt, M.J., & Brem, H. (2006). High-grade astrocytoma/glioblastoma. In J.C. Tonn, M. Westphal, J.T. Rutka, & S.A. Grossman (Eds.), *Neuro-oncology of CNS tumors* (pp. 128–138). Berlin, Germany: Springer.

Wen, P.Y., Teoh, S.K., & McLaren, B.P. (2002). Clinical imaging and laboratory diagnosis of brain tumors. In A.H. Kaye & R.J.L. Edward (Eds.), *Brain tumors: An encyclopedic approach* (pp. 217–226). London, United Kingdom: Churchill Livingstone.

Westcarth, L., & Armstrong, T. (2007). Seizures in people with cancer. *Clinical Journal of Oncology Nursing, 11,* 33–37. doi:10.1188/07.CJON.33-37

Whitehead, W.E., & Illner, A. (2006). Spinal column tumors. In J.C. Tonn, M. Westphal, J.T. Rutka, & S.A. Grossman (Eds.), *Neuro-oncology of CNS tumors* (pp. 583–598). Berlin, Germany: Springer.

Yamada, K., & Sorensen, G.A. (2008). Anatomic imaging. In M. Bernstein & M.S. Berger (Eds.), *Neuro-oncology: The essentials* (2nd ed., pp. 47–69). New York, NY: Thieme.

Yung, W.K.A., Aaron, J., & Aldape, K.D. (2005). Mixed gliomas. In M.S. Berger & M.D. Prados (Eds.), *Textbook of neuro-oncology* (pp. 177–189). Philadelphia, PA: Elsevier Saunders.

CHAPTER 4

Pathology, Histology, and Molecular Markers of Primary Brain Tumors

Annick Desjardins, MD, FRCPC, and
Deborah Hutchinson Allen, RN, MSN, CNS, FNP-BC, AOCNP®

Introduction

Primary brain tumors are divided into mass lesions arising from the brain and its lining. They are further split into two groups: (a) tumors of neuroglial origin (gliomas) and (b) nonglial tumors that are specified by a combination of cell origin and specific location (Okazaki, 1989). This chapter will discuss neuroglial tumors (gliomas) in the context of tumor grading classification, pathology, histology, and molecular markers.

Tumor Grading Classification Systems

Most central nervous system (CNS) tumor histology grading classification systems or schemes are used to predict tumor behavior while minimizing the variations that may be observed between individuals. The histologic typing of tumors was first developed in 1979 (Berger, Leibel, Bruner, Finlay, & Levin, 2002). Immunohistochemistry advances were incorporated into the World Health Organization (WHO) classification schemes in 1993, with the addition of genetics in 2000 and new tumor entities in 2007 (Louis et al., 2007). Histology grading schemes are based on several characteristics: increased cellularity, microcysts, nuclear and cellular pleomorphism, vascular mural cell proliferation, mitotic activity, coagulative tumor necrosis, the proportion of normal tissue mixed with the invading tumor, and the type of tumor at the invading edge into normal tissue. Of the classification schemes listed in Figure 4-1, the WHO classification scheme has been the most widely used to standardize grading for clinical trials across the global research setting. All grading schemes have been associated with clinical prognosis (Berger et al., 2002; Louis et al., 2007).

The WHO grading classification scheme defines primary brain and spinal cord tumors for adults and pediatrics into grades I through IV with increasing aggressiveness of malignancy. Each grade has clearly delineated characteristics

---

Figure 4-1. Examples of Tumor Grading Classification Schemes

- World Health Organization
- Modified Ringertz
- Kernohan
- St. Anne-Mayo

---

of the predefined categories for tumor grade distinction (Tatter, 2005). Grade I tumors have characteristics of well-delineated borders without invasion into local tissue, an absence of vascular proliferation and tumor necrosis, and a reduced amount of cellular pleomorphism. Grade II tumors tend to have well-defined borders (although some invasion into the local tissues may be present), increased cellularity, and nuclear pleomorphism (Tatter, 2005). Both grade I and II tumors are slow growing, may be resectable depending on location, and may recur over time. Grade III tumor characteristics are similar to those seen in grade II tumors except that they demonstrate more local tissue invasion, a faster growth pattern with increased mitotic activity, and possible evidence of vascular proliferation. Grade IV tumors have the most aggressive characteristics of more invasion into local tissues, pronounced vascular proliferation, and central necrosis. Table 4-1 demonstrates these generalized characteristics across the grade classifications for primary brain tumors.

Neuroglial Tumors (Gliomas)

Neuroglial tumors, also called gliomas, are the largest group of primary CNS neoplasms, with approximately half of all primary brain tumors being glial cell neoplasms (Central Brain Tumor Registry of the United States [CBTRUS], 2010). The three most common gliomas are named based on the three histologic groups of the presumed glial cell of origin

Table 4-1. World Health Organization Tumor Grading Classification Scheme Characteristics

Tumor Grade	Cellularity	Microcysts	Pleomorphism	Vascular Proliferation	Necrosis	Invasion	Mitotic Activity
I	+	+	+	−	−	−	+
II	+	+	+	−	−	+	+
III	++	+	++	+	−	++	++
IV	+++	+	+++	++	++	+++	+++

Key: − Does not have this characteristic; + Has this characteristic in incremental expression, with +++ representing the greatest expression.

Note. Based on information from Berger et al., 2002; Kleihues et al., 1995; Louis et al., 2007.

(Kleihues, Soylemezoglu, Schäuble, Scheithauer, & Burger, 1995; Louis et al., 2007; Okazaki, 1989):
1. Astrocytoma
2. Oligodendroglioma
3. Ependymoma.

Historical references describe glial cells as outnumbering the trillions of neurons in the brain by 5–10 times (Angevine, 1988), but recent research suggests that this ratio differs significantly throughout our brain depending on anatomic location and function (Azevedo et al., 2009). Neurons, or nerve cells, primarily provide electrical impulses from the brain or peripheral body for autonomic, sensory, or motor function. The several types of glial cells include astrocytes, oligodendrocytes, microglia, and ependymal cells (see Chapter 2). Glial cells provide a number of functions to brain tissues and neurons, including essential nutrients and oxygen, physical support and maintenance of cellular environment, modulation of neurotransmissions, and destruction and removal of dead neurons (Snell, 2001). These cells retain the ability to undergo cell division, which is observed during injury and repair, and are key in synaptic plasticity and synaptogenesis (Snell, 2001). Thus, they have an enormous potential for abnormal growth, making them the chief source of CNS neoplasms.

Astrocytomas

The several different types of astrocytomas represent more than three-quarters of all gliomas (CBTRUS, 2010). They develop when the star-shaped astrocytes undergo growth and cellular transformation. Figure 4-2 lists the most commonly observed astrocytomas. Using a classification system that places tumors into clearly definable categories, astrocytomas more accurately represent a biologic continuum ranging from histologically well-differentiated tumors to poorly or undifferentiated neoplasms with nuclear and cellular pleomorphism, vascular endothelial proliferation, and necrosis (James, Smith, & Jenkins, 2002; Okazaki, 1989). Of particular importance is that all infiltrating gliomas, including those classified as benign, can be fatal without appropriate treatment because of

the tendency for continued growth and invasion, recurrence, or transformation to a more aggressive tumor (Berger et al., 2002; Hoshino et al., 1988; James et al., 2002; McCormack, Miller, Budzilovich, Voorhees, & Ransohoff, 1992). Thus, the terms *low-grade* or *benign* may falsely reassure the layman of a good outcome and a full life.

Fibrillary (diffuse) astrocytomas are the most common subtype of the white-matter tumors that occur in the brain or spinal cord; however, they occur more often in the frontal lobe (Berger et al., 2002; Felsberg & Reifenberger, 2002). They are composed of slow-growing abnormal astrocytes. The degree of individual cellular fibrillarity influences the tumor characteristics, which range from a spectrum of rare low-grade "benign" astrocytoma to the more common and aggressive form, glioblastoma multiforme (GBM). Fibrillary astrocytomas are also called diffuse astrocytomas because they develop projections that slowly extend or diffuse into surrounding structures.

Pilocytic (hair-like) astrocytoma (WHO grade I) is also called *juvenile pilocytic astrocytoma* because of its higher frequency in childhood and adolescence. It represents only 5%–10% of all cerebral gliomas but accounts for nearly one-third of pediatric glial neoplasms (Berger et al., 2002; CBTRUS, 2010). The most common supratentorial neoplasm in children is the opticochiasmatic-hypothalamic pilocytic astrocytoma, a mass located at the junction of the optic nerve, optic chiasma, and hypothalamus. Controversy exists regard-

---

Figure 4-2. Types of Astrocytomas

- Fibrillary or diffuse
- Pilocytic (hair-like), also known as juvenile pilocytic astrocytoma
- Well-differentiated
- Anaplastic astrocytoma
- Glioblastoma multiforme
- Gliomatosis cerebri
- Gliosarcomas
- Pleomorphic xanthoastrocytoma
- Subependymal giant cell

ing which tumor is the most common posterior fossa tumor in this age group, astrocytoma of the cerebellum or medulloblastoma. Brain stem gliomas are frequent and represent the third most common pediatric infratentorial tumor (CBTRUS, 2010; Zimmerman, 1990).

Pilocytic astrocytoma is generally slow growing with relatively well-defined borders, which allows a complete or almost complete resection of the tumor. Survival rates are very good; those who undergo gross total resection have a survival rate that approaches 100% (Berger et al., 2002; Burger, Scheithauer, & Vogel, 1991). Despite its classification as an astrocytoma (WHO grade I), pilocytic astrocytoma is a morphologically and biologically distinct astrocytoma subtype. It is suggested that pilocytic astrocytomas arise from a class of astrocytes that is inconspicuous in normal brain but may become prominent in reactive gliosis and neoplasia (Berger et al., 2002; Burger et al., 1991). The gross examination of pilocytic astrocytoma varies with its location. Cerebellar pilocytic astrocytoma is normally a well circumscribed mass with typically a large cyst encompassing the small, reddish-tan tumor nidus, also referred to as a mural nodule. Pilocytic astrocytomas of the opticochiasmatic-hypothalamic area are lobulated and grossly well circumscribed but will microscopically infiltrate into the floor or walls of the third ventricle (Berger et al., 2002; Okazaki, 1989). In comparison, brain stem pilocytic astrocytomas are uniform, nonfocal infiltrating neoplasms, which diffusely expand to the pons or medulla.

Two histologic patterns are observed with pilocytic astrocytomas: densely compact regions of elongated cells with hair-like (pilocytic) processes, and more loosely organized spongiform foci with stellate astrocytes and microcystic changes (Berger et al., 2002; Burger et al., 1991). Rosenthal fibers, a histologic feature of small amorphous eosinophilic bead-like or corkscrew-shaped hyaline bodies surrounded by glial filaments, are often prominent in pilocytic astrocytomas (Berger et al., 2002; Burger et al., 1991). The mitotic activity is low or absent in pilocytic astrocytomas, and despite the presence of cysts, there is no associated tumor necrosis. In about 10% of cases, calcification occurs (Lee, Van Tassel, Bruner, Moser, & Share, 1989). Despite demonstrating a clinically aggressive course in up to one-third of the cases, it is very rare for pilocytic astrocytoma to demonstrate frank malignant transformation or leptomeningeal dissemination (Berger et al., 2002; Strong et al., 1993). Although dissemination of this histologically benign tumor may occur without any demonstration of malignant transformation or primary tumor recurrence, the growth rate of distant metastases remains very low (Berger et al., 2002; Mishima et al., 1992).

Well-differentiated astrocytomas (WHO grade II) are tumors that may appear grossly circumscribed but are, in fact, unencapsulated and infiltrate diffusely. Gross appearance reveals a solid, slightly grayish mass that varies in consistency from soft to almost gelatinous (Burger et al., 1991).

Necrosis is absent despite the presence of an occasional cystic degeneration. Microscopically, a proliferation of well-differentiated fibrillary astrocytes demonstrating mild nuclear pleomorphism can be observed. Few mitoses are present with a low-to-moderate cell density. No vascular proliferation is visible, which makes hemorrhage occurrence a rarity. Because of its slow growth, degenerative mineralization within the tumor results in calcification in 15%–20% of cases (Berger et al., 2002). Strong immunoreactivity to the antibody of glial fibrillary acidic protein (also known as GFAP) will be present, which confirms astrocyte differentiation and glioma development (Berger et al., 2002; McCormack et al., 1992). Well-differentiated astrocytomas represent about 10%–15% of gliomas (CBTRUS, 2010; Fan, Kovie, & Earle, 1977). Inactivating *TP53* mutations are found in more than 50% of well-differentiated astrocytomas (James et al., 2002). Many growth factors and their receptors are overexpressed in astrocytomas, including platelet-derived growth factor (PDGF), fibroblast growth factors, vascular endothelial growth factor (VEGF), and epidermal growth factor receptor (EGFR). Loss of chromosome arm 22q(22) and gain of chromosome arm 7q(23) are less common alterations in the genome associated with WHO grade II astrocytomas. Astrocytomas are not histologically or biologically uniform tumors, which makes the distinction between well-differentiated and anaplastic astrocytomas (AAs) difficult to determine at best (Berger et al., 2002; Hoshino et al., 1988). Despite the fact that many patients with well-differentiated astrocytoma survive for extended periods, 50% of surgically treated lesions will evolve into AAs or GBM (Piepmeier, 1987). Death in patients with well-differentiated astrocytoma is most commonly due to a transformation into a higher-grade neoplasm (Berger et al., 2002; Philippon, Clemenceau, Fauchon, & Foncin, 1993). The median survival of patients with a well-differentiated astrocytoma is usually 7–10 years (CBTRUS, 2010; McCormack et al., 1992).

AAs represent 20%–25% of gliomas but only 4% of all brain tumors (CBTRUS, 2010). AAs occupy an intermediate position between well-differentiated astrocytomas and GBM. The degree of anaplasia increases in a graded fashion with the upper extreme merging imperceptibly with GBM (Berger et al., 2002; Burger et al., 1991; Burger, Vogel, Green, & Strike, 1985). On gross examination, AAs are diffusely infiltrating tumors with poorly delineated borders, even if they appear grossly circumscribed. AAs are normally heterogeneous masses with cystic areas and areas of hemorrhage. However, necrosis, the hallmark of GBM, is absent. Histologic evaluation demonstrates a less well-differentiated neoplasm with greater hypercellularity and pleomorphism than well-differentiated astrocytomas. Also, mitoses and vascular endothelial proliferation are present. Calcification is uncommon unless the AA is secondary to the malignant degeneration of a preexisting well-differentiated astrocytoma. Median survival is about two years (CBTRUS, 2010).

GBM is at the far end of the astrocytoma spectrum. It is the most aggressive and malignant of all glial neoplasms, representing 15%–20% of primary brain neoplasms and half of all astrocytomas (CBTRUS, 2010). Its "multiforme" appellation comes from its highly variable gross and microscopic appearance. On gross pathology, necrosis has been the hallmark of GBM for years (Burger et al., 1991); however, the presence of marked vascular endothelial proliferation alone may be sufficient for a diagnosis of GBM (Kleihues et al., 1995, 2000). GBM is usually recognizable by its large, heterogeneous mass or masses with central necrosis, thick irregular "shaggy" walls, and increased vascularity (Berger et al., 2002; Hallani et al., 2010). Commonly, intratumoral hemorrhage will be seen. Severe cerebral edema and tumor burden causes increased intracranial pressure within the tissue, termed *mass effect*. By histology, the cellular composition of GBM is in multiple forms, as the name implies. Distinct subsets of neoplastic astrocytes that differ from each other in morphology, biologic activity, metastatic potential, and radiation sensitivity are typically contained in GBM (Berger et al., 2002; Berkman et al., 1992); varied expression of GBMs has virtually no limit. Some tumor foci seem relatively well differentiated while others contain bizarre pleomorphic or undifferentiated cells. Numerous mitoses are present, and vascular proliferation is severe. On magnetic resonance imaging, the contrast enhancing mass demonstrates only the area of blood-brain barrier disrupted neovessels, while neoplastic cells are present well beyond the area of enhancement. As with AAs, calcification is rare unless the GBM developed secondary to the malignant degeneration of a preexisting well-differentiated astrocytoma. In 0.5%–1% of cases, multifocal or multicentric gliomas occur (Barnard & Geddes, 1987).

Multifocal gliomas are lesions with microscopic parenchymal connections or masses that occur as satellite lesions from cerebrospinal fluid spread, whereas multicentric gliomas represent isolated gliomas arising in distinctly separate sites with no detectable microscopic connections to one another (Leeds, Kumar, & Jackson, 2002). Wide and rapid spread characterizes GBM, most frequently along the white-matter tracts. Bihemispheric spread across the corpus callosum, anterior and posterior commissures (nerve fibers that connect hemispheres), and internal and external capsules is also common. As the disease progresses, most patients will develop satellite lesions grossly separated from but microscopically connected to the parent tumor. Once dissemination occurs at the level of the ependymal, subpial, and throughout the cerebral and spinal subarachnoid spaces, most of the time, it represents a terminal state (Grabb, Albright, & Pang, 1992). Very uncommonly, GBM will develop extracerebral metastases to the lung, liver, bone, and other sites. Aggressively growing GBM cells look very different from normal cells.

Genetic alterations are frequent in GBM. *TP53* mutations and 10q mutations are two examples. GBM is divided into primary GBM (*de novo*) and secondary GBM (arising from lower-grade precursors) (Kanu et al., 2009; Louis & Gusella, 1995) (see Figure 4-3). These subtypes can be stratified genetically based on *TP53* mutations and EGFR amplification or overexpression (Kleihues et al., 2000; Watanabe et al., 1996). The *TP53* gene is mutated in approximately 65% of secondary GBMs but only 10% of primary GBMs (Cavenee et al., 2000). EGFR amplification or overexpression occurs in 40%–60% of primary GBMs but is rare in secondary GBMs (Feldkamp, Lala, Lau, Roncari, & Guha, 1999; James et al., 2002; Watanabe et al., 1996).

Gliomatosis cerebri represents a diffuse overgrowth of the brain with neoplastic glial cells and an extreme form of diffusely infiltrating glioma (Mineura, Sasajima, Kowada, Uesaka, & Shishido, 1991). On gross examination, the cerebral hemispheres, cerebellum, or brain stem is diffusely enlarged, while the normal anatomic landmarks are preserved (Dickson, Horoupian, Thal, & Lantos, 1988). Despite the observation that some areas have more concentrated neoplastic processes, such as the optic nerves and compact white matter pathways (corpus callosum, fornices, and cerebellar peduncles), no grossly discernible focal masses are formed (Okazaki, 1989; Yip, Fisch, & Lamarche, 2003). Histologic evaluation demonstrates a diffuse infiltration of the brain with neoplastic glial cells in varying states of differentiation

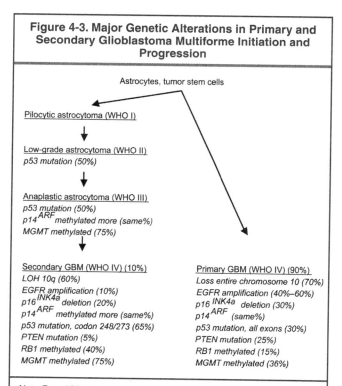

Figure 4-3. Major Genetic Alterations in Primary and Secondary Glioblastoma Multiforme Initiation and Progression

Astrocytes, tumor stem cells

Pilocytic astrocytoma (WHO I)

Low-grade astrocytoma (WHO II)
p53 mutation (50%)

Anaplastic astrocytoma (WHO III)
p53 mutation (50%)
p14^ARF methylated more (same%)
MGMT methylated (75%)

Secondary GBM (WHO IV) (10%)
LOH 10q (60%)
EGFR amplification (10%)
p16^INK4a deletion (20%)
p14^ARF methylated more (same%)
p53 mutation, codon 248/273 (65%)
PTEN mutation (5%)
RB1 methylated (40%)
MGMT methylated (75%)

Primary GBM (WHO IV) (90%)
Loss entire chromosome 10 (70%)
EGFR amplification (40%–60%)
p16^INK4a deletion (30%)
p14^ARF (same%)
p53 mutation, all exons (30%)
PTEN mutation (25%)
RB1 methylated (15%)
MGMT methylated (36%)

Note. From "Glioblastoma Multiforme Oncogenomics and Signaling Pathways," by O.O. Kanu, B. Hughes, C. Di, N. Lin, J. Fu, D.D. Bigner, ... C. Adamson, 2009, *Clinical Medicine Insights: Oncology, 3*, p. 40. Copyright 2009 by Libertas Academica. Reprinted with permission.

and relative preservation of the underlying cytoarchitecture (Ross, Robitaille, Villemure, & Tampieri, 1991). A perineuronal, perivascular, and subpial location of the tumor cells is typically encountered (Spagnoli et al., 1987). Primary leptomeningeal gliomatosis, a form of gliomatosis cerebri, can also occur (Leproux, Melanson, Mercier, Michaud, & Ethier, 1993; Rippe et al., 1990).

Gliosarcomas are rare primary tumors composed of both neoplastic glial cells and spindle-cell sarcomatous elements. Gliosarcomas are most often GBMs, and generally, the sarcomatous component arises from neoplastically transformed vascular elements within the GBM itself. Gliosarcomas have a tendency for a peripheral location, with dural invasion (Berger et al., 2002; Jack et al., 1987) coming in contact with the skull or the falx cerebri (Maiuri, Stella, Benvenuti, Giamundo, & Pettinato, 1990). On gross examination, gliosarcomas are firm, lobulated tumors with central necrotic areas. The sarcomatous portion is sharply demarcated and often separable from the adjacent brain, whereas the astrocytic component is soft and poorly delineated, or defined, from surrounding parenchyma (Jack et al., 1987). On histology, the pathologic diagnosis of gliosarcoma is made by the identification of glial and mesenchymal tumor elements. The mesenchymal component is variable but most often resembles a typical fibrosarcoma or malignant fibrous histiocytoma. Cartilaginous and rhabdomyosarcomatous components have been described (Burger et al., 1991). The infiltrating component of the gliosarcoma is almost always a GBM, consistent with the common observation of pleomorphic cells with vascular endothelial proliferation and necrosis (Berger et al., 2002). Less than 2% of GBMs will undergo sarcomatous transformation (Burger et al., 1991), and they normally affect patients in their fifth to seventh decades. Fifteen to thirty percent of all gliosarcomas will have extracranial metastases and metastases to the visceral organs through hematogenous dissemination (Berger et al., 2002; Jack et al., 1987).

Less common astrocytoma subtypes include *pleomorphic xanthoastrocytoma* and *subependymal giant cell astrocytoma*.

Oligodendrogliomas

Oligodendrogliomas arise from a specific type of glial cell, oligodendrocytes, which make and maintain the myelin of the CNS. Oligodendrogliomas mainly affect middle-aged adults. They occur mostly in the cerebral hemispheres and cortical involvement is common, explaining the high frequency of seizure activity at presentation. On gross examination, they are typically well-circumscribed unencapsulated focal white matter tumors that might involve the cortex and leptomeninges. More rarely, poorly delineated, diffusely infiltrating tumors are seen. Cysts are relatively common; hemorrhage and necrosis are not common (Berger et al., 2002; Okazaki, 1989). Oligodendrogliomas may have a gritty texture because of the high frequency of calcification.

It is the most common intracranial tumor to calcify, and nodular or clumped calcification is present in 70%–90% of cases, as well as scalloped erosion of the inner table of the skull (Berger et al., 2002; Dolinskas & Simeone, 1987). On histology, well-differentiated oligodendrogliomas are characterized by uniform cells with regular spherical nucleoli, surrounded by a clear halo (fried-egg appearance). Mitoses are in small number, but calcospherites are common. Similar to the other glioma types, oligodendrogliomas have a differentiation spectrum that ranges from well differentiated to progressively worsening degrees of anaplasia. Moderate pleomorphism and abundant mitosis are typically seen in anaplastic or malignant oligodendrogliomas (Burger et al., 1991). Forty to eighty percent of oligodendrogliomas present a preferential allelic loss on chromosomes 1p and 19q (James et al., 2002; Louis, 2006).

Mixed gliomas are relatively rare and are histologically heterogeneous neoplasms consisting of at least two different glial cell lines. *Oligoastrocytoma* is the most common mixed glioma (Berger et al., 2002; Kyritsis, Yung, Bruner, Gleason, & Levin, 1993). The prognosis for a patient with an oligoastrocytoma is slightly better than that of a patient with a tumor of a pure astrocytic lineage. On occasion, ependymal elements are also present. Genetic changes typical of astrocytomas (*TP53* mutations) or oligodendrogliomas (1p and 19q loss) are found in oligoastrocytomas. In about one-third of oligoastrocytomas, the astrocytoma genotype predominates, and in one-third, the oligodendroglioma genotype predominates (Berger et al., 2002).

Ependymal Tumors

The ependyma, a thin layer of ciliated cuboidal or columnar epithelium that lines the ventricular walls and central canal of the spinal cord, is formed of ependymal cells, which are embryologically related to other glial cell types. Neoplastically transformed ependymal cells often reflect a dual glial and epithelial heritage (Angevine, 1988; Burger et al., 1991; Packer, Friedman, Kun, & Fuller, 2002) (see Figure 4-4).

Cellular ependymomas are predominantly infratentorial tumors filling the fourth ventricle and extruding through the natural passageways, floor or roof of the fourth ventricle, lateral recesses and foramen of Magendie, into the adjacent cerebrospinal fluid cisterns. They occur mainly in children and adolescents and represent 2%–8% of all primary intra-

Figure 4-4. Types of Ependymal Tumors

- Cellular
- Plastic
- Papillary
- Myxopapillary
- Subependymoma
- Anaplastic

cranial brain tumors. Cellular ependymomas constitute 15% of posterior fossa neoplasms in childhood and are the third most common pediatric brain tumor (CBTRUS, 2010; Nazar et al., 1990).

Ependymomas that have a tendency to extend postero-inferiorly into the cisterna magna, anterolaterally into the cerebellopontine angle cisterns, and down through the foramen magnum into the upper cervical spine behind the cervicomedullary junction are referred to as *plastic ependymomas* (Lee & Van Tassel, 1989). About 60% of intracranial ependymomas are located in the posterior fossa, and more than 90% of them are located in the fourth ventricle, with the medulla and cerebellopontine angle cisterns representing the rest of the posterior fossa sites (Lee & Van Tassel, 1989). Two-thirds to three-quarters of the supratentorial ependymomas are extraventricular (Armington et al., 1985; Packer et al., 2002; Palma, Celli, & Cantore, 1993).

Ependymomas have predominantly glial features; they are lobulated, partly cystic, slow-growing neoplasms. Calcifications are common, but not hemorrhage (Lizak & Woodruff, 1992; Swartz, Zimmerman, & Bilaniuk, 1982). On histologic examination, cellular ependymomas are composed of fusiform cells arranged around small blood vessels. An important microscopic finding is the presence of the so-called perivascular pseudorosettes (Burger et al., 1991; Packer et al., 2002). On occasion, ependymoma forms true ependymal rosettes—miniature reproductions of the lining of a normal ependymal cavity (Okazaki, 1989). A spectrum of anaplasia exists in ependymomas that range from the typical well-differentiated neoplasm with infrequent mitoses, mild cellular pleomorphism, and minimal or no necrosis to lesions with high cell density, high mitotic activity, and extensive cellular pleomorphism, vascular proliferation, and necrosis (Burger et al., 1991). The more aggressive ependymomas, or WHO grade III *anaplastic ependymomas*, occur with nearly equal frequency in both supratentorial and infratentorial locations. Supratentorial ependymomas have a greater tendency to recur at the primary tumor site (Berger et al., 2002). Drop metastasis, also called *spinal seeding*, is relatively uncommon (Lyons & Kelly, 1991; Palma et al., 1993; Perrin, Laperriere, Loblew, & Laxton, 2002).

Papillary ependymomas are uncommon and are single or multilayered neoplastic cells covering glial papillae. *Myxopapillary ependymomas* are rare tumors of the spinal cord that occur almost exclusively in the conus medullaris or filum terminale.

Subependymomas are rare benign CNS tumors. Subependymomas are small, nodular or lobulated, and usually located at the caudal fourth ventricle or the foramen of Monro (Jelenik, Smirniotopoulos, Parisi, & Kanzer, 1990; Packer et al., 2002). They occur predominantly in middle-aged adults and are generally discovered incidentally or at the time of autopsy. On gross examination, they are firm, well-delineated, avascular, white-to-grayish intraventricu-

lar masses attached to the septum pellucidum or inferior fourth ventricle. On microscopic examination, a sparsely cellular neoplasm with a prominent fibrillary background and microcystic changes is seen. However, hypercellularity, ependymal rosette formation, neovascularity, mitosis, and necrosis are absent (Lobato et al., 1986; Okazaki, 1989; Packer et al., 2002).

Choroid Plexus Tumors

More than 90% of tumors involving the choroid plexus are choroid plexus papillomas. They typically affect children younger than five years of age and are mostly found in the atrium of the lateral ventricle (Packer et al., 2002). The fourth ventricle is more commonly affected in adult cases of choroid plexus papilloma, and the third ventricle is an uncommon location at any age. Very rarely, a patient will be diagnosed with a choroid plexus carcinoma rather than a papilloma.

Neuronal and Mixed Neuronal-Glial Tumors

In adults, glial tumors outnumber neuronal neoplasms by approximately 100:1 (Berger et al., 2002; CBTRUS, 2010; Louis, Scheithauer, Budka, von Deimling, & Kepes, 2000). See Figure 4-5 for a list of types of neuronal and mixed neuronal-glial tumors.

Tumors of the Mesenchyme and Meninges

Most primary intracranial mesenchymal tumors develop from meningothelial cells. Meningiomas are the most frequent primary intracranial mesenchymal tumors (McDermott, Quinones-Hinosa, Fuller, & Wilson, 2002).

Meningiomas

Meningiomas are normally slow-growing tumors that are typically well circumscribed and arise from the meningothelial arachnoid cap cells (McDermott et al., 2002). In the majority of the cases, they occur in a specific location around the arachnoid villi. With the exception of children with a diagnosis of neurofibromatosis type 2, meningiomas are usually a supratentorial tumor of the adult (McDermott

---

Figure 4-5. Types of Neuronal and Mixed Neuronal-Glial Tumors

- Gangliocytoma
- Ganglioglioma
- Lhermitte-Duclos disease
- Dysembryoplastic neuroepithelial tumors
- Central neurocytoma
- Olfactory neuroblastoma (esthesioneuroblastoma)

et al., 2002). The WHO grading classification system for meningiomas is shown in Table 4-2.

Table 4-2. World Health Organization Grading Classification for Meningiomas	
WHO Grade	Classification
1	Benign
2	Atypical
3	Anaplastic

Molecular Markers

Recent technologic advances in oncology care have increased knowledge regarding prognostic and predictive gene markers or patterns of gene expression that are observed in tumor development (National Cancer Institute, 2006). These markers may be useful in illuminating how tumors respond to treatment modalities and relevant to discussions regarding survival. Pertinent to cancer development and progression, many concurrent stages of molecular activities occur to promote cellular life, including self-sustaining growth-signaling pathways, unresponsiveness to normal cellular antigrowth signals, inhibited apoptosis and sustained angiogenesis, unlimited replication potential, invasion of local tissues, and metastasis to distant sites (Hanahan & Weinberg, 2000; Hunt, 2008).

Impact of Molecular and Genetic Pathology

The brain is unique from other tissues and organs, which challenges oncology teams in treating tumor development. Historically, the use of histologic classifications has implied tumor homogeneity by grouping tumors into types for the ease of discussing treatment options. Yet, genomic mapping of CNS tumors suggests that a more complex heterogeneous nature exists. This may be one explanation of resistance to treatment (James et al., 2002).

A dynamic interplay of many factors contributes to the development of CNS tumors (James et al., 2002; Rich & Bigner, 2004). Glial invasion occurs through growth of tumor cells into the white-matter and gray-matter tracts of the brain and spine, resulting in subpial spread and perivascular growth. As tumor cells are activated, disruptions in cell-to-cell adhesion occurs, resulting in remodeling of the extracellular matrix permitting cellular motility to other areas of the CNS (James et al., 2002; Mott, Turner, Bigner, & McLendon, 2008). Through chromosomal loss or mutations, growth is encouraged, natural apoptosis becomes affected, the tumor cell life becomes prolonged, and the cell cycle remains activated (Hanahan & Weinberg, 2000; Sathornsumetee, Reardon, et al., 2007).

The two key genetic concepts associated with cancer development and occurring in glioma pathogenesis are oncogenes and tumor suppressor genes. Amplification or mutation to oncogenes will promote cellular proliferation. Just as tumor suppressor gene proteins inhibit cell growth, deletion of tumor suppressor genes will result in unmonitored cellular growth (Pecorino, 2008). Table 4-3 displays commonly observed oncogenes and tumor suppressor genes and their association with specific glioma development (James et al., 2002).

Glial Invasion

One main characteristic of gliomas is their tendency to infiltrate the surrounding brain. This characteristic dramatically reduces the ability for localized therapies to effectively control the disease. This invasive capacity is seen in both well-differentiated or low-grade and high-grade gliomas, implying that the invasive phenotype is acquired early. Preferential invasion along the white-matter tracts, preferential growth around neurons in the gray matter, and perivascular growth and subpial spread are typical features. A dynamic interplay between cell-cell adhesion, remodeling of the extracellular matrix, and cell motility promotes invasion of glioma cells into the brain (Cavenee et al., 2000). Proteases elaborated by glioma cells appear to play a significant role in astrocytoma invasion. Cysteine, serine, and metalloproteinases are selective proteases that degrade the extracellular environment to facilitate migration. It is also possible that proteases remodel the environment to facilitate tumor cell growth. Matrix metalloproteinases MMP2 and MMP9, serine protease urokinase-type plasminogen activator and its receptor, and cysteine protease cathepsin B are observed in glioma development with the level of expression associated with glioma grade, such that more expression means a more aggressively behaving glioma (Rao, 2003). Figure 4-6 displays invasion in glioma tumors.

Integrins are a family of cell adhesion molecules ("Integrin," 2007). Integrin receptors are expressed by most malignant gliomas and mediate interactions with molecules in the extracellular space. Integrin heterodimers, compounds formed by two simpler but different molecules ("Heterodimer," 2007), interact with tenascin, fibronectin, laminin, and vitronectin (Uhm, Gladson, & Rao, 1999). Activation of these integrins through interaction with extracellular ligands results in alterations of the cellular cytoskeleton, promoting locomotion. Focal adhesion kinase, a cytoplasmic tyrosine kinase expressed in high-grade gliomas and activated by EGFR and integrins, signals through different pathways that affect proliferation, survival, and migration (Natarajan, Hecker, & Gladson, 2003).

Most of the growth factors expressed in astrocytomas, such as fibroblast growth factor, epidermal growth factor (EGF), and VEGF, stimulate migration. For example, EGFR-amplified cells are preferentially located at the infiltrating edges of GBM (Okada et al., 2003).

Table 4-3. Commonly Observed Gene or Chromosomal Abnormalities in the Development of Central Nervous System Tumors

Gene or Chromosome	Abnormality	Abnormal Function	Tumor Type	Frequency of Occurrence
CDK2A	Deletion/mutation	Cell cycle progression and proliferation	AA and GBM	50%
CDK4	Amplification	Cell cycle progression	AA and GBM	10%–15%
CMYC	Amplification	Cell cycle arrest, apoptosis	Medulloblastoma	5%–10%
EGFR	Amplification	Cell proliferation, sustainability	AA GBM	10%–15% 40%–60%
MDM2	Overexpression	Cell growth	AA and GBM	5%–10%
MYCN	Amplification	Inactivation of tumor suppressor gene; onco-genesis	Medulloblastoma	5%–10%
NF2	Deletion	Inactivation of tumor suppressor genes; cell proliferation	Meningioma	50%–60%
p16	Deletion	Cell cycle progression	AA and GBM	50%
PTCH	Deletion/mutation	Inactivation of tumor suppressor gene; onco-genesis	Medulloblastoma	10%–20%
PTEN	Deletion/mutation	Cell cycle progression, migration, proliferation	AA and GBM	10%
TP53	Deletion/inactivation	Cell cycle arrest, apoptosis, DNA repair	AA and GBM Low-grade astrocytoma	30%–40% 50%
Chromosome 1p	Deletion	Inactivation of tumor suppressor genes, onco-genesis	Oligodendroglioma GBM	40%–90% 30%
Chromosome 10	Deletion/mutation	Cell cycle progression, migration, proliferation	GBM	60%–95%
Chromosome 17p	Deletion	Loss of *TP53*; accelerated cell growth and survival	Medulloblastoma	30%–50%
Chromosome 17q	Deletion	Inactivation of tumor suppressor genes; onco-genesis	Pilocytic astrocytoma	20%–30%
Chromosome 19q	Deletion	Inactivation of tumor suppressor genes; onco-genesis	Oligodendroglioma	50%–90%
Chromosome 22	Deletion	Inactivation of tumor suppressor genes; onco-genesis	Ependymoma Low-grade astrocytoma	25%–50% 25%–50%

AA—anaplastic astrocytoma; CMYC—myelocytomatosis viral oncogene homolog; CDK—cyclin-dependent kinase; GBM—glioblastoma multiforme; EGFR—epithelial growth factor receptor; LGA—low-grade astrocytoma; MDM2—murine double minute 2; MYCN—neuroblastoma-derived myelocytomatosis viral-related oncogene; PTCH—patched Drosophila homolog; PTEN—phosphatase and tensin homolog

Note. Based on information from Kanu et al., 2009; Louis, 2006.

From "Genetic and Molecular Basis of Primary Central Nervous System Tumors" (p. 241), by C.D. James, J.S. Smith, and R.B. Jenkins in V. Levin (Ed.), *Cancer in the Nervous System* (2nd ed.), 2002, New York, NY: Oxford University Press. Copyright 2002 by Victor Levin. Adapted with permission.

Tumor Progression

Many genetic alterations target cell cycle regulatory genes. The critical cell cycle regulatory complex is where most of these abnormalities occur. p16 inhibits the cyclin-dependent kinase (CDK)/cycle D complexes, which serve to prevent these complexes from phosphorylating the retinoblastoma proteins (pRb). This process ensures that pRb maintains its brake on the cell cycle, slowing or stopping mitosis. Each component of this pathway can be affected in as many as 50% of AAs and nearly 100% of GBMs and can be observed in anaplastic oligodendrogliomas (Rich & Bigner, 2004).

Inactivation of *CDKN2A*, a tumor suppressor gene, is often associated with malignant glioma development. Located on the short arm of chromosome 9, these deletions are observed in about 50% of AAs and GBMs (Rich & Bigner, 2004). Of interest is that the p16[INK4A] protein is encoded by *CDKN2A* and is independently associated with glioma development for some despite having an intact *CDKN2A*. These deletions have been found in the giant cell phenotypes that are more commonly seen in secondary glioblastomas, are more frequently observed in younger individuals, and are associated with longer survivals (Lukas, Boire, & Nicholas, 2007; Rich & Bigner, 2004).

Chromosome 10 loss is a frequent (60%–95%) finding in GBM but is far less common in AA (Louis, 2006). A second tumor suppressor gene inactivation that is highly associated with malignant glioma formation is the inactivation of *PTEN*, also referred to as *MMAC-1*. Located on chromosome 10q23, the inactivation is observed in as many as 44% of all glioblastomas with 60% of these having chromosome 10q deletions (Louis, 2006). The encoded *PTEN* protein, Tep1, regulates cell migration and invasion. Tep1 assists in promoting the activity of Akt, a serine/threonine kinase, which regulates cell proliferation and survival (Holland et al., 2000). Thus, the deletion of *PTEN* has been associated with shorter survival (Louis, 2006).

Loss of chromosomes 1p and 19q are frequently associated with oligodendroglioma oncogenesis. The inactivation

Figure 4-6. Invasion in Glioma Tumors

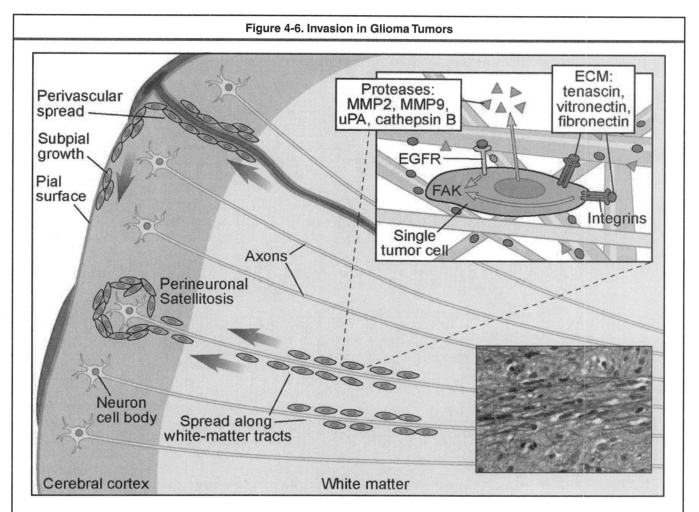

Malignant glioma cells show preferential invasion along the white-matter tracts, around neurons and blood vessels, and in the subpial region. The Luxol fast blue H&E stain, 400X photomicrograph illustrates individual elongated hyperchromatic tumor nuclei oriented along myelinated axons. The inset top right corner illustrates molecular events relating to invasion of single cells: elaboration of proteases such as matrix metalloproteinases MMP2 and MMP9, urokinase-type plasminogen activator (uPA), and cathepsin B; expression of integrins that interact with extracellular matrix (ECM) components such as tenascin, vitronectin, and fibronectin that are themselves expressed by tumor cells; and activation of focal adhesion kinase (FAK)-medicated cellular signaling pathways via epidermal growth factor receptor (EGFR) or integrin signaling.

Note. From "Molecular Pathology of Malignant Gliomas," by D.N. Louis, 2006, *Annual Review of Pathology: Mechanisms of Disease, 1,* p. 103. doi:10.1146/annurev .pathol.1.110304.100043. Copyright 2006 by Annual Reviews, Inc. Reprinted with permission.

of the tumor suppressor genes located on these chromosomal arms is suspected to promote glial development. Although 50%–80% of oligodendrogliomas have loss of 19q (James et al., 2002; Louis, 2006) and are not considered high-grade malignancies, the occurrence of this pathologic event in astrocytic tumors is more likely to indicate malignancy. Loss of 1p most commonly occurs with the combined loss of 19q, occurring in greater than 40% of oligodendrogliomas (Louis, 2006). This combined loss has been indicated in increased chemosensitivity and longer survival rates (Sathornsumetee, Rich, & Reardon, 2007; Yip, Iafrate, & Louis, 2008) (see Figure 4-7).

EGFR is prominent in oncogene amplification. EGFR-amplified cells are preferentially located at the infiltrated edges of the tumor. EGFR's primary responsibility is the encoding of a transmembrane tyrosine kinase that, when activated by EGF, results in cellular growth. EGFR amplification is observed in nearly 40% of GBMs but in few AAs (Camp et al., 2005). As such, lower grade gliomas express little to no EGFR amplification. A mutation of EGFR (EGFRvIII) occurs in 50% of those with EGFR amplification, resulting in upregulation of the metalloproteinases MMP1 and MMP13, which promote increased cellular proliferation and tumorigenesis (James et al., 2002; Rich & Bigner, 2004). This mutant overexpression is associated with a small cell phenotype of primary glioblastoma and is predominantly observed in older adults with shorter survival rates (Mott et al., 2008).

Figure 4-7. Stem Cells and Tumor Differentiation

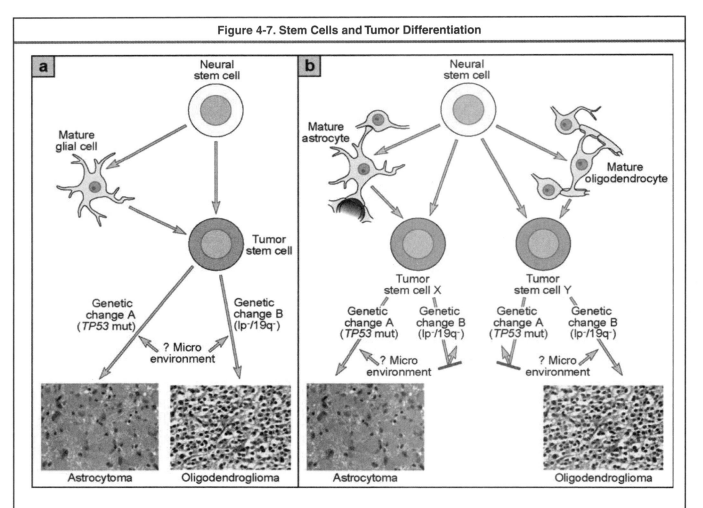

(a) Illustrates a single type of tumor stem cell that can arise either from a neural stem cell or mature glial cell. The end phenotype of glioma depends on the activation of particular cellular pathways, as a result of a genetic change that may be influenced by the micro-environment. (b) illustrates one type of tumor stem cell, X, which is permissive for neoplastic transformation only in the setting of specific genetic changes (*TP53* mutation), whereas other genetic changes (1p & 19q loss) are lethal, which influences the type of glioma phenotype; tumor stem cell Y undergoes tumorigenesis only in the setting of one genetic change (1p & 19q loss), yielding an oligodendroglial tumor.

Note. From "Molecular Pathology of Malignant Gliomas," by D.N. Louis, 2006, *Annual Review of Pathology: Mechanisms of Disease, 1*, p. 100. doi:10.1146/annurev.pathol.1.110304.100043. Copyright 2006 by Annual Reviews, Inc. Reprinted with permission.

Tumor Necrosis and Hypoxia

Necrosis is the single most important histologic feature predicting poor prognosis in patients with primary brain tumors (Louis et al., 2007). A vicious circle involving necrosis-induced hypoxia and various angiogenic and growth factors combined may foster the aggressive nature associated with the highly malignant GBM (see Figure 4-8).

Several factors are responsible for the development of necrosis. Regions of necrosis may develop in areas where (a) metabolic demands exceed the supply, (b) vascular thrombosis occurs secondary to coagulation abnormalities (common in patients with malignant gliomas), or (c) pseudopalisades develop, expressing hypoxia-inducible genes, such as hypoxia-inducible factor 1 alpha (HIF-1α) (Brat et al., 2004; Brat & Van Meir, 2004). Hypoxia-inducible genes further encourage the development of tissue necrosis. Pseudopalisades, a configuration of cells around necrotic foci, not only overexpress HIF-1 but also secrete proangiogenic factors including VEGF and interleukin-8. Thus, these pseudopalisades provide an opportunity for tumor cell migration away from central necrosis. Procoagulant properties of tissue in tumors aid in vaso-occlusion and intravascular thrombosis, which may increase the development of central necrosis (Rong, Durden, Van Meir, & Brat, 2006; Sathornsumetee, Rich, et al., 2007).

Other possible consequences of hypoxia are the possible facilitation of angiogenesis, the release of growth factors, and the emergence of highly malignant clones (Graeber et al., 1996; Kinzler & Vogelstein, 1996). Hypoxia might be able to select those apoptosis-resistant tumor cells bearing inactivated *TP53*. Tumor suppressor gene inactivation is paramount in the differentiation of tumorigenesis, with *TP53* being a major pathway for glioma development. As *TP53* regulates cellular responses to DNA damage, hypoxia, angiogenesis, and apoptosis, among other functions, *TP53* inactivation promotes accelerated cellular growth and prolongs cellular survival. *TP53* deletion has been associated with malignant transformation (James et al., 2002). Located at chromosome 17p13.1, this deletion is frequently observed in astrocytomas (Rich & Bigner, 2004).

Angiogenesis

Another hallmark of glioblastoma is vascular proliferation. It occurs in two forms: a diffuse increase in vascular density provided by more densely arrayed small vessels and the unusual complex form of angiogenesis most commonly known as microvascular proliferation. Most predominantly observed in GBM is an irregular distribution of microvascular proliferation throughout the tissues. Less commonly, microvascular proliferation is found at the invading edge; one explanation for this is the expression of angiogenic molecules expressed by migrating glioma cells in certain tumors (Gilbertson & Rich, 2007; Sathornsumetee et al., 2008).

Figure 4-8. Necrosis/Hypoxia and Angiogenesis in Glioma Development

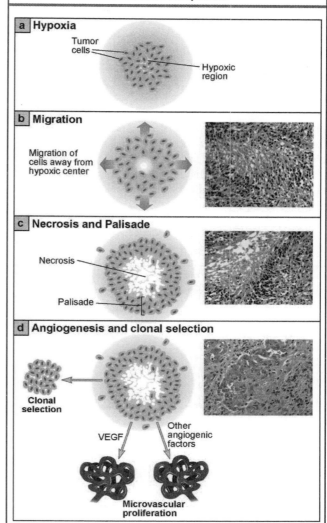

An intriguing hypothesis links tumor hypoxia, necrosis, and angiogenesis. (a) Localized hypoxia appears to upregulate migration-associated genes, (b) leading to migration of tumor cells away from a central hypoxic center (see photomicrograph inset; H&E, 200X). (c) Necrosis then ensues in the central region (see inset), sometimes in association with vascular thrombosis, and a palisade of densely packed tumor cells develops. These palisading cells express abundant angiogenic factors such as vascular endothelial growth factor (VEGF), which leads to (d) adjacent angiogenesis that includes so-called glomeruloid microvascular proliferation (see inset). Another consequence of hypoxia may be clonal selection of malignant cells that are able to survive selection pressures.

Note. From "Molecular Pathology of Malignant Gliomas," by D.N. Louis, 2006, *Annual Review of Pathology: Mechanisms of Disease, 1,* p. 108. doi:10.1146/annurev.pathol.1.110304.100043. Copyright 2006 by Annual Reviews, Inc. Reprinted with permission.

Neogenesis and angiogenesis are stimulated through microvascular proliferation from angiogenic growth factors and receptors, such as VEGF, PDGF, EGF, insulin-like growth factor-1, hepatocyte growth factor/scatter factor, transforming growth factor-beta, and Akt (Mellinghoff et al., 2005; Rich & Bigner, 2004). This vascular proliferation is a primary histopathologic characteristic of malignant gliomas. VEGF is found on the cellular surface and surrounds the glioma. Increased VEGF expression is associated with aggressive tumor characteristics and a poor prognosis. Important to tumor survival is the expression of VEGFR-2 from tumor-associated endothelial cells, creating a paracrine loop of angiogenic activation. These receptors may be prime therapeutic targets as observed in mouse xenografts that demonstrated inhibited growth of malignant gliomas in response to VEGF monoclonal antibodies (Sathornsumetee et al., 2008) (see Figure 4-9).

Summary

Several important molecular markers contribute to CNS tumor development. Understanding the role of these markers aids in predicting which patients may respond to particular treatments or have resistance, thus personalizing their treatment and oncology care (Louis, 2006; Lukas et al., 2007). Scientists are identifying more molecular markers to enhance treatment and outcomes. The future of evidence-based practice for the care of patients with primary brain tumors lies in these discoveries. The clustering of markers or single nucleotide pleomorphisms may yield predictors for the determination of how tumors respond to treatment or how individuals react to treatment with varying side effects. The role of the oncology nurse in the care of patients with CNS tumors will continue to evolve as therapeutic molecular markers provide new venues for patient and family education.

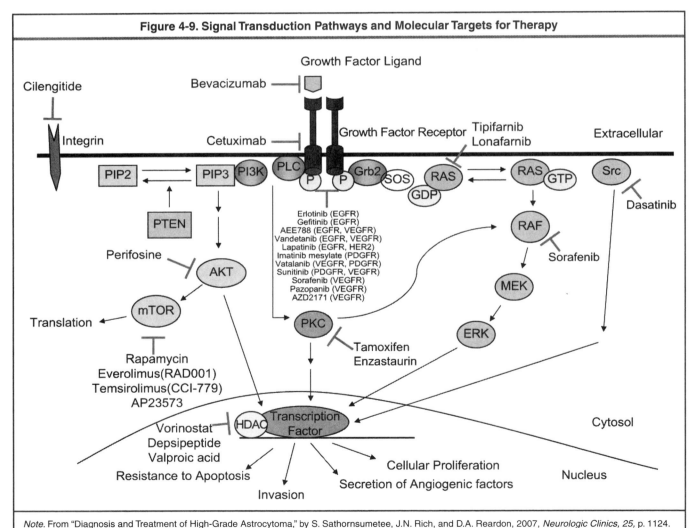

Figure 4-9. Signal Transduction Pathways and Molecular Targets for Therapy

Note. From "Diagnosis and Treatment of High-Grade Astrocytoma," by S. Sathornsumetee, J.N. Rich, and D.A. Reardon, 2007, *Neurologic Clinics, 25,* p. 1124. Copyright 2007 by Elsevier. Reprinted with permission.

References

Angevine, J. (1988). The neuroglia. *BNI Quarterly, 4,* 21–34.

Armington, W.G., Osborn, A.G., Cubberley, D.A., Harnsberger, H.R., Boyer, R., Naidich, T.P., & Sherry, R.G. (1985). Supratentorial ependymoma: CT appearance. *Radiology, 157,* 367–372.

Azevedo, F., Carvalho, L., Grinberg, L., Farfel, J., Ferretti, R., Leite, F., ... Herculano-Houzel, S. (2009). Equal numbers of neuronal and nonneuronal cells make the human brain an isometrically scaled-up primate brain. *Journal of Comparative Neurology, 513,* 532–541. doi:10.1002/cne.21974

Barnard, R.O., & Geddes, J.F. (1987). The incidence of multifocal gliomas: A histologic study of large hemispheric sections. *Cancer, 60,* 1519–1531.

Berger, M., Leibel, S., Bruner, J., Finlay, J., & Levin, V. (2002). Primary cerebral tumors. In V. Levin (Ed.), *Cancer in the nervous system* (2nd ed., pp. 75–148). New York, NY: Oxford University Press.

Berkman, R.A., Clark, W.C., Saxena, A., Robertson, J.T., Oldfield, E.H., & Ali, I.U. (1992). Clonal composition of glioblastoma multiforme. *Journal of Neurosurgery, 77,* 432–437. doi:10.3171/jns.1992.77.3.0432

Brat, D.J., Castellano-Sanchez, A.A., Hunter, S.B., Pecot, M., Cohen, C., Hammond, E.H., ... Van Meir, E.G. (2004). Pseudopalisades in glioblastoma are hypoxic, express extracellular matrix proteases, and are formed by an actively migrating cell population. *Cancer Research, 64,* 920–927. Retrieved from http://cancerres.aacrjournals.org/cgi/reprint/64/3/920

Brat, D.J., & Van Meir, E.G. (2004). Vaso-occlusive and prothrombotic mechanisms associated with tumor hypoxia, necrosis, and accelerated growth in glioblastoma. *Laboratory Investigation, 84,* 397–405. doi:10.1038/labinvest.3700070

Burger, P.C., Scheithauer, B.W., & Vogel, F.S. (1991). *Surgical pathology of the nervous system and its coverings* (3rd ed., pp. 193–405). New York, NY: Churchill Livingstone.

Burger, P.C., Vogel, F.S., Green, S.B., & Strike, T.A. (1985). Glioblastoma multiforme and anaplastic astrocytoma: Pathologic criteria and prognostic implications. *Cancer, 56,* 1106–1111.

Camp, E.R., Summy, J., Bauer, T.W., Liu, W., Gallick, G.E., & Ellis, L.M. (2005). Molecular mechanisms of resistance to therapies targeting the epidermal growth factor receptor. *Clinical Cancer Research, 11,* 397–405. Retrieved from http://clincancerres.aacrjournals.org/content/11/1/397.long

Cavenee, W., Furnari, F., Nagane, M., Huang, H., Newcombe, E., Bigner, D., ... Kleihues, P. (2000). Diffuse astrocytomas. In P. Kleihues & W.K. Cavenee (Eds.), *World Health Organization classification of tumors: Pathology and genetics of tumours of the nervous system* (2nd ed., pp. 10–21). Lyon, France: IARC.

Central Brain Tumor Registry of the United States. (2010). *CBTRUS statistical report: Primary brain and central nervous system tumors diagnosed in the United States in 2004–2006.* Retrieved from http://www.cbtrus.org/2010-NPCR-SEER/CBTRUS -WEBREPORT-Final-3-2-10.pdf

Dickson, D.W., Horoupian, D.S., Thal, L.J., & Lantos, G. (1988). Gliomatosis cerebri presenting with hydrocephalus and dementia. *American Journal of Neuroradiology, 9,* 200–202.

Dolinskas, C.A., & Simeone, F.A. (1987). CT characteristics of intraventricular oligodendrogliomas. *American Journal of Neuroradiology, 8,* 1077–1082.

Fan, K.J., Kovi, J., & Earle, K.M. (1977). The ethnic distribution of primary central nervous system tumors. AFIP, 1958 to 1970. *Journal of Neuropathology and Experimental Neurology, 36,* 41–49.

Feldkamp, M.M., Lala, P., Lau, N., Roncari, L., & Guha, A. (1999). Expression of activated epidermal growth factor receptors, Ras- guanosine triphosphate, and mitogen-activated protein kinase in human glioblastoma multiforme specimens. *Neurosurgery, 45,* 1442–1453.

Felsberg, J., & Reifenberger, G. (2002). Neuropathology and molecular genetics of diffusely infiltrating cerebral gliomas. *Medical Laser Application, 17,* 133–146. doi:10.1078/1615-00056

Gilbertson, R.J., & Rich, J.N. (2007). Making a tumour's bed: Glioblastoma stem cells and the vascular niche. *Nature Reviews Cancer, 7,* 733–736. doi:10.1038/nrc2246

Grabb, P.A., Albright, A., & Pang, D. (1992). Dissemination of supratentorial malignant gliomas via the cerebrospinal fluid in children. *Neurosurgery, 30,* 64–71.

Graeber, T.G., Osmanian, C., Jacks, T., Housman, D.E., Koch, C.J., Lowe, S.W., & Giaccia, A.J. (1996). Hypoxia-mediated selection of cells with diminished apoptotic potential in solid tumours. *Nature, 379,* 88–91. doi:10.1038/379088a0

Hallani, S., Boisselier, B., Peglion, F., Rousseau, A., Colin, C., Idboih, A., ... Sanson, M. (2010). A new alternative mechanism in glioblastoma vascularization: Tubular vasculogenic mimicry. *Brain, 133,* 973–982. doi:10.1093/brain/awq044

Hanahan, D., & Weinberg, R.A. (2000). The hallmarks of cancer. *Cell, 100,* 57–70. doi:10.1016/S0092-8674(00)81683-9

Heterodimer. (2007). *Dorland's illustrated medical dictionary* (31st ed.). Philadelphia, PA: Elsevier Saunders.

Holland, E.C., Celstino, J., Dai, C., Schaefer, L., Sawaya, R.E., & Fuller, G.N. (2000). Combined activation of Ras and Akt in neural progenitors induces glioblastoma formation in mice. *Nature Genetics, 25,* 55–57. doi:10.1038/75596

Hoshino, T., Rodriguez, L.A., Cho, K.G., Lee, K.S., Wilson, C.B., Edwards, M.S., ... Davis, R.L. (1988). Prognostic implication of the proliferative potential of low-grade astrocytomas. *Journal of Neurosurgery, 69,* 839–842. doi:10.3171/jns.1988.69.6.0839

Hunt, J.L. (2008). Molecular testing in solid tumors: An overview. *Archives of Pathology and Laboratory Medicine, 132,* 164–167.

Integrin. (2007). *Dorland's illustrated medical dictionary* (31st ed.). Philadelphia, PA: Elsevier Saunders.

Jack, C.R., Jr., Bhansali, D.T., Chason, J.L., Boulos, R.S., Mehta, B.A., Patel, S.C., & Sanders, W.P. (1987). Angiographic features of gliosarcoma. *American Journal of Neuroradiology, 8,* 117–122.

James, C.D., Smith, J.S., & Jenkins, R.B. (2002). Genetic and molecular basis of primary central nervous system tumors. In V. Levin (Ed.), *Cancer in the nervous system* (2nd ed., pp. 239–251). New York, NY: Oxford University Press.

Jelenik, J., Smirniotopoulos, J.G., Parisi, J.E., & Kanzer, M. (1990). Lateral ventricular neoplasms of the brain: Differential diagnosis based on clinical, CT, and MR findings. *American Journal of Neuroradiology, 11,* 567–574.

Kanu, O.O., Hughes, B., Di, C., Lin, N., Fu, J., Bigner, D.D., ... Adamson, C. (2009). Glioblastoma multiforme oncogenomics and signaling pathways. *Clinical Medicine: Oncology, 3,* 39–52. Retrieved from http://www.ncbi.nlm.nih.gov/pmc/articles/PMC2748278/?tool=pubmed

Kinzler, K.W., & Vogelstein, B. (1996). Life (and death) in a malignant tumor. *Nature, 379,* 19–20. doi:10.1038/379019a0

Kleihues, P., Burger, P.C., Collins, V.P., Newcomb, E.W., Ohaki, H., & Cavenee, W. (2000). Glioblastoma. In P. Kleihues & W.K. Cavenee (Eds.), *World Health Organization classification of tumors: Pathology and genetics of tumours of the nervous system* (2nd ed., pp. 29–39). Lyon, France: IARC.

Kleihues, P., Soylemezoglu, F., Schäuble, B., Scheithauer, B.W., & Burger, P.C. (1995). Histology, classification, and grading of gliomas. *Glia, 15,* 211–221. doi:10.1002/glia.440150303

Kyritsis, A.P., Yung, W.K., Bruner, J., Gleason, M.J., & Levin, V.A. (1993). The treatment of anaplastic oligodendrogliomas and mixed gliomas. *Neurosurgery, 32,* 365–371.

Lee, Y.Y., & Van Tassel, P. (1989). Intracranial oligodendrogliomas: Imaging findings in 35 untreated cases. *American Journal of Roentgenology, 152,* 361–369. Retrieved from http://www.ajronline.org/cgi/reprint/152/2/361

Lee, Y.Y., Van Tassel, P., Bruner, J.M., Moser, R.P., & Share, J.C. (1989). Juvenile pilocytic astrocytomas: CT and MR characteristics. *American Journal of Roentgenology, 152,* 1263–1270. Retrieved from http://www.ajronline.org/cgi/reprint/152/6/1263

Leeds, N., Kumar, A., & Jackson, E. (2002). Diagnostic imaging. In V. Levin (Ed.), *Cancer in the nervous system* (2nd ed., pp. 3–59). New York, NY: Oxford University Press.

Leproux, F., Melanson, D., Mercier, C., Michaud, J., & Ethier, R. (1993). Leptomeningeal gliomatosis: MR findings. *Journal of Computer Assisted Tomography, 17,* 317–320.

Lizak, P.F., & Woodruff, W.W. (1992). Posterior fossa neoplasms: Multiplanar imaging. *Seminars in Ultrasound, CT, and MRI, 13,* 182–206.

Lobato, R.D., Sarabia, M., Casto, S., Esparza, J., Cordobés, F., Portillo, J.M., & Rivas, J.J. (1986). Symptomatic subependymoma: Report of four new cases studied with computed tomography and review of the literature. *Neurosurgery, 19,* 594–598.

Louis, D. (2006). Molecular pathology of malignant gliomas. *Annual Review of Pathology: Mechanisms of Disease, 1,* 97–117.

Louis, D.N., & Gusella, J.F. (1995). A tiger behind many doors: Multiple genetic pathways to malignant glioma. *Trends in Genetics, 11,* 412–415. doi:10.1016/S0168-9525(00)89125-8

Louis, D.N., Ohgaki, H., Wiestler, O.D., Cavenee, W.K., Burger, P.C., Jouvet, A., ... Kleihues, P. (2007). The 2007 WHO classification of tumours of the central nervous system. *Acta Neuropathologica, 114,* 97–109. doi:10.1007/s00401-007-0243-4

Louis, D.N., Scheithauer, B.W., Budka, H., von Deimling, A., & Kepes, J.J. (2000). Meningiomas. In P. Kleihues & W.K. Cavenee (Eds.), *World Health Organization classification of tumors: Pathology and genetics of tumours of the nervous system* (2nd ed., pp. 176–184). Lyon, France: IARC.

Lukas, R.V., Boire, A., & Nicholas, M.K. (2007). Emerging therapies for malignant glioma. *Expert Review of Anticancer Therapy, 7*(Suppl. 12), S29–S36. doi:10.1586/14737140.7.12s.S29

Lyons, M.K., & Kelly, P.J. (1991). Posterior fossa ependymomas: Report of 30 cases and review of the literature. *Neurosurgery, 28,* 659–672.

Maiuri, F., Stella, L., Benvenuti, D., Giamundo, A., & Pettinato, G. (1990). Cerebral gliosarcomas: Correlation of computed tomographic findings, surgical aspects, pathological features, and prognosis. *Neurosurgery, 26,* 261–267.

McDermott, M., Quinones-Hinosa, A., Fuller, G., & Wilson, C. (2002). Meningiomas. In V. Levin (Ed.), *Cancer in the nervous system* (2nd ed., pp. 269–299). New York, NY: Oxford University Press.

McCormack, B.M., Miller, D.C., Budzilovich, G.N., Voorhees, G.J., & Ransohoff, J. (1992). Treatment and survival of low-grade astrocytoma in adults—1977–1988. *Neurosurgery, 31,* 636–642.

Mellinghoff, I.K., Wang, M.Y., Vivanco, I., Haas-Kogan, D.A., Zhu, S., Dia, E.Q., ... Mischel, P.S. (2005). Molecular determinants of the response of glioblastomas to EGFR kinase inhibitors. *New England Journal of Medicine, 353,* 2012–2024. doi:10.1056/NEJMoa051918

Mineura, K., Sasajima, T., Kowada, M., Uesaka, Y., & Shishido, F. (1991). Innovative approach in the diagnosis of gliomatosis cerebri using carbon-11-L-methionine positron emission tomography. *Journal of Nuclear Medicine, 32,* 726–728. Retrieved from http://jnm.snmjournals.org/cgi/reprint/32/4/726

Mishima, K., Nakamura, M., Nakamura, H., Nakamura, O., Funata, N., & Shitara, N. (1992). Leptomeningeal dissemination of cerebellar pilocytic astrocytoma: Case report. *Journal of Neurosurgery, 77,* 788–791. doi:10.3171/jns.1992.77.5.0788

Mott, R.T., Turner, K.C., Bigner, D.D., & McLendon, R.E. (2008). Utility of EGFR and PTEN numerical aberrations in the evaluation of diffusely infiltrating astrocytomas: Laboratory investigation. *Journal of Neurosurgery, 108,* 330–335. doi:10.3171/JNS/2008/108/2/0330

Natarajan, M., Hecker, T.P., & Gladson, C.L. (2003). FAK signaling in anaplastic astrocytoma and glioblastoma tumors. *Cancer Journal, 9,* 126–133.

National Cancer Institute. (2006, February). Tumor markers: Questions and answers. Retrieved from www.cancer.gov/cancertopics/factsheet/Detection/tumor-markers

Nazar, G.B., Hoffman, H.J., Becker, L.E., Jenkin, D., Humphreys, R.P., & Hendrick, E.B. (1990). Infratentorial ependymomas in childhood: Prognostic factors and treatment. *Journal of Neurosurgery, 72,* 408–417. doi:10.3171/jns.1990.72.3.0408

Okada, Y., Hurwitz, E.E., Esposito, J.M., Brower, M.A., Nutt, C.L., & Louis, D.N. (2003). Selection pressures of *TP53* mutation and microenvironmental location influence epidermal growth factor gene amplification in human glioblastomas. *Cancer Research, 63,* 413–416. Retrieved from http://cancerres.aacrjournals.org/cgi/content/full/63/2/413

Okazaki, H. (1989). Neoplastic and related conditions. In H. Okazaki (Ed.), *Fundamentals of neuropathology* (2nd ed., pp. 203–274). Tokyo, Japan: Igaku-Shoin.

Packer, R.J., Friedman, H.S., Kun, L.E., & Fuller, G.N. (2002). Tumors of the brain stem, cerebellum, and fourth ventricle. In V. Levin (Ed.), *Cancer in the nervous system* (2nd ed., pp. 171–192). New York, NY: Oxford University Press.

Palma, L., Celli, P., & Cantore, G. (1993). Supratentorial ependymomas of the first two decades of life: Long-term follow-up of 20 cases (including two subependymoma). *Neurosurgery, 32,* 169–175.

Pecorino, L. (2008). *Molecular biology of cancer: Mechanisms, targets, and therapeutics* (2nd ed.). New York, NY: Oxford University Press.

Perrin, R., Laperriere, N., Loblew, A., & Laxton, A. (2002). Spinal axis metastases. In V. Levin (Ed.), *Cancer in the nervous system* (2nd ed., pp. 341–361). New York, NY: Oxford University Press.

Philippon, J.H., Clemenceau, S.H., Fauchon, F.H., & Foncin, J.F. (1993). Supratentorial low-grade astrocytomas in adults. *Neurosurgery, 32,* 554–559.

Piepmeier, J.M. (1987). Observations in the current treatment of low-grade astrocytic tumors of the cerebral hemispheres. *Journal of Neurosurgery, 67,* 177–181. doi:10.3171/jns.1987.67.2.0177

Rao, J.S. (2003). Molecular mechanisms of glioma invasiveness: The role of proteases. *Nature Reviews Cancer, 3,* 489–501. doi:10.1038/nrc1121

Rich, J.N., & Bigner, D.D. (2004). Development of novel targeted therapies in the treatment of malignant glioma. *Nature Reviews Drug Discovery, 3,* 430–446. doi:10.1038/nrd1380

Rippe, D.J., Boyko, O.B., Fuller, G.N., Friedman, H.S., Oakes, W.J., & Schold, S.C. (1990). Gadopentetate dimeglumine–enhanced MR imaging of gliomatosis cerebri: Appearance mimicking leptomeningeal tumor dissemination. *American Journal of Neuroradiology, 11,* 800–801.

Rong, Y., Durden, D.L., Van Meir, E.G., & Brat, D.J. (2006). "Pseudopalisading" necrosis in glioblastoma: A familiar morphologic feature that links vascular pathology, hypoxia, and angiogenesis. *Journal of Neuropathology and Experimental Neurology, 65,* 529–539.

Ross, I.B., Robitaille, Y., Villemure, J., & Tampieri, D. (1991). Diagnosis and management of gliomatosis cerebri: Recent trends. *Surgical Neurology, 36,* 431–440.

Sathornsumetee, S., Reardon, D.A., Desjardins, A., Quinn, J.A., Vredenburgh, J.J., & Rich, J.N. (2007). Molecularly targeted therapy for malignant gliomas. *Cancer, 110,* 13–24. doi:10.1002/cncr.22741

Sathornsumetee, S., Cao, Y., Marcello, J., Herndon, J., McLendon, R., Desjardins, … Rich, J. (2008). Tumor angiogenic and hypoxic profiles predict radiographic response and survival in malignant astrocytoma patients treated with bevacizumab and irinotecan. *Journal of Clinical Oncology, 26,* 271–278. doi:10.1200/JCO.2007.13.3652

Sathornsumetee, S., Rich, J.N., & Reardon, D.A. (2007). Diagnosis and treatment of high-grade astrocytoma. *Neurologic Clinics, 25,* 1111–1139. doi:10.1016/j.ncl.2007.07.004

Snell, R. (2001). *Clinical neuroanatomy* (5th ed.). Baltimore, MD: Lippincott Williams & Williams.

Spagnoli, M.V., Grossman, R.I., Packer, R.J., Hackney, D.B., Goldberg, H.I., Zimmerman, R.A., & Bilaniuk, L.T. (1987). Magnetic resonance determination of gliomatosis cerebri. *Neuroradiology, 29,* 15–18.

Strong, J.A., Hatten, H.P., Brown, M.T., Debatin, J.F., Friedman, H.S., Oakes, J.W., & Tien, R. (1993). Pilocytic astrocytoma: Correlation between the initial imaging features and clinical aggressiveness. *American Journal of Roentgenology, 161,* 369–372.

Swartz, J.D., Zimmerman, R.A., & Bilaniuk, L.T. (1982). Computed tomography of intracranial ependymomas. *Radiology, 143,* 97–101.

Tatter, S.B. (2005). The new WHO classification of tumors affecting the central nervous system. Retrieved from http://neurosurgery.mgh.harvard.edu/newwhobt.htm

Uhm, J.H., Gladson, C.L., & Rao, J.S. (1999). The role of integrins in the malignant phenotype of gliomas. *Frontiers in Bioscience: A Journal and Virtual Library, 4,* D188–D199.

Watanabe, K., Tachibana, O., Sata, K., Yonekawa, Y., Kleihues, P., & Ohgaki, H. (1996). Overexpression of the EGF receptor and p53 mutations are mutually exclusive in the evolution of primary and secondary glioblastomas. *Brain Pathology, 6,* 217–223.

Yip, M., Fisch, C., & Lamarche, J.B. (2003). Gliomatosis cerebri affecting the entire neuraxis. *RadioGraphics, 23,* 247–253. doi:10.1148/rg.231025113

Yip, S., Iafrate, A.J., & Louis, D.N. (2008). Molecular diagnostic testing in malignant gliomas: A practical update on predictive markers. *Journal of Neuropathology and Experimental Neurology, 67,* 1–15. doi:10.1097/nen.0b013e31815f65fb

Zimmerman, R.A. (1990). Pediatric supratentorial tumors. *Seminars in Roentgenology, 25,* 225–248.

CHAPTER 5

Adult Cancers of the Brain and Spinal Cord

Rosemary Cashman, RN, MA, MSc(A), ACNP

Introduction

A malignant brain tumor diagnosis creates unique challenges for patients and their families. Treatment options have expanded significantly in the last few decades, but these diseases remain obdurately incurable. Despite modest improvements in overall survival, the prognosis for the most common malignant brain tumor is poor, and patients experience a host of treatment side effects as well as profound and progressive disabilities resulting from the disease and treatments. Family members bear a heavy care burden and report disruption of family life and roles, feelings of isolation and helplessness, financial difficulties, and decrements in health and well-being (Catt, Chalmers, & Fallowfield, 2008; Davies, 1997; Fox & Lantz, 1998; Wideheim, Edvardsson, Påhlson, & Ahlström, 2002). Care of those living with a brain tumor requires a broad knowledge base in neuro-oncology and a sensitive and realistic approach that optimizes quality of life and permits a sense of hopefulness to prevail.

Primary Central Nervous System Tumors

Gliomas are the most common type of primary central nervous system (CNS) tumor, accounting for 32% of all CNS tumors (Central Brain Tumor Registry of the United States [CBTRUS], 2010). Historically, gliomas were believed to arise from glial cells (from the Greek word for "glue"), whose function is to support and protect neuronal cells. Subtypes of gliomas include glioblastoma multiforme (GBM), astrocytomas, oligodendrogliomas, oligoastrocytomas, and ependymomas. Most gliomas arise in the cerebrum, especially in the frontal lobes (25%), temporal lobes (19.5%), parietal lobes (13%), and occipital lobes (3.3%) (CBTRUS, 2010). They do not typically disseminate throughout the neural axis or metastasize outside of the CNS, so staging assessments are usually unnecessary. Medulloblastomas and other primitive neuroectodermal tumors and ependymomas, which arise within the ventricles, may be associated with drop metastases in the spine. Contrast-enhanced magnetic resonance imaging (MRI) of the spine and cerebrospinal fluid (CSF) analysis for malignant cells are indicated prior to treatment initiation in these diseases (Adams, 2008).

Primary tumors of the spinal cord and canal are uncommon, and most are benign. They may be classified as extramedullary (outside the spinal cord) or intramedullary (within the spinal cord). Extramedullary tumors account for at least 70% of spinal tumors and include chordomas, sarcomas, meningiomas, and neurofibromas (Stieber, Tatter, Shaffrey, & Shaw, 2005). Intramedullary tumors include primarily ependymomas and, less commonly, astrocytomas, hemangioblastomas, and other gliomas, as well as metastatic tumors (Adams, 2008). For a more detailed description of the presentation of CNS cancers, see Chapter 3.

The precise precursor cells that give rise to glial tumors are uncertain. Growing evidence supports a stem cell hypothesis of brain malignancy. In this model, a few atypical cells possessing dysregulated self-renewal properties are responsible for the growth and recurrence of brain tumors (Reya, Morrison, Clarke, & Weissmann, 2001). This model has been proved in leukemia and solid tumors such as breast cancer, and cells with stem cell characteristics have been identified in pediatric brain tumors (Al-Hajj, Wicha, Benito-Hernandez, Morrison, & Clarke, 2003; Bonnet & Dick, 1997; Hemmati et al., 2003; Singh et al., 2003). Stem cells are immortal in the sense that they possess self-renewal and proliferative capacities throughout the lifetime of an animal. As a result, cancer-promoting mutations may accumulate in the cells over time and can be passed on to mitotically active progenitors with similar proliferation and differentiation capabilities, until they are transformed into malignant cells. Evidence that stem cell progenitors express epidermal growth factor receptor (EGFR) lends further support to the hypothesis because alterations in EGFR activity are found in more than 50% of GBMs and may promote glioma formation (Mellinghoff et al., 2005).

World Health Organization Classification System

Gliomas are classified by the predominant cell type noted in histopathologic analysis (refer to Chapter 4) and by tumor grade. The World Health Organization (WHO) classification system defines four grades of primary brain tumors, with increasing malignancy based on the presence of nuclear atypia, cellular pleomorphism, mitoses, vascular proliferation, and necrosis (Tatter, 2005). Grade I tumors may be completely resectable if they are in a surgically accessible location. Although lower-grade tumors generally confer a better prognosis and may even be curable, all brain tumors can cause disability and death because of their location in critical areas or because of malignant transformation. WHO grade II and III gliomas are invasive tumors that invariably progress to higher-grade lesions and are ultimately fatal. Grade II gliomas are low-grade gliomas (LGGs) and demonstrate increased cellularity and nuclear pleomorphism. Grade III gliomas include anaplastic astrocytomas (AAs), anaplastic oligodendrogliomas, and anaplastic oligoastrocytomas (AOAs) and are distinguished by frequent mitoses. Most pathologists consider the grade IV glioma designation to be interchangeable with GBM. These tumors demonstrate vascular proliferation and areas of necrosis. Histologic subtype alone provides insufficient information about the ultimate biologic behavior of gliomas, and efforts are under way to further characterize these tumors through specific molecular markers (see Table 5-1).

Low-Grade Gliomas

LGGs (grade II) are the most commonly diagnosed tumors during childhood through adulthood, with pilocytic astrocytomas and meningiomas being the two most common benign (grade I) tumor categories. Although outcomes associated with LGGs are variable, a number of prognostic factors for overall survival have been identified. Unfavorable factors include patient age older than 40, tumor diameter larger than 6 cm, tumor crossing the midline on imaging, presence of neurologic deficits, and astrocytic histology (Schiff, Brown, & Giannini, 2007). Younger age, good performance status, and a history of seizures are correlated with a better prognosis (Karim et al., 1996; van Veelen, Avezaat, Kros, van Putten, & Vecht, 1998). Most patients with LGGs are young adults in their 20s and 30s who typically present with seizures. Prognosis varies and is clouded by uncertainties about the natural history of the disease because these tumors may smolder without producing symptoms for a time. Unfortunately, LGGs invariably progress and are ultimately fatal. The management of these tumors is controversial, with ongoing debate about the optimal timing of surgery and radiotherapy and the benefit of aggressive surgical resection. Because no evidence exists to demonstrate that early

Grade	Example	Histopathologic Features
I	Pilocytic astrocytoma	Rosenthal fibers, eosinophilic granular bodies
II	Low-grade astrocytoma	Increased cellularity; nuclear pleomorphism
III	Anaplastic astrocytoma	Features of grade III plus mitotic activity
IV	Glioblastoma multiforme	Features of grade III plus vascular proliferation and necrosis

Table 5-1. World Health Organization Grading of Primary Brain Tumors

Note. Based on information from Berger et al., 2002; Kleihues & Cavenee, 2000.

radiotherapy for LGGs results in improved overall survival, treatment may be deferred until symptomatic tumor growth occurs (van den Bent et al., 2005). Clinical studies are under way to examine the effects of initial treatment of LGGs with chemotherapy, radiotherapy, and concurrent chemoradiation in order to determine the optimal therapeutic approach for these tumors.

Astrocytomas

Astrocytomas are a heterogeneous group of neoplasms that includes low-grade and high-grade tumors composed of proliferating astrocytes. Grade I tumors, such as pilocytic astrocytomas and pleomorphic xanthoastrocytomas, are well circumscribed and usually benign. These uncommon tumors may be cured by surgical resection. Even if the resection is incomplete, these tumors may remain indolent or be successfully treated with adjuvant radiotherapy. By contrast, higher-grade astrocytomas are diffusely infiltrating and thus not curable by local therapies such as radiotherapy and surgery. In addition to tumor grade, other prognostic features specific to astrocytomas may be identified. Although tumor histology is not definitive, it is important. For example, pilocytic histology confers a better prognosis than gemistocytic histology (Kösel, Scheithauer, & Graeber, 2001) (see Table 5-2).

AA and GBM represent approximately 76% of all gliomas (CBTRUS, 2010). The most predictive variable of survival after surgery for recurrent high-grade astrocytomas (HGAs) is a preoperative Karnofsky performance status of 60% or greater (Young et al., 1981). For patients with GBM, median survival after a second surgery ranges from 14 to 36 weeks, which may be perceived as a meaningful outcome for some patients with good quality of life (de Groot, Aldape, & Colman, 2005).

	5-Year Survival by Age Group					10-Year Survival by Age Group				
Diagnosis	**20–44**	**45–54**	**55–64**	**65–74**	**≥ 75**	**20–44**	**45–54**	**55–64**	**65–74**	**≥ 75**
Anaplastic astrocytoma	47.6%	28.2%	9%	4.5%	–	36.1%	13.7%	5.8%	–	–
Glioblastoma multiforme	15.9%	5.2%	2.7%	1.3%	0.6%	10%	2.3%	0.5%	0.6%	–

Table 5-2. Five- and Ten-Year Survival Rates by Diagnosis and Age Groups, SEER 1995–2006 Data

– Too few cases to provide survival rates.

SEER—Surveillance, Epidemiology, and End Results

Note. Adapted from *CBTRUS Statistical Report: Primary Brain and Central Nervous System Tumors Diagnosed in the United States in 2004–2006* (p. 52), by the Central Brain Tumor Registry of the United States, 2010, Hinsdale, IL: Author.

The genetic events that drive the development and progression of gliomas are extensive and complex, involving multiple changes at the level of DNA, RNA, protein, and cellular processes. Further, the distinction between primary and secondary GBMs demonstrates the presence of unique molecular and cytogenetic signatures for these tumors despite their shared histopathology (von Deimling et al., 1993). At the cytogenetic level, among other findings, loss of chromosome 10q has been associated with poor survival in AA and GBM. These molecular and cytogenetic distinctions may have important clinical implications for prognosis and the development of targeted therapies (refer to Chapter 4 for more genetic and molecular review).

In GBM, those patients whose tumors feature a methylated promoter for the gene encoding O-6-methylguanine DNA methyltransferase, also known as *MGMT*, are more likely to benefit from chemotherapy and have a better overall survival regardless of treatment received. The *MGMT* gene removes the methyl group from the O-6 position of guanine, reversing the cytotoxic effects of methylating chemotherapies and facilitating drug resistance of the tumor. When *MGMT* is silenced, a therapeutic response to chemotherapy is facilitated (Hegi et al., 2005). This was observed in a 2004 international randomized phase III trial, which reported improved median and two-year survival for patients with glioblastoma treated with concomitant and adjuvant temozolomide chemotherapy and radiotherapy (Stupp et al., 2005). A recent update demonstrates a persistent benefit for those treated with the concurrent therapy, with 9.8% of patients in that treatment arm alive throughout five years of follow-up compared to 1.9% in the arm receiving radiotherapy alone (Stupp et al., 2009). In patients who received the combination therapy, overall survival was significantly improved in all prognostic subgroups, including older age. Thus, those whose tumor had a methylated promoter for the *MGMT* gene were more likely to benefit from the addition of temozolomide and were more likely to be long-term survivors. This evidence suggests a predictive value of *MGMT* status and may help to identify patients most likely to benefit from chemotherapy. The combined treatment regimen is now the standard of care for patients with WHO grade IV glioma who are younger than 70 years of age and is being investigated in patients with other types of glioma and in patients older than 70.

Pseudoprogression

Since the introduction of concurrent chemoradiation for GBM and the widespread use of MRI to monitor treatment response, the phenomenon of pseudoprogression has been noted in up to 50% of patients treated (Taal et al., 2008). In pseudoprogression, patients with malignant gliomas develop an increase in the size of contrast-enhancing lesions, or new areas of contrast enhancement, with or without edema. Most patients are clinically asymptomatic. Patients with methylated *MGMT* showed more frequent pseudoprogression, suggesting that it may correlate with greater sensitivity to treatment (Brandsma, Stalpers, Taal, Sminia, & van den Bent, 2008). The exact mechanism through which pseudoprogressive changes occur is not fully understood. Current imaging techniques for brain tumors do not differentiate between true progression and pseudoprogression, and further research in this area is needed. Although patient management is not standardized for patients who present with radiographic disease progression in the first months after concurrent therapy, many experts recommend continuation of adjuvant temozolomide until subsequent imaging demonstrates definite disease progression (Brandsma et al., 2008).

Oligodendrogliomas

Oligodendrogliomas were once thought to be a rare subtype of gliomas, most likely because of inherent difficulties in obtaining a definitive histopathologic diagnosis. Current estimates of incidence range from 10% to 50% of all gliomas

(Kros, Zheng, Wolbers, & van den Bent, 2005). Oligodendrocytes normally produce myelin in the CNS, although myelin has not been observed in oligodendroglial tumors. Typical pathologic features of oligodendrogliomas include a honeycomb-like arrangement of cells with round nuclei surrounded by perinuclear halos of cytoplasm and the presence of calcium deposits. The WHO classification system divides these tumors into low grade (grade II) and anaplastic (grade III), but as with astrocytomas, clinicians are increasingly looking beyond the classic histopathologic features and grading system to identify wider diagnostic criteria, especially because some of these tumors may be particularly responsive to treatment (Coons, Johnson, Scheithauer, Yates, & Pearl, 1997; van den Bent & Kros, 2005).

For patients with oligodendroglial-type tumors, codeletion of 1p/19q is a strong prognostic factor in mixed or pure tumors demonstrating classic oligodendroglial histopathology (McDonald et al., 2005). These tumors respond better to chemotherapy and radiation and portend longer overall survival for patients than tumors lacking these features. The prognostic value of 1p/19q codeletion was confirmed in two randomized clinical trials. Patients with codeleted tumors demonstrated a significantly lower risk of tumor progression, with a hazard ratio (HR) of 0.43 and much longer survival (HR for death, 0.31) (Cairncross et al., 2006; van den Bent et al., 2006). The chemosensitivity and prolonged survival associated with these tumors have led to consideration of the use of upfront chemotherapy strategies, which would permit temporary deferral of radiotherapy with its attendant cognitive side effects. However, in the absence of evidence from randomized clinical trials, no firm conclusions can be drawn.

AOA, or mixed tumors, contain morphologic elements of oligodendrogliomas and astrocytomas. Their genetic features include either 1p/19q loss, consistent with an oligodendroglial lineage, or TP53 mutation, suggesting astrocytic lineage. The recognition that some astrocytomas have histologic or molecular genetic features consistent with tumors of oligodendroglial lineage suggests that these particular gliomas may be more responsive to treatment.

Ependymomas

Ependymomas are relatively rare tumors that are thought to derive from the primitive neuroepithelial cells lining the ventricles and central canal of the spinal cord. They are approximately six times more common in children than adults. In adults, 75% of ependymomas arise within the spinal canal (Siffert & Jallo, 2005). The etiology of ependymomas is unknown. The virus SV40 was discovered as a contaminant in poliovirus vaccines administered in Europe and North America between 1955 and 1963 and was hypothesized to be implicated in the pathogenesis of several tumors, including

ependymomas, but this has been disproved (Brenner et al., 2003). A complete surgical resection is the most significant prognostic factor in ependymoma, and postoperative radiotherapy, especially in patients with residual disease, may also improve the outcome. At present, chemotherapy has a limited role in this disease.

Primary Central Nervous System Lymphoma

Primary CNS lymphoma (PCNSL) is a rare form of extranodal non-Hodgkin lymphoma that may affect the brain, leptomeninges, spinal cord, or eyes and typically does not spread outside of the CNS. Diffuse large B-cell lymphoma (DLBCL) is the most common type of systemic lymphoma, and approximately 90% of PCNSLs are DLBCLs (Miller et al., 1994; Non-Hodgkin's Lymphoma Classification Project, 1997). Congenital or acquired immunodeficiency is the only established risk factor for PCNSL, and people who have HIV have a 3,600-fold increased risk of the disease (Coté, Manns, Hardy, Yellin, & Hartge, 1996). Although PCNSL incidence increased dramatically between 1973 and 1984, it has stabilized or slightly decreased and accounted for only 2.7% of primary brain tumors diagnosed in the United States between 1973 and 1984 (Eby et al., 1988; Kadan-Lottick, Skluzacek, & Gurney, 2002).

Patients typically present with neurologic signs and symptoms rather than the classic B symptoms (night sweats, fever, and weight loss) associated with systemic lymphoma. A diagnosis of PCNSL should prompt staging investigations including a contrast-enhanced MRI of the spine and assessment of the CSF (atypical cells are present in one-third of patients) and the eye (malignant spread is present in 20% of patients) (O'Neill & Schiff, 2005). Although widespread disease is uncommon in immunocompetent patients, computed tomography imaging of the chest, abdomen, and pelvis should be performed and a bone marrow examination may be considered in some patients. Because of the high rate of disease in immunodeficiency, serologic testing for HIV should also be performed (Wen, Teoh, Gigas, & MacDonald, 2005).

Treatment options for immunocompetent patients include corticosteroids, surgery, radiotherapy, and chemotherapy. Even when disease is surgically accessible, survival after surgical resection alone is one to four months and offers no benefit over biopsy alone (Bellinzona, Roser, Ostertag, Gaab, & Saini, 2005; Murray, Kun, & Cox, 1986). Corticosteroids may induce a significant transient initial response, but relapse invariably occurs. Because PCNSL is a multifocal disease, whole brain radiation therapy (WBRT) is the most appropriate radiotherapeutic approach. Unfortunately, despite high overall response rates, durable remission is seldom achieved (Nelson et al., 1992). The neurotoxicity risk from WBRT is significantly increased, especially in patients older than 60;

therefore, its use in newly diagnosed patients as a single-treatment modality is often deferred (Batchelor & Loeffler, 2006). Combined modality therapy was developed to optimize response and overall survival. The use of standard chemotherapies for DLBCL is hindered by limited blood-brain barrier penetration of those agents. Methotrexate, a folate antagonist that interrupts DNA biosynthesis, is the most widely used agent in single- or multi-drug therapies for PCNSL. The combination of WBRT and methotrexate-based chemotherapy achieves radiographic responses in 50% of patients and two-year survival in 43%–73% of patients (Ferreri et al., 2003). Most patients will relapse and require salvage therapy. Chemotherapy, including high-dose regimens with autologous stem cell rescue, may be effective, but treatment-related toxicity is common. Studies are under way to examine the effectiveness of temozolomide, methotrexate, and rituximab, an unconjugated monoclonal antibody directed against the CD20 antigen on the surface of B lymphocytes.

Secondary Brain Tumors—Brain Metastases

Brain metastases are malignant tumors that begin outside of the nervous system (Adams, 2008) and are the most common intracranial tumor, roughly 10 times more common than primary brain tumors (Sawaya, Lingon, & Bindal, 1994). Approximately 1.5 million people were expected to be diagnosed with cancer in the United States in 2009, and about 150,000 will develop brain metastases (Altekruse et al., 2009; American Brain Tumor Association, 2009). These data may underrepresent the true incidence of CNS metastases, as 25% of metastases are discovered at autopsy, and the rates of autopsy remain low at roughly 5% (Shojana, Burton, McDonald, & Goldman, 2003). The reported incidence of brain metastases is rising, and this increase has been attributed to advances in cancer therapy leading to longer survival, an aging population that is more likely to develop cancer, and improvements in neuroimaging leading to earlier detection of disease (Adams, 2008; Wen & Loeffler, 1999). In 20% of patients with brain metastases, the disease in the brain precedes the diagnosis of a primary site of cancer (Merchut, 1989). Although any cancer can spread to the brain, certain primary sites such as lung and melanoma have a predilection for intracranial metastasis (Adams, 2008). More than 85% of all brain metastases arise from melanoma, lung, breast, colorectal, or kidney primary sites (Yung, Kunschner, Sawaya, Chang, & Fuller, 2002). Up to 75% of spinal metastases are from lung, breast, and prostate primary cancers (Perrin, Laperriere, Loblaw, & Laxton, 2002). Diffuse infiltration of the leptomeninges is most commonly associated with leukemias and lymphomas, followed by lung and breast carcinoma (DeAngelis, 2002; Nakagawa et al., 1992) (see Table 5-3).

Table 5-3. Incidence of Brain and Spinal Metastases According to Most Common Primary Sites

Cancer	Brain Metastases (%)	Spinal Metastases (%)
Breast	10–30	25–30
Colorectal	3–5	< 10
Lung	35–48	20–25
Melanoma	30–40	< 10
Prostate	< 10	15–20
Renal	10–15	< 10

Note. Based on information from DeAngelis, 2002; Perrin et al., 2002; Schouten et al., 2002; Yung et al., 2002.

Pathophysiology

Metastasis occurs through hematogenous spread. Because the brain receives 15% of cardiac output in its resting state, a proportional amount of circulating tumor cells would be expected to follow blood flow. In fact, the distribution of brain metastases (80% in the cerebral hemispheres, 15% in the cerebellum, and 5% in the brain stem [Adams, 2008]) is consistent with the circulatory flow to these areas, a phenomenon cited in the "mechanical hypothesis" proposed by Ewing (1940). However, blood flow alone does not account for the propensity of specific types of cancer cells to seed within certain organs and not others, nor does it explain why organs with similar blood flow do not equally support the development of metastatic tumors. The "seed and soil" hypothesis proposed by Paget (1889) postulates that genetic changes within the cancer cell (the seed) allow the cells to modify the environment within a metastatic milieu to make it more favorable to the primary cancer cells.

To spread to the brain, cancer cells must complete a complex series of steps termed the *metastatic cascade*. Each step is mediated by molecular mechanisms and fraught with peril for a cancer cell, resulting in less than 0.01% of tumor cells successfully becoming a metastasis (Liotta & Kohn, 2003). Each step in the cascade also represents a potential target to prevent or treat metastases.

After the initial malignant transformation within the primary site, further genetic changes promote some cancer cells' survival and proliferation and confer to some the ability to invade and metastasize. Vascular endothelial growth factor is one of several agents that promote the angiogenesis necessary for the growth of tumor cells and movement of tumor emboli from the primary site into the local circulation. Invasion of the host tissue requires tumor cell attachment to and degradation of the extracellular matrix of the host organ. The degradation process is facilitated by proteolytic enzymes called matrix metalloproteases, and the tumor cells migrate through the extracellular matrix to reach the host circulatory system. Hypoxia in the malignant cells aids in angiogenesis and enhances cell motility. Loss of adhesion molecules on the surface of migrating cells and the action of additional proteolytic enzymes promote tumor cell invasion of normal tissues and entry into the local circulatory system (Gavrilovic & Posner, 2005).

Once in the circulation, most tumor cells are destroyed either by the immune system or via self-destruction through apoptosis (Grossmann, 2002; Nieswandt, Hafner, Echtenacher, & Mannel, 1999). Mechanical damage through shear forces within the bloodstream poses additional threats to the migrating malignant cells. However, tumor cells may form complexes with blood cells to protect against mechanical destruction (Borsig et al., 2001). Lung cancer is the most common primary tumor source of brain metastasis because lung tumor cells may pass directly into the pulmonary veins for direct access of the arterial circulation via the left heart. Once in the capillary bed of the brain parenchyma, malignant cells reproduce and pass into the brain tissue. Disruption of the blood-brain barrier occurs readily and is believed to be achieved through occlusive infarcts in the capillaries caused by tumor emboli (Paillas & Pellet, 1975).

Diagnosis

Gadolinium-enhanced MRI is the most sensitive imaging modality for the detection of metastatic brain lesions (Adams, 2008). Brain metastases are usually spherical, often occur as multiple lesions, are associated with significant vasogenic edema, and tend to displace rather than infiltrate the surrounding brain parenchyma (Delattre, Krol, Thaler, & Posner, 1988; DeYoung & Wick, 2000). The identification of multiple lesions in a patient with a known history of cancer is strongly indicative of brain metastases; however, the appearance of a solitary lesion is less certain and will necessitate investigations to rule out a new primary brain tumor, brain abscess, demyelination, and cerebrovascular accident (Adams, 2008; American College of Surgical Oncology CNS Working Group, 2005). To confirm the diagnosis of cancer in a suspicious brain lesion, surgical resection or a biopsy may be required (Adams, 2008).

Treatment

The status of systemic disease dictates the survival of individuals with brain metastases, and the prognosis is generally very poor, usually less than one year (Markesbery, Brooks, Gupta, & Young, 1978; Ruderman & Hall, 1965). Treatment is aimed at enhancing quality of life and, when possible, controlling the disease. Supportive care includes the use of corticosteroids to treat peritumoral edema and antiepileptics for seizure management. Certain prognostic factors have been identified to select patients who are most likely to survive long enough to benefit from more aggressive treatment of the intracranial disease. Gaspar et al. (1997) performed a recursive partitioning analysis of 1,200 patients with brain metastases who enrolled in WBRT clinical trials from 1979 to 1993. Features of patients with the longest median survival included age younger than 65 years, Karnofsky performance status greater than 70, absence of metastases outside the brain, and control of systemic disease. The number of brain metastases may also influence patient outcome (Alexander et al., 1995; Swift et al., 1993).

WBRT has been the primary active treatment modality for brain metastases for approximately 50 years and extends overall patient survival from two months with steroids alone to three to six months (Cairncross, Chernik, Kim, & Posner, 1979). Prophylactic cranial irradiation may be used in cancer with a very high risk of intracranial metastasis, such as small cell lung cancer. The dosage of radiation varies according to institutional protocol, but 30 Gy in 10 fractions is a common regimen. Side effects of WBRT include fatigue, otitis, alopecia, and transient worsening of neurologic symptoms due to treatment-related increased intracranial pressure. Unfortunately, even if systemic disease remains under control, the majority of patients relapse within a year (refer to Chapter 9 for a more in-depth discussion on radiotherapy). A randomized controlled trial compared outcomes for patients with metastatic brain lesions treated with WBRT alone with outcomes for patients treated with concurrent WBRT and temozolomide chemotherapy. A trend toward a modest improvement in survival was noted in the concurrent treatment arm (Abrey & Christodoulou, 2001).

Stereotactic radiosurgery (SRS) is a technique that uses a single, high-dose fraction of ionizing radiation to a solitary, small (less than 3 cm in diameter), precisely defined target (American College of Surgical Oncology CNS Working Group, 2005). SRS minimizes the radiation delivery to normal brain tissue surrounding the tumor and may be considered for some small tumors that are not amenable to surgical resection and in retreatment of some patients with metastases that progress after WBRT.

In some patients with solitary or multiple brain metastases, neurosurgery may be beneficial, especially if the patient has significant neurologic disease symptoms. However, the risk-to-benefit ratio must be considered. Variables reported in retrospective studies to negatively affect the outcome of patients undergoing surgery for metastatic tumors include age older than 60, Karnofsky performance status less than 70, incomplete surgical removal, and presence of extensive systemic disease (Bindal, Sawaya, Leavens, & Lee, 1993; Iwadate, Namba, & Yamaura, 2000). A recent study found that an SRS boost to the tumor bed of single brain metastases following resection and adjuvant WBRT was safe and provided high rates of disease control (Roberge, Petrecca, El Refae, & Souhami, 2009).

The response to chemotherapies has generally not been impressive, especially in the most common source of brain metastasis, non-small cell lung cancer. However, patients with small metastases from chemosensitive primary tumors, especially breast, small cell lung, and germ cell tumors, have derived benefit from single-agent chemotherapy and multi-modality approaches. For example, the use of chemotherapy in small cell lung cancer yields response rates similar to those seen with the use of WBRT (Landonio et al., 2001). Concurrent chemoradiation produced better response rates, but the overall survival was still determined by systemic disease control (Postmus & Smit, 1999; Pronzato et al., 1995).

Leptomeningeal Disease

The seeding of the leptomeninges with cancer cells is diagnosed in approximately 5% of patients; autopsy reports indicate that the true incidence is higher, especially in certain primary tumor types (Kaplan et al., 1990; Kesari & Batchelor, 2003; Posner, 1995). Many terms are used to indicate the malignant cells' breach of the leptomeninges, including *leptomeningeal carcinomatosis, neoplastic meningitis,* and *leukemic meningitis*; however, the most comprehensive and inclusive term is *leptomeningeal metastasis* (LM).

Primary solid tumor sites most commonly responsible for LM include breast, lung, and melanoma (Kaplan et al., 1990; Kesari & Batchelor, 2003; Posner, 1995). The CNS is a sanctuary site for tumor cells that elude successful treatment of the primary disease site by therapies that do not penetrate the blood-brain barrier. As systemic therapies improve, the risk of leptomeningeal and other brain metastases increases. Although LM incidence from hematologic malignancies has decreased over the past decades because of improved treatments, approximately 10%–30% of patients with acute leukemia will have LM at diagnosis (Peterson et al., 1987). Leptomeningeal dissemination of primary CNS malignancies is relatively rare but is especially relevant for patients with medulloblastoma, PCNSL, and germ cell tumors (Enting, 2005).

Tumor cells reach the leptomeninges after gaining access to the CSF. This occurs through a number of mechanisms, including direct extension from the brain parenchyma, hematogenous spread via the arachnoid vessels, metastasis into the choroid plexus, and hypothetically, iatrogenic spread during surgical resection of parenchymal tumors (Kesari & Batchelor, 2003; Olson, Chernik, & Posner, 1974; van der Ree et al., 1999). Once in the CSF, malignant cells float in the CSF pathways throughout the neural axis and may settle and grow in a diffuse or multifocal pattern (O'Meara, Borkar, Stambuk, & Lymberis, 2007).

Presenting symptoms are varied and will depend on the site of the LM, and patients often have more than one anatomic site of disease (Posner, 1995; Wasserstrom, Glass, & Posner, 1982). Approximately 50% of patients with LM will have involvement of the cerebral hemispheres with the potential for associated signs and symptoms such as headache,

change in mental status, nausea, vomiting, and seizures. Cranial nerve involvement occurs in about 50% of LM cases (Posner, 1995). Diplopia is the most common cranial nerve symptom, but other abnormalities include facial numbness and loss of visual acuity. More than 75% of patients with proven LM have involvement of the spine (Posner, 1995). Spinal symptoms include weakness, paresthesias, bowel and bladder dysfunction, and nuchal rigidity. MRI and CSF analysis via lumbar puncture are complementary diagnostic evaluations. The detection of malignant cells in the CSF provides a definitive diagnosis of LM; however, cytology may yield false-negative results.

LM treatment includes palliative radiotherapy to bulky or symptomatic disease. Systemic treatment may be indicated, including high-dose chemotherapy regimens or intrathecal chemotherapy. The most commonly used systemic agents, methotrexate, cytarabine, and thiotepa, are active against a limited range of primary tumor types. Median survival for patients with LM ranges from a few weeks to a few months (O'Meara et al., 2007).

Paraneoplastic Syndromes: A Related Neuro-Oncologic Topic

A paraneoplastic syndrome (PNS) is a remote effect of cancer that is not due to the local presence of cancer cells or cancer treatment (Adams, 2008). The symptoms are variable and may occur in several body systems, including endocrine, neurologic (central and peripheral nervous systems), hematologic, and mucocutaneous, as well as others that do not fit into any of these categories. These syndromes are mediated by humoral factors (hormones or cytokines) excreted by tumor cells, or by an immune response against the tumor or its metastases. The exact incidence is unknown; however, some authors classify generalized conditions such as anorexia-cachexia, tumor fever, and anemia of chronic disease as PNSs. If these relatively common conditions are included in the overall incidence, a very large proportion of patients with cancer will experience a PNS. Paraneoplastic endocrine disorders are typically caused by malignant cells that produce naturally occurring hormones or hormone precursors (Mazzone & Arroliga, 2003). An example is hypercalcemia, which occurs in approximately 10% of individuals with cancer, especially in cancers of the lung, head and neck, and esophagus (Bollanti, Riondino, & Strollo, 2001). Other endocrine PNSs include paraneoplastic adrenocorticotropic hormone syndrome and syndrome of inappropriate antidiuretic hormone.

Paraneoplastic neurologic disorders are diverse and can affect any part of the central or peripheral nervous systems (Adams, 2008). They may be confined to a single area or cell type or may involve abnormalities at multiple levels of the nervous system. In general, they are rare and present with a rapid onset of disabling symptoms before any cancer diagnosis is made (Adams, 2008). Among the more common neurologic PNSs are Lambert-Eaton myasthenic syndrome, which affects 3% of patients with small cell lung cancer; myasthenia gravis, which affects 15% of patients with thymoma; and demyelinating peripheral neuropathy, which affects about 50% of patients with a rare form of plasmacytoma (Darnell & Posner, 2003). Unlike the endocrine PNSs, which occur when the tumor produces substances that mimic hormones, most neurologic PNSs occur when the tumor expresses an antigen that is normally produced solely by the nervous system. The immune system recognizes the antigen as foreign and responds with antibody production. Identification of antibodies in serum and CSF permits the diagnosis of the PNS (Adams, 2008). The antibodies, named by using the first two letters of the index patient, also help to identify the site of the underlying cancer. For example, the presence of anti-Yo antibodies (so designated because the name of the index patient with this PNS began with the letters YO) in the serum of a woman presenting with cerebellar symptoms strongly suggests a paraneoplastic cerebellar syndrome and implicates an underlying gynecologic cancer, usually ovarian.

PNSs most commonly present with lung cancers, but any malignancy may be associated with them. In general, the development of PNS is a poor prognostic indicator; however, its severity may not be correlated with the extent of the malignancy. Treatment is aimed at the underlying malignancy although effects of the PNS may be permanent. The use of plasma exchange, IV immunoglobulin, and other immunosuppressive agents to treat PNS is currently under investigation (Adams, 2008).

Summary

CNS malignancies cause significant disruption and psychological hardship in the lives of patients and their families. Nurses play an important role in helping patients and their caregivers acquire information and skills to monitor for treatment side effects and disease response or progression. They provide critical support to caregivers who may feel isolated and overwhelmed by the changes they see in an afflicted loved one and by the relentless burden of care imposed by the disease. Nurses can assist patients to identify and work toward realistic goals that may restore a sense of hopefulness and control. The satisfaction gained in meeting the challenges associated with this diagnosis may mitigate its accompanying distress and help patients and their caregivers achieve a sense of integrity and coherence in the experience.

References

Abrey, L., & Christodoulou, C. (2001). Temozolomide for treating brain metastases. *Seminars in Oncology, 28*(4, Suppl. 13), 34–42.

Adams, A.C. (2008). *Mayo Clinic essential neurology*. Rochester, MN: Mayo Foundation for Medical Education and Research.

Alexander, E., 3rd, Moriarty, T.M., Davis, R.B., Wen, P.Y., Fine, H.A., Black, P.M., ... Loeffler, J.S. (1995). Stereotactic radiosurgery for the definitive, noninvasive treatment of brain metastases. *Journal of the National Cancer Institute, 87,* 34–40. doi:10.1093/jnci/87.1.34

Al-Hajj, M., Wicha, M.S., Benito-Hernandez, A., Morrison, S.J., & Clarke, M.F. (2003). Prospective identification of tumorigenic breast cancer cells. *Proceedings of the National Academy of Sciences of the United States of America, 100,* 3893–3988. doi:10.1073/pnas.0530291100

Altekruse, S.F., Kosary, C.L., Krapcho, M., Neyman, N., Aminou, R., Waldron, W., ... Edwards, B.K. (Eds.). (2009, November). SEER stat factsheets: All sites. *SEER Cancer Statistics Review, 1975–2007.* Retrieved from http://seer.cancer.gov/statfacts/html/all.html

American Brain Tumor Association. (2009). Facts and statistics, 2009. Retrieved from http://www.abta.org/siteFiles/pdflibrary/ABTA%20Facts%20and%20Statistics%202009.pdf

American College of Surgical Oncology CNS Working Group. (2005). The management of brain metastases. In D. Schiff & B.P. O'Neill (Eds.), *Principles of neuro-oncology* (pp. 553–580). New York, NY: McGraw-Hill.

Batchelor, T., & Loeffler, J.S. (2006). Primary CNS lymphoma. *Journal of Clinical Oncology, 24,* 1281–1288. doi:10.1200/JCO.2005.04.8819

Bellinzona, M., Roser, F., Ostertag, H., Gaab, R., & Saini, M. (2005). Surgical removal of primary central nervous system lymphomas (PCNSL) presenting as space occupying lesions: A series of 33 cases. *European Journal of Surgical Oncology, 31,* 100–105. doi:10.1016/j.ejso.2004.10.002

Berger, M., Leibel, S., Bruner, J., Finlay, J., & Levin, V. (2002). Primary cerebral tumors. In V. Levin (Ed.), *Cancer in the nervous system* (2nd ed., pp. 75–148). New York, NY: Oxford University Press.

Bindal, R.K., Sawaya, R., Leavens, M.E., & Lee, J.J. (1993). Surgical treatment of multiple brain metastases. *Journal of Neurosurgery, 79,* 210–216. doi: 10.3171/jns.1993.79.2.0210

Bollanti, L., Riondino, G., & Strollo, F. (2001). Endocrine paraneoplastic syndromes with special reference to the elderly. *Endocrine, 14,* 151–157. doi:10.1385/ENDO:14:2:151

Bonnet, D., & Dick, J.E. (1997). Human acute myeloid leukemia is organized as a hierarchy that originates from a primitive hematopoietic cell. *Nature Medicine, 3,* 730–737. doi:10.1038/nm0797-730

Borsig, L., Wong, R., Feramisco, J., Nadeau, D.R., Varki, N.M., & Varki, A. (2001). Heparin and cancer revisited: Mechanistic connections involving platelets, P-selectin, carcinoma mucins, and tumor metastasis. *Proceedings of the National Academy of Sciences of the United States of America, 98,* 3352–3357. doi: 10.1073/pnas.061615598

Brandsma, D., Stalpers, L., Taal, W., Sminia, P., & van den Bent, M.J. (2008). Clinical features, mechanisms, and management of pseudoprogression in malignant gliomas. *Lancet Oncology, 9,* 453–461. doi: 10.1016/S1470-2045(08)70125-6

Brenner, A.V., Linet, M.S., Selker, R.G., Shapiro, W.R., Black, P.M., Fine, H.A., & Inskip, P.D. (2003). Polio vaccination and risk of brain tumors in adults: No apparent association. *Cancer Epidemiology, Biomarkers and Prevention, 12,* 177–178.

Cairncross, G., Berkey, B., Shaw, E., Jenkins, R., Scheithauer, B., Brachman, D., ... Curran, W. (2006). Phase III trial of chemotherapy plus radiotherapy compared with radiotherapy alone for pure and mixed anaplastic oligodendroglioma: Intergroup Radiation Therapy Oncology Group Trial 9402.

Journal of Clinical Oncology, 24, 2707–2714. doi:10.1200/JCO.2005.04.3414

Cairncross, J.G., Chernik, N.L., Kim, J.H., & Posner, J.B. (1979). Sterilization of cerebral metastases by radiation therapy. *Neurology, 29*(9, Pt. 1), 1195–1202.

Catt, S., Chalmers, A., & Fallowfield, L. (2008). Psychosocial and supportive-care needs in high-grade glioma. *Lancet Oncology, 9,* 884–891. doi: 10.1016/S1470-2045(08)70230-4

Central Brain Tumor Registry of the United States. (2010). *CBTRUS statistical report: Primary brain and central nervous system tumors diagnosed in the United States in 2004–2006.* Retrieved from http://www.cbtrus.org/2010-NPCR-SEER/CBTRUS -WEBREPORT-Final-3-2-10.pdf

Coons, S.W., Johnson, P.C., Scheithauer, B.W., Yates, A.J., & Pearl, D.K. (1997). Improving diagnostic accuracy and interobserver concordance in the classification and grading of primary gliomas. *Cancer, 79,* 1381–1393. doi: 10.1002/(SICI)1097 -0142(19970401)79:7<1381::AID-CNCR16>3.0.CO;2-W

Coté, T.R., Manns, A., Hardy, C.R., Yellin, F.J., & Hartge, P. (1996). Epidemiology of brain lymphoma among people with or without acquired immunodeficiency syndrome. AIDS/Cancer Study Group. *Journal of the National Cancer Institute, 88,* 675–679. doi:10.1093/jnci/88.10.675

Darnell, R.B., & Posner, J.B. (2003). Paraneoplastic syndromes involving the nervous syndrome. *New England Journal of Medicine, 349,* 1543–1554. doi:10.1056/NEJMra023009

Davies, E. (1997). Patients' perceptions of follow-up services. In E. Davies & A. Hopkins (Eds.), *Improving care for patients with malignant cerebral glioma* (pp. 81–91). London, United Kingdom: Royal College of Physicians.

DeAngelis, L.M. (2002). Leukemia and lymphoma metastases. In V. Levin (Ed.), *Cancer in the nervous system* (2nd ed., pp. 362–374). New York, NY: Oxford University Press.

de Groot, J.F., Aldape, K.D., & Colman, H. (2005). High grade astrocytomas. In D. Schiff & B.P. O'Neill (Eds.), *Principles of neuro-oncology* (pp. 260–288). New York, NY: McGraw-Hill.

Delattre, J.Y., Krol, G., Thaler, H.T., & Posner, J.B. (1988). Distribution of brain metastases. *Archives of Neurology, 45,* 741–744.

DeYoung, B.R., & Wick, M.R. (2000). Immunohistologic evaluation of metastatic carcinomas of unknown origin: An algorithmic approach. *Seminars in Diagnostic Pathology, 17,* 184–193.

Eby, N.L., Grufferman, S., Flannelly, C.M., Schold, S.C., Jr., Vogel, F.S., & Burger, P.C. (1988). Increasing incidence of primary brain lymphoma in the U.S. *Cancer, 62,* 2461–2465.

Enting, R.H. (2005). Leptomeningeal neoplasia: Epidemiology, clinical presentation, CSF analysis and diagnostic imaging. *Cancer Treatment Research, 125,* 17–30.

Ewing, J. (1940). *Neoplastic diseases: A treatise on tumors* (4th ed.). Philadelphia, PA: Saunders.

Ferreri, A.J., Abrey, L.E., Blay, J.Y., Borisch, B., Hochman, J., Neuwelt, E.A., ... Batchelor, T. (2003). Summary statement on primary central nervous system lymphomas from the Eighth International Conference on Malignant Lymphoma, Lugano, Switzerland, June 12 to 15, 2002. *Journal of Clinical Oncology, 21,* 2407–2414. doi: 10.1200/JCO.2003.01.135

Fox, S., & Lantz, C. (1998). The brain tumor experience and quality of life: A quality of life study. *Journal of Neuroscience Nursing, 30,* 245–252.

Gaspar, L., Scott, C., Rotman, M., Asbell, S., Phillips, T., Wasserman, T., ... Byhardt, R. (1997). Recursive partitioning analysis (RPA) of prognostic factors in three Radiation Therapy Oncology Group (RTOG) brain metastases trials. *International Journal of Radiation Oncology, Biology, Physics, 37,* 745–751.

Gavrilovic, I.T., & Posner, J.B. (2005). Brain metastases: Epidemiology and pathophysiology. *Journal of Neuro-Oncology, 75,* 5–14. doi:10.1007/s11060-004-8093-6

Grossmann, J. (2002). Molecular mechanisms of "detachment-induced apoptosis—Anoikis." *Apoptosis, 7,* 247–260. doi:10.1023/A:1015312119693

Hegi, M.E., Diserens, A.C., Gorlia, T., Hamou, M.F., de Tribolet, N., Weller, M., ... Stupp, R. (2005). *MGMT* gene silencing and benefit from temozolomide in glioblastoma. *New England Journal of Medicine, 352,* 997–1003. doi:10.1056/NEJMoa043331

Hemmati, H.D., Nakano, I., Lazareff, J.A., Masterman-Smith, M., Geschwind, D.H., Bronner-Fraser, M., & Kornblum, H.I. (2003). Cancerous stem cells can arise from pediatric brain tumors. *Proceedings of the National Academy of Sciences of the United States of America, 100,* 15178–15183. doi:10.1073/pnas.2036535100

Iwadate, Y., Namba, H., & Yamaura, A. (2000). Significance of surgical resection for the treatment of multiple brain metastases. *Anticancer Research, 20,* 573–577.

Kadan-Lottick, N.S., Skluzacek, M.C., & Gurney, J.G. (2002). Decreasing incidence rates of primary central nervous system lymphoma. *Cancer, 95,* 193–202. doi:10.1002/cncr.10643

Kaplan, J.G., DeSouza, T.G., Farkash, A., Shafran, B., Pack, D., Rehman, F., ... Portenoy, R. (1990). Leptomeningeal metastases: Comparison of clinical features and laboratory data of solid tumors, lymphomas and leukemias. *Journal of Neuro-Oncology, 9,* 225–229.

Karim, A.B.M.F., Maat, B., Hatlevoll, R., Menten, J., Rutten, E.H.J.M., Thomas, D.G.T., ... van Glabbeke, M. (1996). A randomized trial on dose-response in radiation therapy of low-grade cerebral glioma: European Organization for Research and Treatment of Cancer (EORTC) study 22844. *International Journal of Radiation Oncology, Biology, Physics, 36,* 549–556.

Kesari, S., & Batchelor, T.T. (2003). Leptomeningeal metastases. *Neurologic Clinics, 21,* 25–66.

Kleihues, P., & Cavenee, W. (2000). *World Health Organization classification of tumours of the nervous system.* Lyon, France: IARC.

Kösel, S., Scheithauer, B., & Graeber, M. (2001). Genotype-phenotype correlation in gemistocytic astrocytomas. *Neurosurgery, 48,* 187–193.

Kros, J.H., Zheng, P., Wolbers, J.G., & van den Bent, M.J. (2005). Oligodendroglial tumors. In M.S. Berger & M.D. Prados (Eds.), *Textbook of neuro-oncology* (pp. 167–176). Philadelphia, PA: Elsevier Saunders.

Landonio, G., Sartore-Bianchi, A., Giannetta, L., Renga, M., Riva, M., & Siena, S. (2001). Controversies in the management of brain metastases: The role of chemotherapy. *Forum, 11,* 59–74.

Liotta, L.A., & Kohn, E.C. (2003). Cancer's deadly signature. *Nature Genetics, 33,* 10–11. doi:10.1038/ng0103-10

Markesbery, W.R., Brooks, W.H., Gupta, G.D., & Young, A.B. (1978). Treatment for patients with cerebral metastases. *Archives of Neurology, 35,* 754–756.

Mazzone, P.J., & Arroliga, A.C. (2003). Endocrine paraneoplastic syndromes in lung cancer. *Current Opinion in Pulmonary Medicine, 9,* 313–320.

McDonald, J.M., See, S.J., Tremont, I.W., Colman, H., Gilbert, M.R., Groves, M., ... Aldape, K. (2005). The prognostic impact of histology and 1p/19q status in anaplastic oligodendroglial tumors. *Cancer, 104,* 1468–1477. doi:10.1002/cncr.21338

Mellinghoff, I.K., Wang, M.Y., Vivanco, I., Haas-Kogan, D.A., Zhu, S., Dia, E.Q., ... Mischel, P.S. (2005). Molecular determinants of the response of glioblastomas to EGFR kinase inhibitors. *New England Journal of Medicine, 353,* 2012–2024. doi:10.1056/NEJMoa051918

Merchut, M.P. (1989). Brain metastases from undiagnosed systemic neoplasms. *Archives of Internal Medicine, 149,* 1076–1080.

Miller, D.C., Hochberg, F.H., Harris, N.L., Gruber, M.L., Louis, D.N., & Cohen, H. (1994). Pathology with clinical correlations of primary central nervous system non-Hodgkin's lymphoma. The Massachusetts General Hospital experience 1958–1989. *Cancer, 74,* 1383–1397.

Murray, K., Kun, L., & Cox, J. (1986). Primary malignant lymphoma of the central nervous system. Results of treatment of 11 cases and review of the literature. *Journal of Neurosurgery, 65,* 600–607. doi:10.3171/jns.1986.65.5.0600

Nakagawa, H., Murasawa, A., Kubo, S., Nakajima, S., Nakajima, Y., & Izumoto, S. (1992). Diagnosis and treatment of patients with meningeal carcinomatosis. *Journal of Neuro-Oncology, 13,* 81–89.

Nelson, D.F., Martz, K.L., Bonner, H., Nelson, J.S., Newall, J., Kerman, H.D., ... Murray, K.J. (1992). Non-Hodgkin's lymphoma of the brain: Can high dose, large volume radiation therapy improve survival? Report on a prospective trial by the Radiation Therapy Oncology Group (RTOG): RTOG 8315. *International Journal of Radiation Oncology, Biology, Physics, 23,* 9–17.

Nieswandt, B., Hafner, M., Echtenacher, B., & Mannel, D.N. (1999). Lysis of tumor cells by natural killer cells in mice impeded by platelets. *Cancer Research, 59,* 1295–1300.

Non-Hodgkin's Lymphoma Classification Project. (1997). A clinical evaluation of the International Lymphoma Study Group classification of non-Hodgkin's lymphoma. *Blood, 89,* 3909–3918. Retrieved from http://bloodjournal.hematologylibrary.org/cgi/content/full/89/11/3909

Olson, M.E., Chernik, N.L., & Posner, J.B. (1974). Infiltration of the leptomeninges by systemic cancer. A clinical and pathologic study. *Archives of Neurology, 30,* 122–137.

O'Meara, W.P., Borkar, S.A., Stambuk, H.E., & Lymberis, S.C. (2007). Leptomeningeal metastasis. *Current Problems in Cancer, 31,* 367–424. doi:10.1016/j.currproblcancer.2007.07.001

O'Neill, B.P., & Schiff, D. (2005). Primary central nervous system lymphoma. In D. Schiff & B.P. O'Neill (Eds.), *Principles of neuro-oncology* (pp. 343–367). New York, NY: McGraw-Hill.

Paget, S. (1889). The distribution of secondary growths in cancer of the breast. *Lancet, 1,* 571–573.

Paillas, J.E., & Pellet, W. (1975). Brain metastases. In P.J. Vinken, & G.W. Bruyn (Eds.), *Handbook of clinical neurology* (Vol. 18, pp. 210–232). New York, NY: Elsevier.

Perrin, R.G., Laperriere, N.J., Loblaw, D.A., & Laxton, A.W. (2002). Spinal axis metastases. In V. Levin (Ed.), *Cancer in the nervous system* (2nd ed., pp. 341–361). New York, NY: Oxford University Press.

Peterson, B.A., Brunning, R.D., Bloomfield, C.D., Hurd, D.D., Gau, J.A., Peng, G.T., & Goldman, A.L. (1987). Central nervous system involvement in acute non-lymphocytic leukemia: A prospective study of adults in remission. *American Journal of Medicine, 83,* 464–470.

Posner, J.B. (1995). *Neurologic complications of cancer.* New York, NY: Oxford University Press.

Postmus, P.E., & Smit, E.F. (1999). Chemotherapy for brain metastases of lung cancer: A review. *Annals of Oncology, 10,* 753–759.

Pronzato, P., Bruna, F., Neri, E., Roveri, D., Trabucchi, A., Vanoli, M., ... Bertelli, G. (1995). Radiotherapy plus carboplatin and teniposide in patients with brain metastases from non small cell lung cancer. *Anticancer Research, 15,* 517–519.

Reya, T., Morrison, S.J., Clarke, M.F., & Weissmann, I.L. (2001). Stem cells, cancer and cancer stem cells. *Nature, 414,* 105–111. doi:10.1038/35102167

Roberge, D., Petrecca, K., El Refae, M., & Souhami, L. (2009). Whole-brain radiotherapy and tumor bed radiosurgery following resection of solitary brain metastases. *Journal of Neuro-Oncology, 95,* 95–99. doi:10.1007/s11060-009-9899-z

Ruderman, N.B., & Hall, T.C. (1965). Use of glucocorticoids in the palliative treatment of metastatic brain tumors. *Cancer, 18,* 298–306.

Sawaya, R., Lingon, B.L., & Bindal, R.K. (1994). Management of metastatic brain tumors. *Annals of Surgical Oncology, 1,* 169–178.

Schiff, D., Brown, P., & Giannini, C. (2007). Outcomes in low grade glioma: The impact of prognostic factors and treatment. *Neurology, 69,* 1366–1373.

Schouten, L.J., Rutten, J., Huveneers, H.A., & Twijnstra, A. (2002). Incidence of brain metastases in a cohort of patients with carcinoma of the breast, colon, kidney, and lung and melanoma. *Cancer, 94,* 2698–2705. doi:10.1002/cncr.10541

Shojana, K.G., Burton, E.C., McDonald, K.M., & Goldman, L. (2003). Changes in rates of autopsy-detected diagnostic errors over time: A systematic review. *JAMA, 289,* 2849–2856. doi:10.1001/jama.289.21.2849

Siffert, J., & Jallo, G. (2005). Ependymomas and intraventricular tumor. In D. Schiff & B.P. O'Neill (Eds.), *Principles of neuro-oncology* (pp. 431–445). New York, NY: McGraw-Hill.

Singh, S.K., Clarke, M.F., Terasaki, M., Bonn, V.E., Hawkins, C., Squire, J., & Dirks, P.B. (2003). Identification of a stem cell in human brain tumors. *Cancer Research, 63,* 5821–1528.

Stieber, V.W., Tatter, S.B., Shaffrey, M.E., & Shaw, E.G. (2005). Primary spinal tumors. In D. Schiff & B.P. O'Neill (Eds.), *Principles of neuro-oncology* (pp. 503–504). New York, NY: McGraw-Hill.

Stupp, R., Hegi, M.E., Mason, W.P., van den Bent, M.J., Taphoorn, M.J., Janzer, R.C., ... Mirimanoff, R.O. (2009). Effects of radiotherapy with concomitant and adjuvant temozolomide versus radiotherapy alone on survival in glioblastoma in a randomised phase III study: 5-year analysis of the EORTC-NCIC trial. *Lancet Oncology, 10,* 459–466. doi:10.1016/S1470-2045(09)70025-7

Stupp, R., Mason, W.P., van den Bent, M.J., Weller, M., Fisher, B., Taphoorn, M.J., ... Mirimanoff, R.O. (2005). Radiotherapy plus concomitant and adjuvant temozolomide for glioblastoma. *New England Journal of Medicine, 352,* 987–996. doi:10.1056/NEJMoa043330

Swift, P.S., Phillips, T., Martz, K., Wara, W., Mohiuddin, M., Chang, C.H., & Asbell, S.O. (1993). CT characteristics of patients with brain metastases treated in RTOG study 79-16. *International Journal of Radiation Oncology, Biology, Physics, 25,* 209–214.

Taal, W., Brandsma, D., de Bruin, H.G., Bromberg, J.E., Swaak-Kragten, A.T., Smitt, P.A., ... van den Bent, M.J. (2008). Incidence of early pseudo-progression in a cohort of malignant glioma patients treated with chemoirradiation with temozolomide. *Cancer, 113,* 405–410. doi:10.1002/cncr.23562

Tatter, S.B. (2005). The new WHO classification of tumors affecting the central nervous system. Retrieved from http://neurosurgery.mgh.harvard.edu/newwhobt.htm

van den Bent, M.J., Afra, D., de Witte, O., Ben Hassel, M., Schraub, S., Hoang-Xuan, K., ... Mirimanoff, R.O. (2005). Long-term efficacy of early versus delayed radiotherapy for low-grade astrocytoma and oligodendroglioma in adults: The EORTC 22845 randomised trial. *Lancet, 366,* 985–990. doi:10.1016/S0140-6736(05)67070-5

van den Bent, M.J., Carpentier, A.F., Brandes, A.A., Sanson, M., Taphoorn, M.J., Bernsen, H.J., ... Gorlia, T. (2006). Adjuvant procarbazine, lomustine, and vincristine improves progression-free survival but not overall survival in newly diagnosed anaplastic oligodendrogliomas and oligoastrocytomas: A randomized European Organisation for Research and Treatment of Cancer phase III trial. *Journal of Clinical Oncology, 24,* 2715–2722. doi:10.1200/JCO.2005.04.6078

van den Bent, M.J., & Kros, J.M. (2005). Oligodendroglioma and mixed gliomas. In D. Schiff & B.P. O'Neill (Eds.), *Principles of neuro-oncology* (pp. 311–332). New York, NY: McGraw-Hill.

van der Ree, T.C., Dipped, D.W., Avezaat, C.J., Sleeves Smitt, P.A.S., Vecht, C.J., & van den Bent, M.J. (1999). Leptomeningeal metastasis after surgical resection of brain metastases. *Journal of Neurology, Neurosurgery and Psychiatry, 66,* 225–227. doi:10.1136/jnnp.66.2.225

van Veelen, M.L.C., Avezaat, C.J.J., Kros, J.M., van Putten, W., & Vecht, C. (1998). Supratentorial low grade astrocytoma: Prognostic factors, dedifferentiation, and the issue of early versus late surgery. *Journal of Neurology, Neurosurgery and Psychiatry, 64,* 581–587. doi:10.1136/jnnp.64.5.581

von Deimling, A., von Amman, K., Schoenfeld, D., Wiestler, O.D., Seizinger, B.R., & Louis, D.N. (1993). Subsets of glioblastoma multiforme defined by molecular genetic analysis. *Brain Pathology, 3,* 19–26.

Wasserstrom, W.R., Glass, J.P., & Posner, J.B. (1982). Diagnosis and treatment of leptomeningeal metastasis from solid tumors: Experience with 90 patients. *Cancer, 49,* 759–772.

Wen, P., & Loeffler, J.S. (1999). Management of brain metastases. *Oncology, 13,* 941–954, 957–961.

Wen, P.Y., Teoh, S.K., Gigas, D.G., & MacDonald, L. (2005). Presentation and approach to the patient. In D. Schiff & B.P. O'Neill (Eds.), *Principles of neuro-oncology* (pp. 37–51). New York, NY: McGraw-Hill.

Wideheim, A.K., Edvardsson, T., Påhlson, A., & Ahlström, G. (2002). A family's perspective on living with a highly malignant brain tumor. *Cancer Nursing, 25,* 236–244.

Young, B., Oldfield, E.H., Markesbery, W.R., Haack, D., Tibbs, P.A., McCombs, P., … Meacham, W.F. (1981). Reoperation for glioblastoma. *Journal of Neurosurgery, 55,* 917–921. doi:10.3171/jns.1981.55.6.0917

Yung, W.K.A., Kunschner, L.J., Sawaya, R., Chang, E.L., & Fuller, G.N. (2002). Intracranial metastases. In V. Levin (Ed.), *Cancer in the nervous system* (2nd ed., pp. 321–340). New York, NY: Oxford University Press.

CHAPTER 6

Pediatric Cancers of the Brain and Spinal Cord

Melody Ann Watral, MSN, RN, CPNP-PC, CPON®

Introduction

Pediatric central nervous system (CNS) tumors are the most common solid tumor of childhood and are second only to the childhood leukemias in terms of incidence in childhood. The Central Brain Tumor Registry of the United States (CBTRUS, 2010) estimated that 4,030 new cases of childhood primary nonmalignant and malignant CNS tumors are expected to be diagnosed in the United States in 2010, with 2,880 of these tumors in children younger than 15 years old.

Overall Incidence

The overall incidence rate of CNS tumors in children ages 0–19 is 4.71 per 100,000 person-years (CBTRUS, 2010). Children ages 0–4 years have the highest incidence rate at 5.13 per 100,000 person-years, with the lowest incidence rate of 4.22 per 100,000 person-years in children ages 10–14 years (CBTRUS, 2010). The incidence rate is higher in males than females at 4.75:4.66 per 100,000 person-years (CBTRUS, 2010).

Incidence by Histology

When examining the histology of CNS tumors in childhood, the embryonal tumors, which include medulloblastoma and primitive neuroectodermal tumors (PNETs), are most common in young children (ages 0–4) (CBTRUS, 2010). Pilocytic astrocytoma is the most common type of CNS tumor found in children ages 5–14. Pituitary tumors are the most common tumor type in adolescents and young adults ages 15–19 (see Figure 6-1).

Incidence by Location

As illustrated in Figure 6-2, tumors located in the frontal, temporal, parietal, and occipital lobes account for 17.2% of the CNS tumors that occur in childhood (ages 0–19) (CBTRUS, 2010).

Unlike CNS tumors in adults, pediatric CNS tumors tend to be located below the tentorium. The tentorium is a thick membrane that separates the upper two-thirds of the brain from the lower third, shown in Figure 6-3. Tumors located above the tentorium are supratentorial, and tumors located below the tentorium are infratentorial. The majority of pediatric CNS tumors are located in the posterior fossa (below the tentorium), which is composed of the cerebellum and brain stem (26.8%) and the fourth ventricle (CBTRUS, 2010).

Primary Tumors of the Brain in Childhood

Astrocytomas

This group of tumors represents approximately 50% of the CNS tumors diagnosed in childhood (ages 0–19) (Strickler & Phillips, 2000). The cell of origin, the astrocyte, is a star-shaped glial cell. The glial cells are considered the "glue cells" of the CNS. These cells provide structure and support to nerve cells and capillaries within the CNS, but their exact function is unknown (Strickler & Phillips, 2000). Oligodendrogliomas are included among the astrocytomas. This tumor type originates from the oligodendrocyte cell, another glial cell type that insulates the nerve fibers within the brain.

The World Health Organization (WHO) grading system is used to classify astrocytomas based on their histology (appearance under the microscope) (Tatter, 2005). Low-grade, or grade I, astrocytomas include pilocytic astrocytomas, pleomorphic xanthoastrocytomas, subependymal giant cell astrocytomas, and subependymomas. These tumors appear well differentiated and are slow growing. Grade II tumors, usually fibrillary astrocytomas or oligodendrogliomas, are considered more infiltrative and are able to penetrate into the surrounding tissues.

Figure 6-1. Distribution of Childhood Primary Brain and Central Nervous System Tumors by Histology

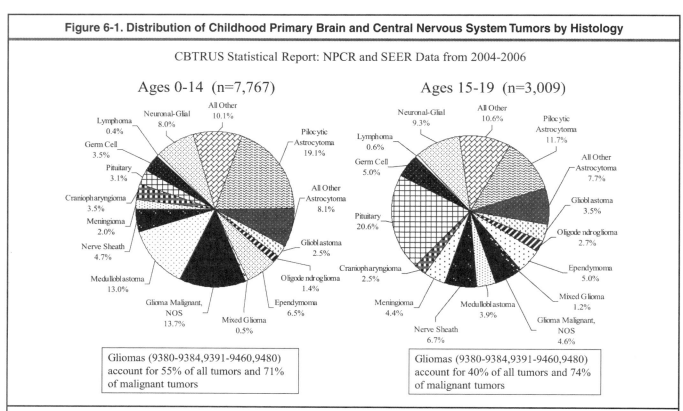

CBTRUS Statistical Report: NPCR and SEER Data from 2004-2006

Ages 0-14 (n=7,767)

Ages 15-19 (n=3,009)

Gliomas (9380-9384,9391-9460,9480) account for 55% of all tumors and 71% of malignant tumors

Gliomas (9380-9384,9391-9460,9480) account for 40% of all tumors and 74% of malignant tumors

Note. From *CBTRUS Statistical Report: Primary Brain and Central Nervous System Tumors Diagnosed in the United States in 2004–2006* (p. 24), by the Central Brain Tumor Registry of the United States, 2010, Hinsdale, IL: Author. Retrieved from http://www.cbtrus.org/2010-NPCR-SEER/CBTRUS-WEBREPORT -Final-3-2-10.pdf.

Anaplastic astrocytomas are considered grade III tumors, which are more aggressive with increased anaplasia and mitotic activity without necrosis and microvascular proliferation. These tumors can spread into the surrounding tissue and other parts of the brain and spinal cord.

The grade IV status of glioblastoma multiforme reflects this tumor's highly aggressive nature. Microscopic evaluation shows both increased cell division and the presence of necrotic tissue within the tumor—evidence of this tumor's predilection for rapid growth and spread through the cerebrospinal fluid (CSF) to other parts of the brain and spinal cord.

Embryonal Tumors

Embryonal tumors, such as medulloblastoma, PNET, and pineoblastoma tumors, originate from primitive (embryonal) cells. Medulloblastomas are the most common type of malignant pediatric brain tumor, usually arising infratentorially in the posterior fossa. Medulloblastomas span a histologic spectrum ending in overtly malignant large-cell/anaplastic lesions characterized by increased nuclear size, marked cytologic anaplasia, and increased mitotic and apoptotic rates (Eberhart & Burger, 2003). Medulloblastomas account for approximately 16.9% of all pediatric CNS tumors (CBTRUS, 2010).

The term *supratentorial embryonal tumor* is used for every undifferentiated, small, round, blue cell tumor located above the tentorium (Marec-Berard et al., 2002). Pineoblastomas arise from the parenchyma of the pineal gland and are considered to be another type of supratentorial PNET (Gururangan et al., 2003). Supratentorial PNETs account for 2.5% of cerebral tumors in childhood (Marec-Berard et al., 2002) (see Figure 6-4).

Ependymomas

This type of tumor arises from the ependymal cells, which line the ventricles of the brain and comprise the center of the spinal cord. This tumor type accounts for 9% of all pediatric CNS tumors (Stiefbold & Thompson, 2006). They are usually located infratentorially, with the most common location being the posterior fossa for childhood ependymomas. However, these tumors may occur in other parts of the brain and in the spinal cord. Of note, spinal cord tumors are more common in teenagers, whereas brain tumors tend to occur in younger children.

Ependymomas are graded based on how closely they resemble the normal ependymal cell. Myxopapillary ependymomas and subependymomas are both considered low-grade

Figure 6-2. Distribution of All Childhood (Ages 0–19 Years) Primary Brain and Central Nervous System Tumors by Site (N = 10,776)

CBTRUS Statistical Report: NPCR and SEER Data from 2004-2006

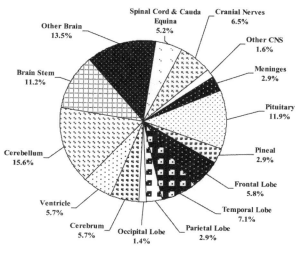

Note. From *CBTRUS Statistical Report: Primary Brain and Central Nervous System Tumors Diagnosed in the United States in 2004–2006* (p. 23), by the Central Brain Tumor Registry of the United States, 2010, Hinsdale, IL: Author. Retrieved from http://www.cbtrus.org/2010-NPCR-SEER/CBTRUS-WEBREPORT-Final-3-2-10.pdf.

Figure 6-3. The Tentorium

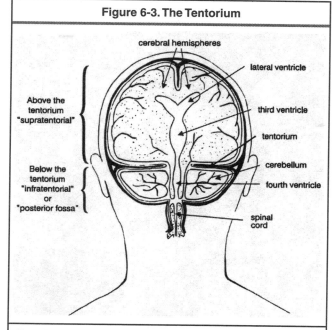

Note. Figure courtesy of the American Brain Tumor Association. Used with permission.

Figure 6-4. Head Cross Section, Sagittal View

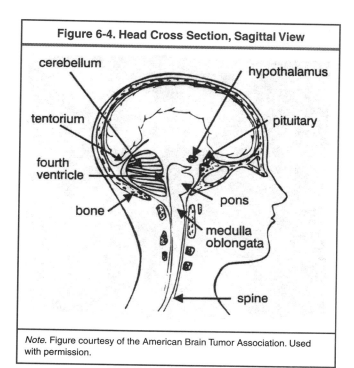

Note. Figure courtesy of the American Brain Tumor Association. Used with permission.

tumors (grade I). Ependymoma variants (cellular, papillary, epithelial, clear cell, and mixed), which are the most common of the ependymal tumors, are considered grade II tumors. Anaplastic ependymomas (grade III) are considered high-grade aggressive tumors (Binning, Klimo, Gluf, & Goumnervoa, 2007; Tatter, 2005).

In terms of location, grade I ependymomas are usually located in the lower spine or near a ventricle. Grade II ependymomas may be located along the lining of a ventricle, particularly within the posterior fossa or within the spinal cord. Grade III ependymomas are most commonly found within the posterior fossa.

Brain Stem Gliomas

Brain stem tumors account for approximately 11.2% of all pediatric brain tumors (CBTRUS, 2010). The median age at occurrence of pediatric brain stem gliomas is six to seven years. Brain stem tumors develop because abnormal glial cells invade the brain stem, which subsequently infiltrate between the normal neural structures. More than 80% of these tumors occur in the pons and are diffusely infiltrative (Ryan-Murray & Petriecione, 2002). The other forms are more localized and may have an exophytic component that protrudes outside the brain stem. A magnetic resonance imaging (MRI) scan of the brain is performed to identify the extent of disease and to assess for the presence of vasogenic edema (Jallo, Biser-Rohrbaugh, & Freed, 2004). Patients diagnosed with a diffusely infiltrative lesion of the brain stem usually die to their disease within a year from diagnosis (median survival time). Survival rates at two years after diagnosis are less than 10%–20% (Rosenblum, 2005).

Craniopharyngioma

Craniopharyngiomas are rare epithelial tumors that arise along the path of the craniopharyngeal duct (Karavitaki, Cudlip, Adams, & Wass, 2006). They account for 5%–13% of all pediatric brain tumors (American Brain Tumor Association [ABTA], 2007). This tumor may also involve the pituitary gland, optic nerve, and third ventricle.

Diencephalic Tumors

Tumor types in this region of the brain include hypothalamic tumors, tumors of the chiasma, and thalamic tumors. These tumors are considered low-grade (grade I and II astrocytomas) because of their slow-growing nature (see Figure 6-5).

Optic Chiasma or Nerve Pathway Gliomas

Optic chiasma or nerve pathway gliomas are tumors that can occur anywhere along the optic pathway. They are usually considered grade I tumors because of their slow growth. Biopsy of these tumors is often deferred because of the potential for loss of sight related to the surgery. They have the capacity to spread along the optic pathway. Of note, these tumors in childhood are more commonly associated in patients with a diagnosis of neurofibromatosis type 1.

Germ Cell Tumors

This group of rare tumors includes germinoma (the most common in this group), teratoma, yolk-sac, embryonal carcinoma, choriocarcinoma, and mixed germ cell tumors. Germ cell tumors represent only 1%–3% of all childhood brain tumors (ABTA, 2007). They are the only tumors that may be diagnosed by tumor markers (beta-human chorionic gonadotropin and alpha-fetoprotein) found in the CSF (ABTA, 2007). These tumors may spread via the CSF to other locations in the CNS.

Choroid Plexus Papilloma and Carcinoma

Choroid plexus papilloma and carcinoma arise from the choroid plexus epithelium, exhibiting papillary and intraventricular growth (Gopal, Parker, Debski, & Parker, 2008).

Figure 6-5. Hypothalamic Tumor, Before and After Chemotherapy

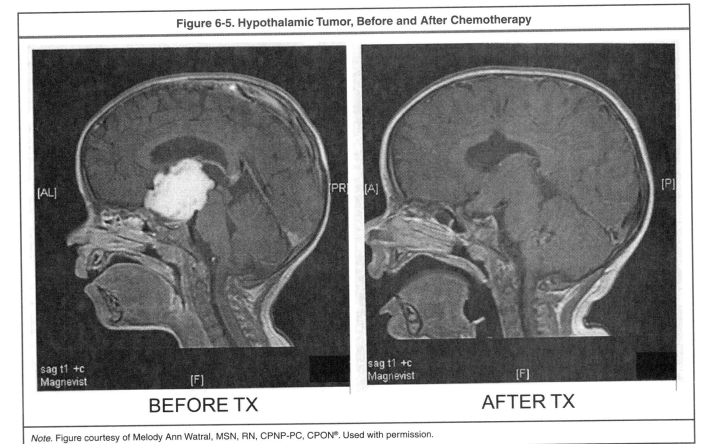

BEFORE TX   AFTER TX

Note. Figure courtesy of Melody Ann Watral, MSN, RN, CPNP-PC, CPON®. Used with permission.

They typically arise in the lateral ventricles. Papilloma is the benign variant, and carcinoma the malignant variant. These neoplasms are more common in children than adults, representing 1%–4% of all pediatric brain tumors, with 10%–20% occurring during infancy (Paulus & Brander, 2007).

Atypical Teratoid Rhabdoid Tumor

Atypical teratoid rhabdoid tumors (ATRTs) are aggressive high-grade tumors that are usually found in the cerebellum of the brain but can occur outside the CNS. ATRT was once identified as a PNET or medulloblastoma but was recognized in the late 1980s to be a completely different histologic entity (Strother, 2005). This tumor type is usually limited to children younger than the age of two but occasionally occurs in older children.

Benign Pediatric Brain Tumors

These types of tumors may be found in the CNS and are considered benign by histologic or radiographic evaluation. The mass may be followed by serial MRI scanning and clinical evaluation. Although the tumor is considered histologically benign, surgical intervention may be required if the mass causes obstructive hydrocephalus. Examples of these tumors include lipoma and cyst types such as arachnoid, colloid, dermoid, and epidermoid (ABTA, 2007).

Pediatric Spinal Tumors

Location

Spinal cord tumors account for 5.2% of all pediatric primary CNS tumors (CBTRUS, 2010). Occurrence of these tumors is sporadic throughout childhood, with the median age at occurrence being 10 years. In pediatric patients with intrinsic tumor of the spinal cord, "male patients are slightly more commonly affected than female patients, in a 1.3:1.0 ratio" (Blaney et al., 2006, p. 847). Figure 6-6 shows a cross section of the spine.

Extradural spinal tumors are localized between the bony structures and the dura. These tumors may arise from bony elements, the meninges, or the soft tissues. They account for approximately 30% of all pediatric spinal cord tumors (Wetjen & Raffel, 2008). The most common extradural spinal cord tumors are sarcomas, neuroblastomas, teratomas, lymphomas, and metastatic tumors (Binning et al., 2007). As an example, neuroblastomas arise from the neural crest cell derivatives of the sympathetic nervous system. If the tumor arises in the paraspinal location in the abdomen, it can extend into the spinal canal through the intervertebral foramina, resulting in a dumbbell-shaped mass. Neuroblastoma is the most common cause of extradural spinal cord compression in pediatric patients (Sciubba, Hsieh, McLoughlin, & Jallo, 2008).

Figure 6-6. Cross Section of the Vertebrae and Spine

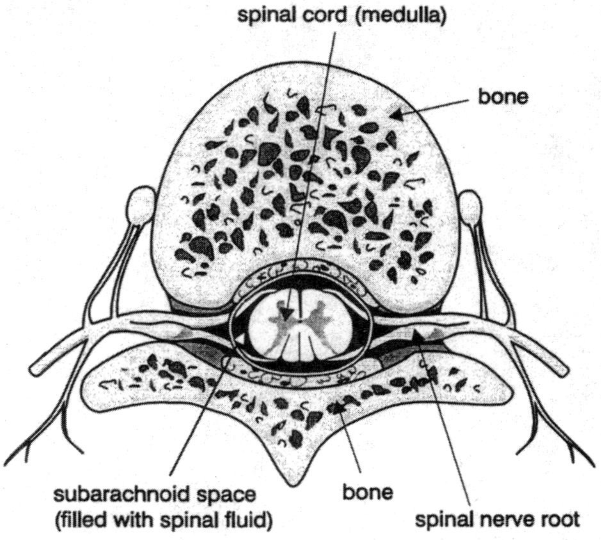

spinal cord (medulla)

bone

subarachnoid space (filled with spinal fluid)

bone

spinal nerve root

Note. Figure courtesy of the American Brain Tumor Association. Used with permission.

Chordoma is a tumor of the axial skeleton that is distinctly uncommon in children and adolescents (Ridenour, Ahrens, Folpe, & Miller, 2009). These tumors may occur in the sacrum, along the spinal axis or at the base of the skull, or at the clivus (shallow depression), which is the most common presentation site in childhood. They account for only 0.2% of all CNS tumors for both adult and pediatric diseases combined (Palmer & Harrison, 2008). Chordomas are thought to arise from primitive notochordal (backbone) remnants (Palmer & Harrison, 2008).

Intradural spinal tumors (see Figure 6-7) are either extramedullary (within the dura but not part of the spinal cord) or intramedullary (within the spinal cord parenchyma). The most common intradural-extramedullary spinal tumors in childhood are neurofibroma, schwannoma, meningioma, myxopapillary ependymoma, and dermoid/epidermoid cysts (Binning et al., 2007). The majority of intradural-intramedullary spinal cord tumors in children and young adults are low-grade gliomas (Constantini et al., 2000), such as astrocytomas and gangliogliomas. Much less commonly reported intradural-intramedullary tumors include developmental tumors (teratomas), oligodendrogliomas, schwannomas, neurofibromas, subependymomas, neurocytomas, dermoid/epidermoid cysts, and metastases (Auguste & Gupta, 2006).

Histology

Spinal cord tumor classification is based on the histology of the tumor and is not different from the classification used for primary brain tumors.

Secondary (Transformative) Tumors of the Brain and Spine

Secondary CNS tumors are those that may originate as benign or low-grade tumors but over time transform into more malignant variants of the original tumor. This change in tumor histology may be related to the natural course of the tumor or as a result of or response to previous tumor therapy (i.e., as a side effect of radiation or chemotherapy). Examples include the progression of a low-grade ependymoma into an anaplastic ependymoma or a low-grade astrocytoma into an anaplastic astrocytoma or glioblastoma multiforme.

Metastatic Central Nervous System Disease in Childhood

The spread of primary tumors within the CNS is a result of the tumor cells seeding via the CSF. The term *drop metastasis* refers to tumors of the spinal cord identified in the presence of a posterior fossa tumor or intraventricular tumor. The most common offenders in this process are medulloblastoma, ependymoma, and supratentorial PNET. Although considered uncommon, tumors within the spinal cord or canal may be responsible for tumor seeding to the brain. Rarely, some CNS tumors may spread outside the CNS into the bones or bone marrow (Stiefbold & Thompson, 2006).

Hematologic malignancies such as leukemias and lymphomas may spread to the epidural space. Up to 5% of pediatric patients who have solid malignant tumors outside the spine have been shown to develop spinal metastases (Klein, Sanford, & Muhlbauer, 1991). Neuroblastoma may metastasize to both the brain and spine. Sarcomas such as Ewing sarcoma may present in the CNS of children, with 5%–10% of Ewing sarcomas originating in the spine (Sciubba et al., 2008). Malignant melanoma possibly can infiltrate into the CNS of children as it is known to do in adult patients.

Leptomeningeal Spread of Central Nervous System Disease

This metastatic process refers to the involvement of the meninges and may be associated with either brain or spinal tumors. Malignant cells can be disseminated via the CSF along the meninges and may involve the cranial nerves and/or the cauda equina. Although high-grade tumors account for most tumor spread along the meninges, low-grade gliomas may also serve as a disease source for tumor spread. Leptomeningeal dissemination is similar in children and adults (Blaney & Poplack, 2005).

Figure 6-7. Intradural Tumor of the Spine, Sagittal Images

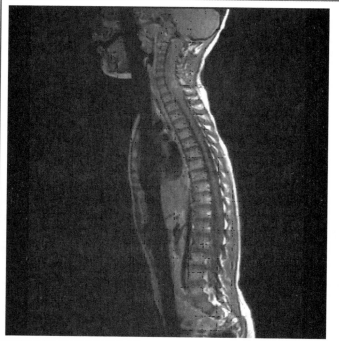 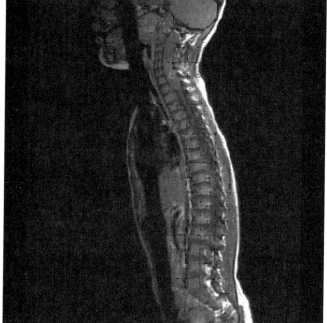

Note. Figures courtesy of Melody Ann Watral, MSN, RN, CPNP-PC, CPON®. Used with permission.

Summary

CNS tumors are the most common solid tumors in childhood, the second leading cause of cancer in children, and the leading cause of death among pediatric patients with cancer (ABTA, 2007). As evidenced in this text, a variety of CNS tumors, both benign and malignant, occur in children. The persistently high morbidity and mortality rates in these patients warrants strong research efforts toward their treatment and cure.

References

American Brain Tumor Association. (2007). *A primer of brain tumors: A patient's reference manual* (8th ed.). Des Plaines, IL: Author.

Auguste, K.I., & Gupta, N. (2006). Pediatric intramedullary spinal cord tumors. *Neurosurgery Clinics of North America, 17,* 51–61.

Binning, M., Klimo, P., Jr., Gluf, W., & Goumnervoa, L. (2007). Spinal tumors in children. *Neurosurgery Clinics of North America, 18,* 631–658. doi:10.1016/j.nec.2007.07.001

Blaney, S.M., Kun, L.E., Hunter, J., Rorke-Adams, L.B., Lau, C., Strother, D., & Pollack, I.F. (2006). Tumors of the central nervous system. In P.A. Pizzo & D.G. Poplack (Eds.), *Principles and practice of pediatric oncology* (5th ed., pp. 786–866). Philadelphia, PA: Lippincott Williams & Wilkins.

Blaney, S.M., & Poplack, D.G. (2005). Leptomeningeal metastases and dural/skull metastases. In D. Schiff & B.P. O'Neill (Eds.) *Principles of neuro-oncology* (5th ed., pp. 607–628). New York, NY: McGraw-Hill.

Central Brain Tumor Registry of the United States. (2010). *CBTRUS statistical report: Primary brain and central nervous system tumors diagnosed in the United States in 2004–2006.* Retrieved from http://www.cbtrus.org/2010-NPCR-SEER/CBTRUS -WEBREPORT-Final-3-2-10.pdf

Constantini, S., Miller, D.C., Allen, J.C., Rorke, L.B., Freed, D., & Epstein, F.J. (2000). Radical excision of intramedullary spinal cord tumors: Surgical morbidity and long-term follow-up evaluation in 164 children and young adults. *Journal of Neurosurgery, 93*(Suppl. 2), 183–193.

Eberhart, C.G., & Burger, P.C. (2003). Anaplasia and grading in medulloblastomas. *Brain Pathology, 13,* 376–385.

Gopal, P., Parker, J.R., Debski, R., & Parker, J.C., Jr. (2008). Choroid plexus carcinoma. *Archives in Pathology and Laboratory Medicine, 132,* 1350–1354.

Gururangan, S., McLaughlin, C., Quinn, J., Rich, J., Reardon, D., Halperin, E.C., ... Martin, P.L. (2003). High-dose chemotherapy with autologous stem-cell rescue in children and adults with newly diagnosed pineoblastomas. *Journal of Clinical Oncology, 21,* 2187–2191. doi:10.1200/JCO.2003.10.096

Jallo, G.I., Biser-Rohrbaugh, A., & Freed, D. (2004). Brain stem gliomas. *Child's Nervous System, 20,* 143–153. doi:10.1007/ s00381-003-0870-6

Karavitaki, N., Cudlip, S., Adams, C.B., & Wass, J.A. (2006). Craniopharyngiomas. *Endocrine Reviews, 27,* 371–397. doi:10.1210/er.2006-0002

Klein, S.L., Sanford, R.A., & Muhlbauer, M.S. (1991). Pediatric spinal epidural metastases. *Journal of Neurosurgery, 74,* 70–75. doi:10.3171/jns.1991.74.1.0070

Marec-Berard, P., Jouvet, A., Thiesse, P., Kalifa, C., Doz, F., & Frappaz, D. (2002). Supratentorial embryonal tumors in children under 5 years of age: An SFOP study of treatment with postoperative chemotherapy alone. *Medical and Pediatric Oncology, 38,* 83–90. doi:10.1002/mpo.1277

Palmer, C.A., & Harrison, D.K. (2008, June). Chordoma. Retrieved from http://emedicine.medscape.com/article/250902-overview

Paulus, W., & Brander, S. (2007). Choroid plexus tumors. In D. Louis, H. Ohgaki, O. Weister, & W. Cavanee (Eds.), *WHO classification of tumours of the central nervous system* (4th ed., pp. 81–85). Lyon, France: IARC.

Ridenour, R., III, Ahrens, W.A., Folpe, A., & Miller, D.V. (2009). Clinical and histopathologic features of chordomas in children and young adults. *Pediatric and Developmental Pathology, 13,* 9–17. doi:10.2350/09-01-0584.1

Rosenblum, R.K. (2005). Brain stem glioma: Two case studies. *Journal of Pediatric Oncology Nursing, 22,* 114–118. doi:10.1177/1043454204273813

Ryan-Murray, J., & Petriecione, M.M. (2002). Central nervous system tumors. In C.R. Baggott, K.P. Kelly, D. Fochtman, & G.V. Foley (Eds.), *Nursing care of children and adolescents with cancer* (4th ed., pp. 503–523). Philadelphia, PA: Saunders.

Sciubba, D.M., Hsieh, P., McLoughlin, G.S., & Jallo, G.I. (2008). Pediatric tumors involving the spinal column. *Neurosurgery Clinics of North America, 19,* 81–92. doi:10.1016/j.nec.2007.09.008

Stiefbold, A.M., & Thompson, S.J. (2006). *Central nervous system tumors: A handbook for families.* Retrieved from http://www. association-office.com/Files/APHON/materials/2004-260.pdf

Strickler, R., & Phillips, M. (2000). Astrocytomas: The clinical picture. *Clinical Journal of Oncology Nursing, 4,* 153–158.

Strother, D. (2005). Atypical teratoid rhabdoid tumors of childhood: Diagnosis, treatment and challenges. *Expert Review of Anticancer Therapies, 5,* 907–915. doi:10.1586/14737140.5.5.907

Tatter, S.B. (2005). The new WHO classification of tumors affecting the central nervous system. Retrieved from http://neurosurgery. mgh.harvard.edu/newwhobt.htm

Wetjen, N.M., & Raffel, C. (2008). Spinal extradural neoplasms and intradural extramedullary neoplasms. In A. Albright, I. Pollack, & P. Adelson (Eds.), *Principles and practice of pediatric neurosurgery* (2nd ed., pp. 694–705). New York, NY: Thieme.

Treatment Modalities: Surgical Treatments

Sharon S. Cush, RN, OCN®, and Kara Penne, RN, MSN, ANP, AOCNP®

Introduction

Surgery is usually the first step in treating many types of cancer, and neoplasms of the brain and spinal cord are no exception. Many things are considered when making a decision to proceed with surgery, including the type or extent of resection that can be recommended. As with any medical treatment, the patient's medical history, physical examination, and performance status play key roles in surgical decision making. However, a primary reason to undergo any surgery is to obtain tissue for diagnosis (biopsy). Other reasons to consider surgery are for decompression of the mass to relieve symptoms, implanting devices to provide treatment, and in some cases, cure by complete resection.

This chapter is divided into two portions that separately address brain surgery and spinal cord surgery.

Brain Surgery

Introduction

The development of modern microsurgical techniques has made surgical resection of brain neoplasms the usual first step in treatment of both malignant and benign lesions. Increased intracranial pressure resulting from tumor growth and surrounding vasogenic edema often dictate the extent and urgency of brain surgery. Surgical resection of a brain lesion should accomplish several essential things, including (a) obtaining tissue diagnosis for future treatment planning, (b) maximizing resection to relieve mass effect, and (c) minimizing damage to normal brain that would produce neurologic deficits.

Preoperative Management

Most tumors are identified through magnetic resonance imaging (MRI) with gadolinium enhancement after clinical assessment of focal signs or symptoms (Adams, 2008). In many instances, the surgeon will need additional imaging studies in order to obtain more precise surgical planning. Computed tomography (CT) scans are often used to evaluate bony anatomy for erosion, calcification, or involvement of bony pathology. Magnetic resonance spectroscopy may be used to provide a chemical analysis of the tumor, which differs significantly from normal brain tissue and varies greatly with the degree of malignancy within tumors. Positron-emission tomography (PET) scans provide metabolic analyses, which are useful for estimating tumor activity and malignancy (Ojemann, 1995b). If the surgeon is concerned about abnormal vascular supply, proximity to major vessels, or the status of venous sinuses, angiography (magnetic resonance or conventional) can be used to provide this essential information (Ojemann, 1995b).

A common finding on MRI or CT is the presence of vasogenic edema. This can be quite significant with high-grade tumors and cause severe neurologic deficits. Initiation of high-dose steroids, usually dexamethasone, decreases the edema, thus improving symptoms prior to surgical intervention (Enam & Rock, 1999). The decrease of intracranial swelling and pressure allows for a safer operation with less retraction and manipulation of the brain during the procedure.

If a patient should present with a seizure, antiepileptic drugs (AEDs) are initiated. The selection of AED and dosage depends on the type, severity, and frequency of seizure activity. The use of prophylactic AEDs in patients who are seizure-free has become a less common practice but still is used during the immediate perioperative period to decrease the risk of seizures.

Surgical Procedures

Biopsy is a procedure to remove tissue from a tumor for microscopic examination by a pathologist to determine the type and degree of malignancy. Of the two reasons for a biopsy, the first is for the sole purpose of confirming a diagnosis. This type of surgery is usually a stereotactic procedure requiring a small incision, a single burr hole, and a minimal hospital stay. The second is an open biopsy where tissue sampling is taken at the beginning of an open craniotomy in anticipation of further debulking or total resection of the tumor (Rock, Naftzger, & Rosenblum, 1999).

Gross total resection is usually reserved for tumors that can be totally cured by surgical resection, including but not limited to meningiomas, craniopharyngiomas, pituitary adenomas, pilocytic astrocytomas, and low-grade gliomas. The majority of these are resected through an open craniotomy; however, a transsphenoidal or transnasal endoscopic approach to benign tumors in the sella or near the skull base has become increasingly popular. Endoscopic surgery affords the patient a complete resection with minimal time spent in the hospital and recovery process while providing the same or fewer complications as an open surgical procedure. Meningiomas lend themselves to total resection, as they usually occur between dural linings on the surface of the brain. Even those found deep in the brain in the cerebellar pontine angle, sphenoid wing, or olfactory groove can be totally removed along with dural attachment and bony invasion while preserving or improving neurologic function (Ojemann, 1995a). Pilocytic astrocytomas, frequently found in the pediatric population, are also amenable to total resection. It is the treatment of choice for this tumor, as it is generally sharply demarcated from surrounding parenchyma and located in easily accessible regions in the brain (Rock et al., 1999).

Other low-grade gliomas that may not be as demarcated as the pilocytic astrocytoma can also be completely resected but often present a greater challenge to perform the resection safely with negative margins. Technologic innovations that reduce operative morbidity while maximizing tumor removal include interactive image-guided systems and awake craniotomy techniques combined with electrophysiologic cortical mapping (to be discussed later) (Bampoe, Bauman, Cairncross, & Bernstein, 1999). Single metastatic lesions to the brain are frequently treated solely with gross total resection. Metastatic lesions are also generally well demarcated and located in surgically accessible areas of the brain. Fifty percent of patients who present with a single lesion in the brain are treated with resection alone (McDonnell, Flanigin, & Yaghmai, 1995). Comorbidities preventing a major surgery or unresectable location are usually the reasons causing a high-risk status for the other 50% (McDonnell et al., 1995). These patients are generally treated with radiation therapy alone consisting of whole brain radiation therapy with a radiosurgery boost to the tumor or stereotactic radiosurgery (McDonnell et al., 1995).

Partial resection or tumor debulking is usually offered to patients who will benefit from decompression by means of improving neurologic deficits, decreasing tumor burden for adjuvant therapy, and insertion of devices to decrease intracranial pressure or provide treatment access. An open craniotomy is the usual method, but the amount of tumor resected and the extent of retraction and manipulation is less than when this procedure is used for total resection. Debulking the tumor can reduce vasogenic edema and the subsequent need for the use of steroids, diminishing the risk of steroid-induced complications such as diabetes, muscle atrophy, and immune suppression. Likewise, neurologic deficits caused by pressure of the growing mass or surrounding edema will frequently improve when the mass is reduced (Enam & Rock, 1999).

Special devices can be implanted at the time of partial resection with the intention of accessing them for withdrawing fluid or instilling chemotherapy agents. Ommaya and Rickham® (Medtronic PS Medical) reservoirs are devices used to withdraw fluid or instill chemotherapy. Another device frequently used to divert cerebrospinal fluid (CSF) is a shunt that normally goes from the ventricle or the cystic component of a tumor to the abdomen. Shunts are most frequently required when the tumor is located within or near the ventricular system and impedes the normal flow of CSF (Yaşargil, 1996). Resection is also necessary when regional or intratumoral treatment is planned. Gliadel® Wafers (Eisai Inc.), polymer wafers impregnated with bischloroethylnitrosourea (commonly known as BCNU or carmustine), are placed around the edges of the tumor bed at the time of resection and slowly release the drug over three to four weeks. This is demonstrated in the section of pictures in Figure 7-1 outlining a surgical resection with the polymer wafer insertion. Clinical trials are ongoing using monoclonal antibodies tagged with radioisotopes, viral or bacterial endotoxins, and substances such as a gel containing paclitaxel. The primary goal of these therapies is to provide maximum tumor control through local administration with minimum systemic side effects (Stupp, Hegi, Gilbert, & Chakravarti, 2007).

Intraoperative Technology

Interactive image-guided systems make precise maximum resection possible. The current computer-assisted methods are used for surgical targeting and navigation. The use of neuroimaging data can be divided into four main categories: (a) planning a procedure, (b) guiding the procedure, (c) monitoring the progress of resection, and (d) controlling the procedure intraoperatively. All of this promotes minimally invasive procedures that reduce patient risk and morbidity (Yaşargil, 1996).

Awake craniotomy with functional mapping has provided surgeons with another means of resecting tumors that involve eloquent areas (areas that control vital functions) in the cerebral cortex. The lesion is identified anatomically, as well as the adjacent or overlying eloquent cortex. This allows for the planning of surgical trajectories and techniques that promote complete resection as safely as possible (Black, 2001). Awake-craniotomy is usually reserved for patients with lesions in the sensory and motor speech areas of the dominant hemisphere or in the sensorimotor cortex in either hemisphere. The procedure

Figure 7-1. Surgical Insertion of Carmustine Wafers for Localized Chemotherapy

The following images show operative preparation and tumor resection with carmustine-coated wafer insertion and pre- and postoperative magnetic resonance imaging (MRI) scans showing tumor resection.

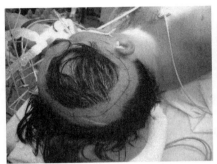

(a) Patient's head is positioned, and operative area is cleansed and shaved.

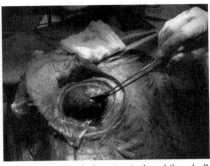

(b) Once the scalp is retracted and the skull removed, the dura is opened to prepare for tumor resection.

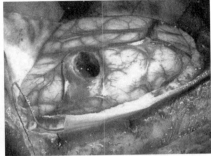

(c) The tumor is resected as closely as possible to avoid harming other structures.

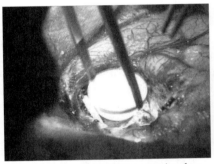

(d) In this case, carmustine-coated wafers are fitted along the surgical cavity borders to provide local chemotherapy.

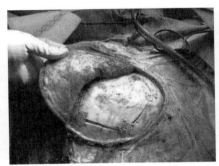

(e) After dural closure and sealants are provided, the skull is attached and secured with special bolts to provide optimal healing.

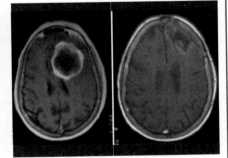

(f) Preoperative MRI on the left shows the enhancing malignant glioma, and the postoperative MRI on the right shows the fluid-filled surgical cavity with some blood products and outlines of the wafers.

Note. Photos courtesy of M. Ewend, MD, Division of Neurosurgery, University of North Carolina. Used with permission.

usually involves short-acting sedative agents and an infusion of local anesthetic to perform the craniotomy. Sedation is allowed to wear off once the dura is open, facilitating the patient to awaken. Once the patient is awake and able to cooperate fully, cortical stimulation and mapping is performed, which allows assessment of strength and speech throughout the procedure. This process reduces the likelihood of excising functional neural tissue. Sedation is resumed for closure once resection is completed (Tan & Black, 2001).

Postoperative Management

Leaking CSF may manifest as rhinorrhea (runny nose) or may seep directly from the wound, causing wound healing problems. Regardless of the site, it is essential to identify and repair it as soon as possible to avoid the risk of meningitis. Several methods are available to repair the leak. The use of a fat graft cemented in an acrylate is one of the most effective methods for smaller leak repair, whereas an anterior repair using a pericranial flap has been found to be effective for larger defects. This flap, harvested from nearby cranial periosteum or temporalis muscle, is well vascularized from adjacent blood vessels, thus promoting better healing than artificial materials. In the case of large defects of the frontal sinus, mobilization of the mucous membrane is used to occlude the orifice, after which it is packed with autologous muscle and cemented in place (Yaşargil, 1996).

Cerebral edema is a problem preoperatively, intraoperatively, and postoperatively. As was discussed in preoperative management, high-dose steroids can effectively reduce swelling and permit a larger cranial opening at the time of surgery. This provides the surgeon with better access and limits manipulation and retraction on the brain, which contributes to postoperative edema even when adequate resection has been performed. Additional agents, such as mannitol, are often required to control postoperative edema. In some instances, reoperation with craniectomy becomes necessary in the management of an edematous brain (Rock et al., 1999).

The incidence of early postoperative seizures ranges from 4% to 19% (Yaşargil, 1996). The presence of preoperative seizures has been associated with an increased incidence of postoperative seizures. Furthermore, the prevalence of postoperative epilepsy has been more associated with gliomas and meningiomas (Yaşargil, 1996). These patients require careful postoperative monitoring with pharmacologic therapy adjusted judiciously. If seizures persist despite therapeutic levels of anticonvulsants, an imaging scan should be considered to rule out hemorrhage, infarction, or edema. All of these conditions may require further surgical management.

Pituitary axis dysfunction manifests most frequently as central diabetes insipidus or syndrome of inappropriate antidiuretic hormone secretion (Yaşargil, 1996). Monitoring of minor electrolyte imbalance and urine and serum osmolality is essential. In conscious patients, urine output can be replaced by fluid intake, orally and intravenously, thus avoiding the use of hypertonic saline and desmopressin acetate (DDAVP®, sanofi-aventis), a synthetic vasopressin. Other more severe cases of endocrine dysfunction may present as panhypopituitarism. For those with panhypopituitarism, hormone replacements and monitoring by an endocrinologist are essential to postoperative management (Yaşargil, 1996).

Hemorrhage and infarction still occur despite advanced methods of coagulation and bleeding control during the operation. Bleeding may occur in subgaleal, epidural, subdural, and intraparenchymal vessels. Some of the reasons for postoperative hemorrhage or infarct include abnormal clotting mechanisms, thrombocytopenia, perioperative hypertension, inadequate hemostasis, direct vessel injury, and undetected retraction injury (Yaşargil, 1996). Early discovery and treatment of hematoma are essential to ensure a good postoperative outcome.

Infection continues to be a postoperative complication even in an era with state-of-the-art sterilization techniques, operative field preparation and maintenance, and perioperative use of antibiotics. Patients with malignant gliomas are known to have suppressed immune systems, and most require high-dose steroids, which further suppress the immune system. The currently recommended regimen of adjuvant therapy with temozolomide concomitant with radiation therapy even suggests prophylactic use of antibiotics to avoid treatment-related infections associated with myelosuppression in patients with glioma (Stupp et al., 2005).

Spinal Surgery

Introduction

Spinal cord tumors are lesions that can occur within or next to the spinal cord. Primary spinal cord tumors account for approximately 3% of all primary central nervous system tumors (Samii & Klekamp, 1994). Extradural tumors are present outside of the dura. Intradural extramedullary tumors arise from the dura but are outside the spinal cord. Intramedullary tumors arise within the spinal cord. All of these can be addressed with surgical intervention but are associated with varying risks and outcomes. Surgical intervention is often necessary for establishing a diagnosis and optimum resection in order to minimize symptoms. Surgical intervention is warranted for all primary spinal cord tumors if safe, given the location of the tumor (see Figures 7-2 and 7-3).

Preoperative Management

Prior to surgery, appropriate radiographic evaluation is warranted and may include plain films, CT, MRI, myelography, and PET. Plain films will show osteolytic changes including compression fracture and pathologic fracture from metastatic disease. CT is helpful in showing involvement of vertebral bodies. CT is combined with myelography to evaluate CSF flow and to better identify the location of the tumor (e.g., extradural, intradural, intramedullary, extramedullary). MRI is the gold standard of imaging for evaluation of spinal cord tumors (Adams, 2008), especially in surgical planning. It allows the physician to evaluate tumor location and involvement of vertebral bodies.

Figure 7-2. Spinal Surgery Considerations

Goals
- Establish pathologic diagnosis
- Surgical debulking
- Curative resection

Tumor Types
- Intradural
  - Extramedullary
  - Intramedullary
- Extradural
- Vascular spinal cord tumors or metastases

Tumor Location and Proximity to Critical Structures/Areas
- Determines type of surgery
- Involves assessing risk of increasing problems with neurologic function

Note. Based on information from Adams, 2008; Epstein et al., 1991; Roessler et al., 1998.

Figure 7-3. Indications for Spinal Surgery

- Intramedullary tumor
- Diagnosis of tumor
- Worsening neurologic status
- Cord compression
- Pathologic fracture dislocation

Baseline neurologic evaluation is critical to determine the rate of progression of neurologic deterioration (Adams, 2008). Surgical resection of certain types of spinal cord tumors can involve the risk of worsening neurologic symptoms but is often necessary to prevent progression of symptoms. If the patient is having rapid worsening of neurologic function and deficits, surgery is indicated emergently. Angiography or tumor embolization may be required prior to surgery if the tumor has a significant vascular supply. The presence of a lesion on the spinal cord can cause symptoms of cord compression. This is a medical emergency and should be treated immediately with high-dose steroids to slow the progression of neurologic deficits and to protect the patient from any permanent deficits (Adams, 2008).

Surgical Considerations

The goal of surgery is to establish pathologic diagnosis, as well as surgical debulking if medically indicated (Adams, 2008). These goals can be accomplished through biopsy and partial or complete resection. Surgical options vary based on tumor type and tumor location. For instance, surgical resection is recommended for intramedullary astrocytomas because it has been shown to improve overall outcome and carries the same surgical risk as a biopsy alone (Epstein, Farmer, & Schneider, 1991). One study demonstrated 100% 10-year survival in patients after radical resection of intramedullary ependymomas compared with 62% of those with incomplete resection followed by radiation therapy (Epstein et al., 1991; McCormick, Torres, Post, & Stein, 1990). Similar to surgical procedures for brain tumors, if the location of the tumor is adjacent to a critical area of the brain or spinal cord, partial resection will be pursued for confirming a diagnosis or for debulking. Recent techniques with intraoperative imaging and guidance technology allow resection with preservation of normal tissue. This is extremely helpful for treating lesions in close proximity to the brain stem or at the cervicomedullary junction (Roessler et al., 1998). Treatment modalities of chemotherapy, radiation therapy, stereotactic radiosurgery, or any combination thereof may be used to primarily debulk the tumor and then followed up with surgical resection for macroscopic clearance of the remaining malignant tissue. Surgery is based on location and proximity to critical areas, as well as risk of worsening neurologic function (Adams, 2008).

Intradural Tumors

Intradural tumors can be intramedullary or extramedullary. Intramedullary tumors arise from the spinal cord cells themselves and are within the parenchyma of the spinal cord, such as ependymomas (see Figure 7-4). Extramedullary tumors are outside the parenchyma of the spinal cord and within the dura mater. Tumors within the dural sac are best treated surgically via wide posterior laminectomy. Layers of the lamina (roof

Figure 7-4. Ependymoma at L3

A 40-year-old male presented with lower back pain radiating into right thigh. Pathology demonstrates ependymoma.

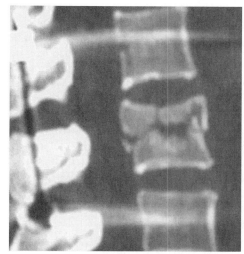

(a) Compression fracture secondary to tumor

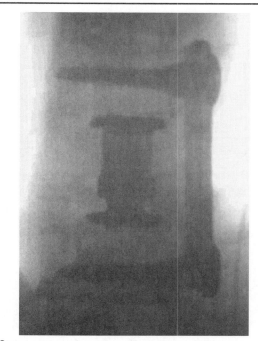

(b) Status postvertebrectomy with posterior stabilization

Note. Images courtesy of R. Isaacs, MD, Duke University Health System, Department of Neurosurgery. Used with permission.

of the spinal cord) are removed to access the spinal cord to expose the tumor. If the tumor is intradural-intramedullary, the surgeon will open the dura and spinal cord to access the tumor. If the lesion is intradural-extramedullary, then the surgeon will open the dura only to resect the tumor (Freeman & Cahill, 1996).

Extradural Tumors

These tumors often arise in the vertebral bodies and are usually metastatic. Given the bony involvement, resection of entire vertebral bodies is often warranted. Anterior or anterolateral approaches allow for more direct access to the lesion than other approaches would provide. Anterior decompression allows decompression of a large portion of the dural sac. Reconstruction involves use of a bone graft with or without a stabilizing plate (see Figure 7-5) and prosthetic devices such as rods and screws (Cahill, 1996). However, anterior decompression of three or more levels increases risk of instability. In such cases, posterolateral decompression and posterior fixation with instrumentation may be warranted. Instrumentation may include a prosthetic construct or sublaminar wires if the integrity of the vertebral body is poor. Posterolateral decompression and stabilization involves resection of affected vertebral bodies. Stabilization is completed with use of bone struts, steel rods, and methyl methacrylate (Cahill, 1996).

Vascular Spinal Cord Tumors and Metastases

Certain types of cancers have a higher likelihood of bleeding because of the tumor's vascularity. Examples include renal cell and thyroid cancers. In these settings, preoperative tumor embolization is warranted to reduce vascularity, therefore reducing the risk of bleeding and allowing for improved tumor resection (see Figure 7-6) (Cahill, 1996).

Figure 7-6. Thoracic Tumor With Extension Into Chest Cavity

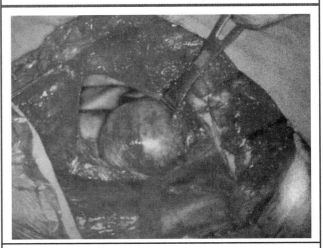

Note. Photo courtesy of R. Isaacs, MD, Duke University Health System, Department of Neurosurgery. Used with permission.

Intraoperative Technology

Methods of intraoperative monitoring assist the surgeon with resection and preservation of neurologic function. Ultrasound is frequently used to ensure enough bone has been removed to achieve safe resection. It is also used to confirm placement of the myelotomy, where the nerve fibers of the spinal cord will be severed to allow for resection. Ultrasound is also used after resection prior to closing the incision to evaluate for any residual macroscopic tumor cells (Epstein et al., 1991).

For surgical resection of intramedullary tumors, intraoperative somatosensory-evoked potentials (SSEPs) may be used to monitor sensory pathways to prevent injury or further damage. Some research suggests that although SSEPs confirm known nerve injury, the potentials are not reliable for predicting impending nerve injury, thus limiting intraoperative usefulness (Cooper, 1996). Likewise, motor-evoked potential monitoring is used intraoperatively to directly measure motor pathways. It has been shown to provide improved functional outcomes but has not been proved to improve overall surgical outcome (Morota et al., 1997).

Surgical Complications

The typical postoperative period for patients with spinal cord tumors involves a change in baseline neurologic status. Neurologic function recovery to the preoperative state varies from days to months (Samii & Klekamp, 1994). If the patient has significant neurologic deficits preoperatively, he or she is more likely to have higher occurrence of neurologic deterioration during postoperative recovery. It is also more

---

Figure 7-5. Lateral Plate Placement for Stabilization in Lumbar Vertebrectomy

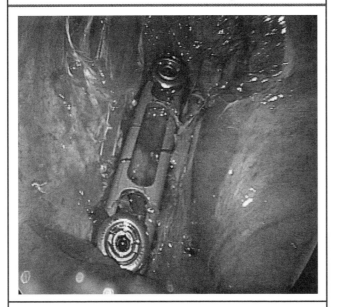

Note. Photo courtesy of R. Isaacs, MD, Duke University Health System, Department of Neurosurgery. Used with permission.

likely that the patient will have minimal improvement in preoperative symptoms. CSF leak is also seen intraoperatively and may be associated with subsequent infection. Patients with a history of prior irradiation as well as those who are immunocompromised are at higher risk (Cooper, 1996). These patients should be monitored closely for signs of neurologic compromise and infection.

Summary

Surgery remains the first treatment of choice for most neoplasms in the brain and spine (Adams, 2008). The type of surgical procedure and subsequent plans for treatment are essential parts of the preoperative discussion between the patient and surgeon. Diligent perioperative and postoperative monitoring, appropriate patient selection, and state-of-the-art modern technology are essential for the best surgical outcomes for this patient population. Recent technologic advances have further improved patient outcomes and the quality of life of patients with brain and central nervous system tumors.

References

Adams, A.C. (2008). *Mayo Clinic essential neurology*. Rochester, MN: Mayo Foundation for Medical Education and Research.

Bampoe, J.O., Bauman, G., Cairncross, J.G., & Bernstein, M. (1999). Adult low-grade gliomas: Natural history, prognostic factors, and timing of treatment. In J.P. Rock, M.L. Rosenblum, E.G. Shaw, & J.G. Cairncross (Eds.), *The practical management of low-grade primary brain tumors* (pp. 135–148). Philadelphia, PA: Lippincott Williams & Wilkins.

Black, P.M. (2001). Illustrative case. *Techniques in Neurosurgery, 7*, 2–3. Retrieved from http://www.techs-neurosurgery .com/pt/re/techneurosurg/fulltext.00127927-200103000-00002 .htm;jsessionid=LsNHMx6wyvYpMG5qXGw5pG2GTl sV2pNdzltdylkFymLM2zrZzcsl!-761347985!181195628!8091!-1

Cahill, D.W. (1996). Malignant tumors of the bony spine. In A.H. Menezes, V.K.H. Sonntag, E.C. Benzel, D.W. Cahill, P. McCormick, & S.M. Papadopoulos (Eds.), *Principles of spinal surgery* (pp. 1408–1422). New York, NY: McGraw-Hill.

Cooper, P.R. (1996). Management of intramedullary spinal cord tumors. In G.T. Tindall, P.R. Cooper, & D.L. Barrow (Eds.), *The practice of neurosurgery* (pp. 1335–1346). Baltimore, MD: Lippincott Williams & Wilkins.

Enam, S.A., & Rock, J.P. (1999). Uncommon low-grade primary brain tumors. In J.P. Rock, M.L. Rosenblum, E.G. Shaw, & J.G. Cairncross (Eds.), *The practical management of low-grade primary brain tumors* (pp. 111–131). Philadelphia, PA: Lippincott Williams & Wilkins.

Epstein, F.J., Farmer, J.-P., & Schneider, S.J. (1991). Intraoperative ultrasonography: An important surgical adjunct for intramedullary tumors. *Journal of Neurosurgery, 74*, 729–733. doi:10.3171/ jns.1991.74.5.0729

Freeman, T.B., & Cahill, D.W. (1996). Tumors of the meninges, cauda equina, and spinal nerves. In A.H. Menezes, V.K.H. Sonntag, E.C. Benzel, D.W. Cahill, P. McCormick, & S.M. Papadopoulos (Eds.), *Principles of spinal surgery* (pp. 1371–1386). New York, NY: McGraw-Hill.

McCormick, P.C., Torres, T., Post, K.D., & Stein, B.M. (1990). Intramedullary ependymoma of the spinal cord. *Journal of Neurosurgery, 72*, 523–532. doi:10.3171/jns.1990.72.4.0523

McDonnell, D.E., Flanigin, H.F., & Yaghmai, F. (1995). Diagnosis and treatment of intraaxial tumors in adults. In M.B. Allen Jr. & R.H. Miller (Eds.), *Essentials of neurosurgery: A guide to clinical practice* (pp. 155–182). New York, NY: McGraw-Hill.

Morota, N., Deletis, V., Constantini, S., Kofler, M., Cohen, H., & Epstein, F.J. (1997). The role of motor evoked potentials during surgery for intramedullary spinal cord tumors. *Neurosurgery, 41*, 1327–1336.

Ojemann, R. (1995a). Surgical management of olfactory groove meningiomas. In H.H. Schmidek & W.H. Sweet (Eds.), *Operative neurosurgical techniques* (3rd ed., Vol. 1, pp. 393–401). Philadelphia, PA: Saunders.

Ojemann, R.G. (1995b). Surgical principles in the management of brain tumors. In A.H. Kaye & E.R. Laws (Eds.), *Brain tumors* (pp. 293–304). Edinburgh, United Kingdom: Churchill Livingstone.

Rock, J.P., Naftzger, M.E., & Rosenblum, M.L. (1999). Surgery for adult low-grade primary brain tumors. In J.P. Rock, M.L. Rosenblum, E.G. Shaw, & J.G. Cairncross (Eds.), *The practical management of low-grade primary brain tumors* (pp. 71–80). Philadelphia, PA: Lippincott Williams & Wilkins.

Roessler, K., Ungersboeck, K., Aichholzer, M., Dietrich, W., Goerzer, H., Matula, C., ... Koos, W. (1998). Frameless stereotactic lesion contour-guided surgery using a computer-navigated microscope. *Surgical Neurology, 49*, 282–289.

Samii, M., & Klekamp, J. (1994). Surgical results of 100 intramedullary tumors in relation to accompanying syringomyelia. *Neurosurgery, 35*, 865–873.

Stupp, R., Hegi, M.E., Gilbert, M., & Chakravarti, A. (2007). Chemotherapy in malignant glioma: Standard of care and future directions. *Journal of Clinical Oncology, 25*, 4127–4136. doi:10.1200/JCO.2007.11.8554

Stupp, R., Mason, W.P., van den Bent, M.J., Weller, M., Fisher, B., Taphoorn, M.J., ... Mirimanoff, R.O. (2005). Radiotherapy plus concomitant and adjuvant temozolomide for glioblastoma. *New England Journal of Medicine, 352*, 987–996. doi:10.1056/ NEJMoa043330

Tan, T.-C., & Black, P.M. (2001). Awake craniotomy for excision of brain metastases involving eloquent cortex. *Techniques in Neurosurgery, 7*, 85–90. Retrieved from http://www.techs-neurosurgery.com/pt/ re/techneurosurg/fulltext.00127927-200103000-00010.htm;jsess ionid=LsWKBghRNxPd6wCVlbGtJWt1zg02RDNZTNJ1bDp2g DBwdxNyvBqW!1947086508!181195629!8091!-1

Yaşargil, M.G. (1996). *Microneurosurgery in 4 volumes: Microneurosurgery of CNS tumors* (Vol. IVB). New York, NY: Thieme.

CHAPTER 8

Treatment Modalities: Chemotherapy

Alixis Van Horn, RN, CHPN

Introduction

Cancers of the central nervous system (CNS), which is composed of the brain and spinal cord; spinal, peripheral, and cranial nerves; the cerebrospinal fluid (CSF); and supporting structures such as the meninges, accounts for slightly less than 2% of all adult cancers (National Cancer Institute Surveillance, Epidemiology, and End Results [NCI SEER], 2010). An average of approximately 19,000 individuals are diagnosed with a primary CNS malignancy annually (NCI SEER, 2010). The incidence has not significantly changed in the past 7–10 years.

Malignant CNS diseases are currently categorized into grades I–IV by the World Health Organization (WHO), with higher grades corresponding to more aggressive tumors and lower grades associated with more indolent disease (Tatter, 2005). Tumors are also classified by the cells from which they originate, by location, or by histologic features. These cancers originate in the supporting cells of the brain and rarely metastasize outside of the CNS.

The triad of modalities employed to combat CNS tumors is (a) surgical removal (debulking) of the tumor, (b) radiation therapy, and (c) chemotherapy. However, despite aggressive multimodal treatment regimens, two-year survival for adults 20–44 years of age with a WHO grade IV glioblastoma multiforme is 34% (Central Brain Tumor Registry of the United States [CBTRUS], 2010). This chapter will focus on first and second lines of chemotherapies commonly administered for control of CNS cancers.

Chemotherapy

Chemotherapy has been a cornerstone of cancer treatment since nitrogen mustard was found to have antineoplastic activity in the 1940s (Goodman, Messinger, & White, 1946). Over the ensuing 70 years, the understanding of cancer genesis and physiology has evolved, and with that increasing knowledge base, medications have been developed, employed, and refined at a staggering rate. Much of the central mystery of malignancy—its appearance, development, spread, and virulence—remains elusive. To further distinguish itself, CNS cancer treatment is made more difficult by the presence of the blood-brain barrier. This was first described by the medical scientist Paul Ehrlich in the late 19th century, who also coined the term *chemotherapy* (Hirsch, 2006; Vein, 2008). This anatomic and physiologic feature of the brain is formed by a network of closely sealed endothelial cells within the capillaries, which express a high level of proteins that pump foreign molecules away from the brain, preventing or slowing the passage of some chemical compounds and pathogens into the CNS circulation (Pritchard, Sweet, Miller, & Walden, 1999) (see Figure 8-1). This complicates delivery of chemotherapy to the actual site of tumor activity, and only a small percentage of available chemotherapies actually penetrate the blood-brain barrier in efficacious concentrations.

Although the blood-brain barrier affects which chemotherapy agents gain access to the CNS structures and the potential doses that will cross this selective barrier, more subtle and individualized characteristics have an equal or greater influence on an individual's response to treatment. These characteristics lie in the genes. To date, specific genetic characteristics have not been identified that can predict an increased risk of developing brain cancer, yet some genetic markers indicate the likelihood of positive response to treatment once a brain tumor is diagnosed. Research on these markers is very much in its infancy, but significant progress has been made in at least two tumor types. The first, oligodendroglioma, is most commonly a low-grade tumor with an indolent course. However, the use of a fluorescence in situ hybridization (commonly known as FISH) test on the biopsied or resected tumor tissue can identify those patients with a deletion on chromosomes 1p and 19q, as described in Chapter 4. This correlates with a higher incidence of response to treatment and improved outcomes overall (Scheie et al., 2006). In the more aggressive and common grade IV glioblastoma, a tissue assay can provide

Figure 8-1. Cellular Constituents of the Blood-Brain Barrier

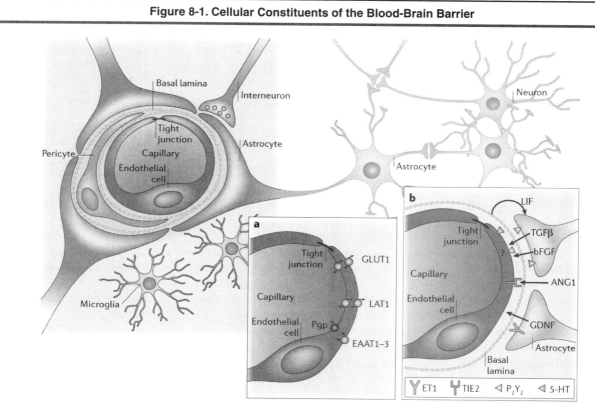

The barrier is formed by capillary endothelial cells, surrounded by basal lamina and astrocytic perivascular end feet. Astrocytes provide the cellular link to the neurons. **Insert a** features a brain endothelial cell in culture. The cells express a number of transporters and receptors, some of which are shown. **Insert b** demonstrates the bidirectional astroglial-endothelial induction processes necessary to establish and maintain the blood-brain barrier.

ANG1—angiopoetin1; bFGF—basic fibroblast growth factor; EAAT1–3—excitatory amino acid transports 1–3; ET1—endothelin 1; 5-HT—5-hydroxytryptamine (serotonin); GDNF—glial cell line-derived neurotrophic factor; GLUT1—glucose transporter 1; LAT1-L-system for large neutral amino acids; LIF—leukemia inhibitory factor; Pgp—P-glycoprotein; P_2Y_2—purinergic receptor; TFGß—transforming growth factor ß; TIE2—endothelium-specific receptor tyrosine kinase 2

Note. From "Astrocyte-Endothelial Interactions at the Blood-Brain Barrier," by N.J. Abbott, L. Rönnbäck, and E. Hansson, 2006, *Nature Reviews Neuroscience, 7*, p. 43. Copyright 2006 by Nature Publishing Group. Reprinted with permission.

an analysis of methylguanine methyltransferase (MGMT) methylation status (Hau, Stupp, & Hegi, 2007). MGMT is a cellular DNA repair protein, sited at the O-6 position of guanine, which neutralizes the cytotoxic effects of alkylators such as temozolomide. A high level of MGMT activity has shown to be a determinant in treatment failure (Hau et al., 2007). This assay is not yet widely available and a real-time test is in development (Vlassenbroeck et al., 2008), and the implications for how this may alter treatment strategies is yet to be determined.

In general, available chemotherapeutic agents for CNS malignancy can be divided into two categories, cytotoxic medications and targeted agents. The distinction rests primarily on the mechanism of action and on the specificity of the agent. Drugs from other classes, such as immunosup-

pressants, cyclooxygenase-2 (COX-2) inhibitors, thiazolidinediones, and even arsenic, have been employed to combat CNS cancers. Rarely used alone, most of these agents are used in combination with existing agents demonstrating some increased degree of efficacy. Many of these novel agents, which are often developed for other non-oncology diagnoses, show promise and continue in clinical trials as well as in clinical practice. Most notably is that of the COX-2 inhibitor celecoxib (Celebrex®, Pfizer Inc.), which is used as an adjuvant treatment with many chemotherapies for malignant high-grade primary glioma (Bajetta, Del Vecchio, Bajetta, & Canova, 2007; Kesari et al., 2008). However, for our purposes the focus shall be on the cytotoxic and targeted agent chemotherapy categories commonly used to treat primary CNS disease.

Cytotoxic Medications

Cytotoxic (cell-killing) drugs are most active during cell division. As compared to a malignant lesion, which is marked by aggressive growth patterns even in an inhospitable environment, the normal adult has only a few systems that are actively growing new cells—primarily, the gastrointestinal (GI) tract, bone marrow, skin, hair, and mucous membranes. Malignant cells are more susceptible to cytotoxic chemotherapies than normal cells, and as a larger percentage of malignant cells are dividing at any given time, the malignant cells are killed in higher proportions. This speaks to why the body sites most often involved in adverse reactions to cytotoxins are the systems that share the characteristic of ongoing reproduction as neoplasms: the bone marrow (myelosuppression), GI tract (nausea, vomiting, anorexia, constipation), hair (alopecia), skin (rash), and mucous membranes (mucositis) (Polovich, Whitford, & Olsen, 2009).

Cytotoxic drugs used in CNS malignancy include temozolomide, irinotecan (CPT-11), lomustine (CCNU) and carmustine (BCNU), bendamustine, and platinum agents, such as oxaliplatin and carboplatin. Lomustine is also available as a wafer (Gliadel® Wafers, Eisai Inc.), designed to be applied directly to the walls and margins of the brain tissue in the intracranial resection cavity (see Chapter 7).

Targeted Agents

In contrast, the second category of chemotherapeutic agents is targeted to disable only a specific kind of cell, working much like a lock and key mechanism. The cell is "locked" during most of its lifetime, but a targeted agent possesses the "key" that allows penetration of the drug and disruption of the cell processes without relying on the random occurrence of cell division (see Figure 8-2).

Growth factor pathways to angiogenesis were first hypothesized in the early 1970s by Judah Folkman (Zhong & Bowen, 2006). Less than 10 years later, researchers showed that malignant cells secrete hormonal messengers signaling the development of new blood vessels, and by the late 1980s those messengers, or factors, had been cloned for study in the laboratory. The first clinical trials on these compounds were performed in the early 1990s. The approach works via the presence of specific targets, called receptors, on the surface of individual cells, which the drug is designed to selectively recognize. Although some nonmalignant cells in the body share these receptors, the percentage of susceptible cells overall is lower, and hence the drugs are better tolerated in terms of side effects. However, like cytotoxic agents, most targeted chemotherapeutic agents have some significant potential adverse effects, which are discussed as follows in detail.

The most common types of targeted agents currently in use for CNS malignancy are monoclonal antibodies (MoAbs) that inhibit the formation of new blood vessels, which a tumor needs to support its aggressive growth. This class of drugs functions as antiangiogenesis agents. They inhibit the activity of endothelial growth factors, especially vascular endothelial growth factor (VEGF), thereby restricting or retarding the tumor's ability to develop supportive blood supply. The tumor, although not directly attacked, is dependent on a constant and adequate source of oxygen and nutrients, and if this process is interrupted, cell death will eventually occur (Fred Hutchinson Cancer Research Center, 2009). The recently U.S. Food and Drug Administration (FDA)-approved MoAb for glioma treatment, bevacizumab (Avastin®, Genentech, Inc.) is the most commonly used drug in this category, but other agents, including cilengitide and sunitinib, are currently in clinical trials.

Malignant Grades III and IV Primary Brain Tumors

Treatment Overview

WHO grades III (anaplastic gliomas) and IV (glioblastoma) are the most aggressive types of adult malignant primary brain tumor, and they occur with the highest frequency, comprising more than 40% of newly diagnosed CNS tumors (CBTRUS, 2010). They are associated with a poor prognosis, complicated treatment courses involving multiple regimens and modalities, and the rapid development of cognitive and functional deficits that affect all domains of a patient's life. Although more common in people older than the age of 65, a significant percentage of those diagnosed are middle aged and younger (Gorlia et al., 2008). Treatment for this grave diagnosis had been largely ineffective in controlling tumor growth or progression until 2005, when Stupp and colleagues reported their groundbreaking research on a new treatment regimen involving the combination of external beam cranial irradiation with concurrent daily temozolomide administration, followed by six months of temozolomide administered in a monthly regimen for patients with newly diagnosed glioblastoma (Kim & Glantz, 2006; Stupp et al., 2005). Although temozolomide has demonstrated a modest survival benefit by extending the time to disease progression or recurrence, the overall outlook for most aggressive primary brain tumors remains grim. Thus, other chemotherapy agents, such as BCNU and irinotecan, or combinations such as PCV (procarbazine, lomustine, and vincristine) that were common regimens prior to the introduction of temozolomide remain options for concurrent administration with newer drugs or as salvage therapy. Much research is focused on exploring dosing regimens of temozolomide that may enhance survival benefit, as well as maintain a tolerable level of toxicity. Additional research focuses on chemotherapy regimens or combinations that include temozolomide for synergistic antitumor benefits, thus improving survival. Temo-

Figure 8-2. Pathways Across the Blood-Brain Barrier (BBB) Demonstrating Key-Lock Mechanisms

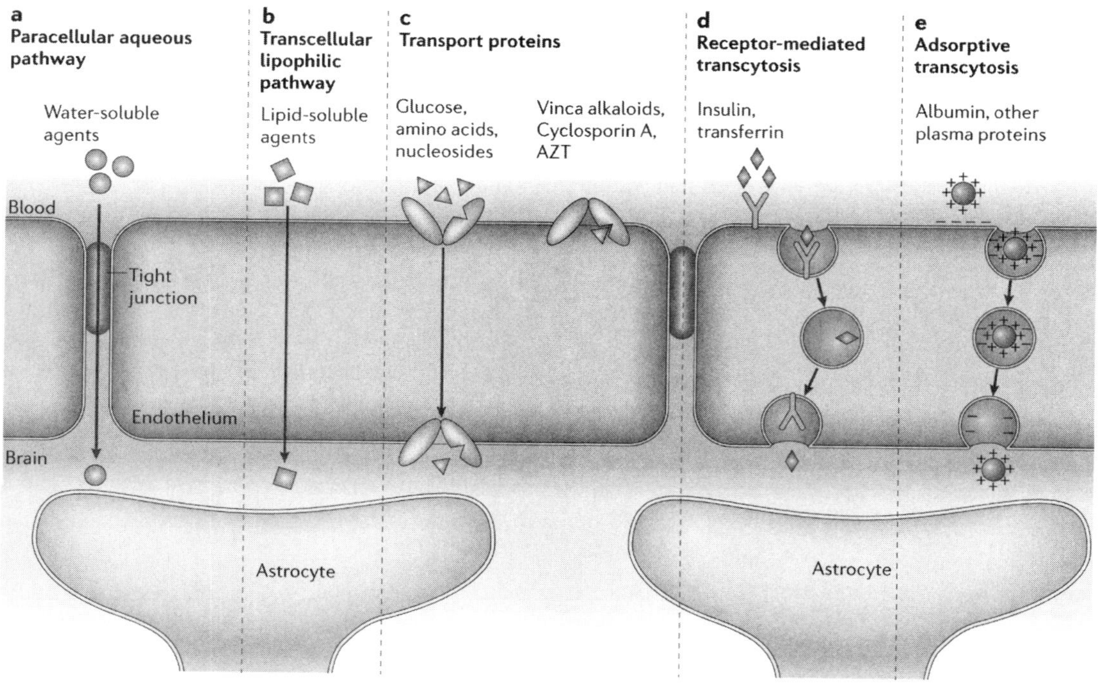

A schematic diagram of the endothelial cells that form the BBB and their associations with the perivascular end feet of astrocytes. The main routes for molecular traffic across the BBB are shown. (a) Tight junctions severely restrict penetration of water-soluble compounds, including polar drugs. (b) Large surface areas of lipid membranes of the endothelium offer an effective diffusive route for lipid-soluble agents. (c) Endothelium contains transport proteins (carriers) for glucose, amino acids, purine bases, nucleosides, choline and other substances. (d) Certain proteins, such as insulin and transferrin, are taken up by specific receptor-mediated endocytosis and transcytosis. (e) Native plasma proteins such as albumin are poorly transported, but cationization can increase their uptake by adsorptive-mediated endocytosis and transcytosis. Drug delivery occurs primarily through routes **b–e** with most CNS drugs entering through route **b**.

Note. From "Astrocyte-Endothelial Interactions at the Blood-Brain Barrier," by N.J. Abbott, L. Rönnbäck, and E. Hannson, 2006, *Nature Reviews Neuroscience, 7,* p. 44. Copyright 2006 by Nature Publishing Group. Reprinted with permission.

zolomide administered concurrently with radiation followed by 6–12 monthly cycles is now standard first-line treatment in North America for newly diagnosed high-grade malignant gliomas (Gorlia et al., 2008). For progressive and recurrent disease, targeted chemotherapies, such as MoAbs and other antiangiogenic agents, as well as a temozolomide rechallenge in alternative dosing patterns, are commonly used. With this first-line treatment now being established, the second, third, and salvage therapies are less well defined and more subject to individual practitioners' experience and habits.

First-Line Therapy

Temozolomide (Temodar®, Schering Plough) is an alkylating agent that is rapidly converted by hydrolysis to the active metabolite MTIC (3-methyl (triazen-1-yl) imidazole-4-carboxamide) in the body. The cytotoxicity of MTIC is thought to be caused by the methylation of DNA at the O-6 and N-7 positions of guanine, inhibiting the MGMT pathway (Hegi et al., 2004). As mentioned previously (and reviewed in Chapter 5), MGMT methylation status has been shown to have correlative value in predicting improved response to this cytotoxic agent although the test is neither widely available nor a stand-alone predictor of overall response or survival. Similar to most cytotoxic agents, it is cell-cycle specific, disrupting cell functions only at a specific time point in cell division. As an oral agent, it is available in 5 mg, 20 mg, 100 mg, 140 mg, 180 mg, and 250 mg capsules, and an IV formulation has been recently approved (Polovich et al., 2009).

For newly diagnosed high-grade primary brain tumors, temozolomide is first used concurrently with radiation at a daily dose of 75 mg/m² orally. Stupp et al. (2005) demonstrated in a large, randomized clinical trial that concurrent administration of temozolomide with external beam cranial irradiation increased overall survival, as well as time to recurrence or progression. In a five-year follow-up, the survival benefit was long-standing (Stupp et al., 2009). Temozolomide is taken on an empty stomach every day from the day radiation starts to the day it ends, including days when not receiving a radiation treatment, ranging from 42 to 49 consecutive days. Patients should be carefully counseled regarding this schedule. After this, a treatment-free interval of two to four weeks is observed, followed by a clinical and radiographic patient reassessment prior to continuing any further therapy (Kim & Glantz, 2006). If tumor response is evident and the daily regimen was tolerated, patients typically begin the standard 28-day regimen of 5 days of taking temozolomide followed by 23 days off treatment at a daily dose of 150–200 mg/m^2 (Stupp et al., 2005, 2009). In the event of a grade 3 or 4 hematologic adverse event (NCI Cancer Therapy Evaluation Program, 2009) (see Table 8-1), dose reductions are done in increments, from 200 mg/m^2 down to 150 mg/m^2, and from 150 mg/m^2 to 100 mg/m^2. An absolute neutrophil count (ANC) less than 1.0×10^9 and a platelet count $50–100 \times 10^9$ is cause for a dose reduction of one level. Persistent or further reductions or an initial ANC greater than 1.0×10^9 and platelet count greater than 50×10^9 is cause for considering discontinuation of the drug (Polovich et al., 2009).

Although the majority of the research thus far has centered on this monthly dosing pattern, other dosing regimens have been reported and include metronomic (daily) dosing: 7 days on, 7 days off; 21 days on, 7 days off; and 5 days on, 23 days off with twice-daily dosing (Balmaceda et al., 2008; Lin & Kleinberg, 2008; Tosoni et al., 2008). Regimens of higher individual doses or more frequent dosing are associated with a greater likelihood of a grade 3 or 4 hematologic adverse event and a higher incidence of side effects. Older adult patients, patients with comorbidities, or those who experienced toxicity on the 75 mg/m^2 daily dose

may be considered for alternative dose-dense regimens to minimize toxicities (Brandes et al., 2009; Neyns, Tosoni, Hwu, & Reardon, 2010).

Clinical trials are being conducted for those in whom radiation is not a feasible or recommended therapy, thereby using temozolomide alone or in combination with a targeted agent upfront.

Patients may receive treatment for 6–36 months depending on their tolerance and the tumor response to therapy. Khasraw, Bell, and Wheeler (2009) reported case studies on three patients who were maintained on standard-dosed temozolomide for five, seven, and eight years.

Rash is the most common allergic reaction to temozolomide therapy and may respond to premedication with antihistamines, steroids, or adjustments to metronomic regimens. However, in rare cases, life-threatening skin reactions of Stevens-Johnson syndrome or toxic epidermal necrolysis have been reported (Sarma, 2009), thereby warranting close monitoring of the patient and thorough examination of all potential drug interactions.

The most common side effects of temozolomide include nausea and vomiting, constipation, and myelosuppression. As temozolomide falls into a very low emetogenic category (Polovich et al., 2009), ondansetron 8 mg given orally 30–60 minutes prior to temozolomide is generally recommended for prevention of GI side effects; adjustments in dosing may be made if nausea occurs. Patients are typically instructed to use laxatives and bowel stimulants during treatment cycles to prevent constipation (Bisanz et al., 2009). Neutropenia and thrombocytopenia are the most common hematologic events, with anemia occurring infrequently; the nadir for myelosuppression is 14–21 days (Trinh, Patel, & Hwu, 2010). In the

Table 8-1. National Cancer Institute Common Terminology Criteria for Adverse Events: Selected Investigations					
	Grade				
Adverse Event	1	2	3	4	5
White blood cell count decreased	< LLN–3,000/mm³; < LLN–3.0 × 10e9/L	< 3,000–2,000/mm³; < 3.0–2.0 × 10e9/L	< 2,000–1,000/mm³; < 2.0–1.0 × 10e9/L	< 1,000/mm³; <1.0 ×10e9/L	–
Definition: A finding based on laboratory test results that indicate a decrease in the number of white blood cells in a blood specimen.					
Neutrophil count decreased	< LLN–1,500/mm³; < LLN–1.5 × 10e9/L	< 1,500–1,000/mm³; < 1.5–1.0 × 10e9/L	< 1,000–500/mm³; < 1.0–0.5 × 10e9/L	< 500/mm³; < 0.5 × 10e9/L	–
Definition: A finding based on laboratory test results that indicate a decrease in the number of neutrophils in a blood specimen.					
Platelet count decreased	< LLN–75,000/mm³; < LLN–75.0 × 10e9/L	< 75,000–50,000/ mm³; < 75.0–50.0 × 10e9/L	< 50,000–25,000/ mm³; < 50.0–25.0 × 10e9/L	< 25,000/mm³; < 25.0 × 10e9/L	–
Definition: A finding based on laboratory test results that indicate a decrease in the number of platelets in a blood specimen.					

LLN—lower limit of normal

Note. From *Common Terminology Criteria for Adverse Events* (Version 4.03, pp. 112–113), by the National Cancer Institute Cancer Therapy Evaluation Program, 2009. Retrieved from http://evs.nci.nih.gov/ftp1/CTCAE/About.html.

5-days-on, 23-days-off dosing regimen, a complete blood count with differential (CBCD) is checked in the third and fourth weeks of therapy for a review of hematologic tolerance; the fourth-week CBCD is usually performed within 48 hours of beginning the next cycle. Anorexia, alopecia, headache, and fatigue are the other common adverse effects cited across the cumulative temozolomide experience (Stupp et al., 2005, 2009). Standard measurements of efficacy include stable disease or reduction in residual tumor, and in those patients with no evidence of recurrent disease at the advent of maintenance therapy, no recurrence of tumor would satisfy criteria for efficacy. Patients are usually clinically observed monthly, with radiographic evaluations (magnetic resonance imaging with and without gadolinium) performed every other month or as needed.

Second-Line Therapies

Patients with recurrent or progressive glioblastoma or refractory anaplastic gliomas, including astrocytoma and oligodendrogliomas, have several options for continued chemotherapeutic treatment outside of clinical trial.

By far the most heavily researched and prescribed secondary therapy for progressive, recurrent, or treatment-resistant high-grade gliomas is bevacizumab (Avastin), the first FDA-approved antiangiogenic agent. This MoAb binds to and inhibits VEGF activity, the critical component of blood vessel formation. Because neoplastic progression is dependent on angiogenesis, anti-VEGF therapy can be successful at slowing or retarding tumor growth. Combined with a cytotoxic agent, such as irinotecan, bevacizumab has been shown to improve progression-free survival in this population (Vredenburgh et al., 2007). Administered intravenously biweekly at an initial dose of 10 mg/kg, bevacizumab is generally well tolerated.

The most commonly reported adverse effect is hemorrhage; therefore, patients may experience epistaxis, hemoptysis, vaginal and rectal bleeding, GI hemorrhage, or intracranial hemorrhage (Polovich et al., 2009). Nasal septal and GI perforation and fistula formation have also been reported. Because of the drug's ability to interfere with blood vessel formation, it has a negative effect on wound and surgical healing and should be withheld postoperatively for a minimum of 14 days, with most clinicians withholding treatment for 28 days or until surgical wound is completely healed (Polovich et al., 2009). A second significant common side effect is thromboembolic events, with myocardial and cerebral infarctions being the most frequently reported in clinical trials. Hypertension may occur, and if not medically controlled, discontinuation of bevacizumab should be considered. The drug may also cause proteinuria. Monitor with renal function studies to check for nephritic syndrome by a dipstick urine test prior to each administration. The drug should be temporarily held for greater than 2+ proteinuria. Skin reactions may also occur, ranging from dryness to exfoliative dermatitis. Dose reductions may be undertaken beginning with 25% to mitigate these reactions (Polovich et al., 2009).

Another targeted agent with some activity in primary brain tumor is irinotecan, also referred to as its clinical trial name CPT-11 (Camptosar®, Pfizer Inc.). Although irinotecan has shown no improvement in overall or progression-free survival when used as a single agent, some data support its use as a second-line therapy when combined with bevacizumab (Friedman et al., 2009). Irinotecan is a cell cycle–specific cytotoxic agent that disrupts DNA replication to cause cell death. The dose is 125 mg/m^2 and is administered intravenously immediately prior to bevacizumab every two or three weeks. Dosing is adjusted up to 340 mg/m^2 in patients on enzyme-inducing antiepileptic drugs, and some studies used this higher dose when patients were also taking dexamethasone (Vredenburgh et al., 2007).

The most common and dose-limiting toxicity is an immediate cholinergic reaction, which occurs during administration and is characterized by flushing, diaphoresis, lacrimation, excess salivation, rhinitis, abdominal cramping, nausea, and diarrhea during or immediately after infusion (Polovich et al., 2009). Atropine 0.25–1 mg IV is the treatment of choice. Late diarrhea, defined as beginning 24 hours after infusion, is very common and can be mitigated with loperamide. Patients should be educated to recognize causes and signs of dehydration, maintain fluid intake, and treat these symptoms aggressively. Dose reductions can be undertaken for patients who have refractive side effects, but more commonly the drug is discontinued from the regimen. Myelosuppression can also be a side effect of irinotecan, and the CBCD should be monitored before each dose or more frequently if counts indicate suppression (Polovich et al., 2009).

Lomustine, also called CCNU (CeeNU®, Bristol-Myers Squibb Co.), is a nitrosourea-based DNA and RNA alkylating agent. This drug was originally first-line therapy for high-grade primary malignant brain tumors in combination with procarbazine and vincristine but is now largely used in salvage therapy combinations (Nieder, Mehta, & Jalali, 2009). It is available in 100 mg, 40 mg, and 10 mg capsules. Standard initial dosing is 110–130 mg/m^2 given every six weeks, and titration of dosing is dependent on degree of myelosuppression, the most common adverse effect.

Hematologic toxicity is both delayed and cumulative, and blood counts should be obtained weekly (Polovich et al., 2009). Hepatic and renal function tests should be performed within the last couple of weeks prior to subsequent administration. Dose reductions begin at 75% and continue to 50% per NCI Common Terminology Criteria for Adverse Events grade for leukocyte and platelet count (Elting et al., 2009). Leukopenia typically occurs five to six weeks after the dose and persists for 7–14 days. Thrombocytopenia is generally more common and severe, but both can be dose-limiting toxicities. Thrombocytopenia begins at four weeks after the dose and persists for 7–14 days. Cumulative effects may also be present with depressed indices or longer duration of suppression. Administering the dose on an empty stomach may reduce the occurrence of nausea and vomiting, which have a typical onset of three to six hours and last less than 24 hours (Polovich et al., 2009). Antiemetic premedication can reduce the occurrence, severity, and duration of this side effect. A small percentage of patients may develop alopecia, stomatitis, visual disturbances, lethargy, disorientation, and ataxia. All other medications should be reviewed, and patients should be cautioned regarding medication contraindications.

Other chemotherapy agents that demonstrate no or low efficacy as single agents in this disease state have been or are being investigated as companion drugs with newer agents, especially combinations of older standard cytotoxic drugs with targeted agents. These include platinum compounds such as oxaliplatin and carboplatin; alkylating agents such as procarbazine; and hydroxyurea. Some targeted agents, in addition to irinotecan, can also be used in combination with standard first-line therapy temozolomide for progression or recurrence, including erlotinib and imatinib, both of which are epidermal growth factor receptor–inhibiting agents that function as antiangiogenics. However, since the advent of bevacizumab and especially in light of its recent FDA approval as a second-line therapy, these combinations are less common in clinical practice, but they remain theoretically useful.

World Health Organization Grades I and II (Low-Grade) Gliomas

Overview

Low-grade gliomas (LGGs) include astrocytomas, oligo-dendrogliomas, and tumors with features of both of these, called mixed (see Chapters 4 and 5 for more details on LGGs). Even when counted as an aggregate, these types of primary brain tumors occur with less frequency than the aggressive WHO grades III and IV tumors and in general have a better prognosis for overall survival, time to progression, and recurrence (CBTRUS, 2010). LGGs are typically treated first with aggressive surgical resection if possible, and most receive radiation therapy if the lesion is diffuse or suboptimally resected or has enhancing components, but subsequent therapeutic recommendations are less standardized. Monitoring, often called "watchful waiting," with routinely scheduled radiographs and clinical examinations versus instituting upfront chemotherapy has long been a controversial area in neuro-oncology (Frenel, Botti, Loussouarn, & Campone, 2009; Piepmeier, 2009). Prognostic factors such as tumor histology, chromosomal deletion status, location and size of the tumor, mitotic index (a measure of cell division expressed as a percentage), age, and presenting symptoms are considered when making treatment decisions (see Chapter 4 for details). The National Comprehensive Cancer Network (NCCN) Central Nervous System Panel has developed treatment guidelines using prognostic factors to assist in decisions when treatment may appear equivocal (NCCN, 2010).

Treatment for Low-Grade Gliomas

The two primary types of LGG arise from different source cells, and their nomenclature reflects this. Astrocytic cells are supportive cells in the brain, and they take their name from their star-like shape. Tumors arising from astrocytes in adults occur most often in the cerebral hemispheres, and if they recur, often do so as a higher-grade, or more aggressive, histology (see Figure 8-3).

Oligodendroglioma is a rarer tumor, arising from the white matter of the cerebral hemispheres, and tends to be diffuse and infiltrating. Presentation of low-grade oligodendroglioma is characterized by seizure, and its indolent course correlates to a relatively positive prognosis (Kanamori et al., 2009). They have a tendency not to recur as frequently as higher-grade tumors or other subtypes of LGG. A chromosomal deletion of both 1p and 19q is associated with their increased sensitivity to chemotherapy (Kanamori et al., 2009). Mixed oligoastrocytomas are those with features of both astrocytomas and oligodendrogliomas. Although treatment does not differ significantly between the astrocytic and dendritic tumor types, mixed tumors are treated by how they behave rather than strictly by histology.

In all subtypes of LGG, upfront chemotherapy is a reasonable course when prognostic indicators are not favorable. Because the number of chemotherapeutic agents available to treat CNS tumors is small, similar agents are used. Overall survival has improved and time to progression has increased in LGGs, including oligodendroglioma, with the use of the cytotoxic alkylating agent temozolomide (Frenel et al., 2009; Tilleul et al., 2009; Wyss et al., 2009). As seen with high-grade gliomas, temozolomide has a variety of dosing levels and schedules. It appears the standard dosing of 150 mg/m^2 for 5 days on in a 28-day cycle for 6–12 cycles is the most widely used regimen in clinical practice. Temozolomide acts on LGGs similarly to high-grade gliomas by disrupting DNA replication, thus causing cell death. Common side effects include nausea, fatigue, constipation, and myelosuppression. Premedication with ondansetron 8 mg orally up to one hour prior to oral or IV temozolomide dosing is given to prevent or manage nausea; constipation is prevented or relieved with increased fluids and fiber, laxatives, bulking agents, and physical activity. CBC should be conducted at 14–21 day nadir with each cycle. Fatigue can be mitigated with energy conservation techniques, adequate nutritional intake, and frequent rest periods. If fatigue persistently inhibits an individual's ability to perform activities of daily living or causes distress, stimulants such as methylphenidate or modafinil can be used.

Meningioma

The meninges, a three-layered structure between the skull and brain, function as a fibrous sheath that encloses and cushions the main structures of the CNS. Also referred to

Figure 8-3. Astrocytic Tumor Demonstrating Classic Star-Shaped Appearance

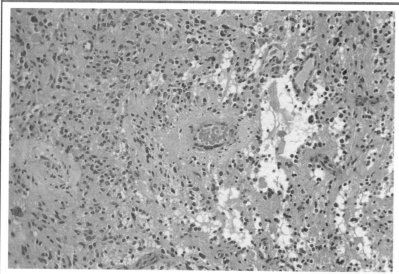 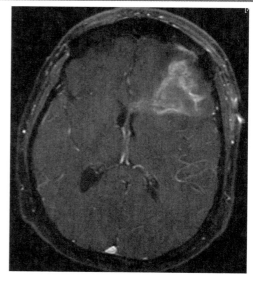

Microscopic examination of World Health Organization grade III anaplastic astrocytoma with typical imaging presentation on T1-weighted contrasted magnetic resonance imaging.

Note. From "Molecular Pathology of Malignant Gliomas," by D.N. Louis, 2006, *Annual Review of Pathology: Mechanisms of Disease, 1,* p. 108. doi:10.1146/annurev.pathol.1.110304.100043. Copyright 2006 by Annual Reviews, Inc. Reprinted with permission.

Magnetic resonance image courtesy of Deborah H. Allen, MSN, RN, CNS, FNP-BC, AOCNP. Used with permission.

as the dura, this extremely vascular component of the CNS is susceptible to a different basis for CNS malignancy. Meningiomas are the most common CNS malignancy in adults. Meningiomas are not discrete, uniformly bordered, or even solid lesions and are not intraparenchymal but instead may range from a few layers of neoplastic cells adhering to the meningeal surface to a thick rind that encases, surrounds, or penetrates adjacent structures, including nerve fibers and bone. Although surgical resection is first-line therapy, it can be challenging, and it is not uncommon that residual tumor remains after resection (Norden, Drappatz, & Wen, 2009). Most meningiomas are slow growing, and although they may eventually become large enough to cause functional deficits, they often have a low impact on life expectancy (Marosi et al., 2008; Newton, 2007). A small percentage, called atypical or malignant meningioma, is aggressive and associated with a poor prognosis (Rosenberg et al., 2009). If significant residual tumor is present after surgical intervention or if the histology is greater than grade I, radiation therapy is also employed (Rosenberg et al., 2009). Chemotherapeutic options are limited but include the following agents.

Hydroxyurea, an antimetabolite, is given at a dose of 15–20 mg/kg/day orally, with reported treatment lengths of 8–150 weeks (Newton, 2007). In the literature, only modest benefits have been shown in slowly progressive tumors with no cases of tumor regression reported (Newton, 2007). Additionally,

several studies cite high incidence of adverse events, including neutropenia and thrombocytopenia (Newton, 2007). Other common side effects include GI and dermatologic symptoms.

Some meningiomas are susceptible to the chemotherapeutic effect of somatostatin, and the presence of receptors can be verified with an octreotide scintigraphy scan, a nuclear medicine diagnostic tool using the radionuclide indium-111 (Chamberlain & Raizer, 2009; Nathoo et al., 2007). Somatostatin is available as a short-acting subcutaneous injection, given at 100 mcg three times daily after a trial of two weeks with 50 mcg given subcutaneously three times daily. Sensitivity to drug is determined by serum measurement of growth hormone and insulin-like growth factor-1 before the patient receives the long-acting formulation (Chamberlain, Glantz, & Fadul, 2007). Most patients or primary caregivers can be taught to administer subcutaneous injections at home. If sensitivity to drug is demonstrated, somatostatin is available in a long-acting intramuscular injection, given every four weeks intragluteally. This administration requires the dose to be mixed with a diluent that is included in the packaging. Administration instructions provided for reconstitution and administration must be strictly followed. Dosing begins at 10 mg intramuscularly every month and may increase in 10 mg increments at three-month intervals, up to 40 mg intramuscularly every month depending on the patient's tolerance and response. Tumor response is measured by routinely scheduled neurologic and radiographic examination.

Somatostatin may contribute to gallbladder abnormalities, and patients should be monitored periodically. Serum glucose levels can also be affected by this treatment and should be checked at drug initiation and with dosage changes. If chronic therapy is planned, thyroid-stimulating hormone (TSH) and total and free thyroxine should be assessed at baseline and periodically, as TSH production can be suppressed. B_{12} levels should also be monitored. GI symptoms, including diarrhea, abdominal pain, cholelithiasis, nausea, flatulence, and less frequently constipation, were reported in the clinical trials. Dose adjustments in the concomitant medications bromocriptine, beta-blockers, oral hypoglycemics, and insulin may be necessary. A clinical trial is under way for a somatostatin analog.

Ependymomas

Although certainly more common in pediatric patients, ependymomas also occur in adults. Classified as grade I (myxopapillary and subependymoma), grade II (ependymoma), and grade III (anaplastic ependymoma), these tumors of the brain or spinal cord arise from the neuroectoderm and are most commonly infratentorial. Surgical gross total resection is typically undertaken if possible, followed by external beam cranial irradiation for the higher-grade ependymomas or for residual tumor (Rodriguez et al., 2009). Chemotherapy has not been shown to have significant benefit for overall survival or time to progression or recurrence, but it is occasionally employed (Rudà, Gilbert, & Soffietti, 2008). Nitrosoureas, platinum-based agents, or temozolomide in standard-dose regimens are all options for chemotherapeutic treatment (Vitanovics, Balint, Hanzely, Banczerowski, & Afra, 2010).

Summary

Chemotherapy remains an integral component of medical care for adult primary CNS malignancy. Depending on the tumor histology and a host of other prognostic factors, chemotherapy can improve overall survival and lengthen time to progression or recurrence in a significant proportion of these disease states. Although all chemotherapy is associated with side effects, therapies available to treat CNS cancers are generally well tolerated, and many can be maintained for extended periods to increase intervals between remission and progression or recurrence.

References

Bajetta, E., Del Vecchio, M., Bajetta, R., & Canova, S. (2007). Medical treatment and other combination regimens. *Tumori, 93*(Suppl. 3), 22–26.

Balmaceda, C., Peereboom, D., Pannullo, S., Cheung, Y., Fisher, P., Alavi, J., ... Fine, R.L. (2008). Multi-institutional phase II study of temozolomide administration twice daily in treatment of recurrent high-grade glioma. *Cancer, 112,* 1139–1146. doi:10.1002/cncr.23167

Bisanz, A.K., Woolery, M.J., Lyons, H.F., Gaido, L., Yenulevich, M., & Fulton, S. (2009). ONS PEP resource: Constipation. In L.H. Eaton & J.M. Tipton (Eds.), *Putting evidence into practice: Improving patient outcomes* (pp. 93–104). Pittsburgh, PA: Oncology Nursing Society.

Brandes, A.A., Franceschi, E., Tosoni, A., Benevento, F., Scopece, L., Mazzocchi, V., ... Ermani, M. (2009). Temozolomide concomitant and adjuvant to radiotherapy in elderly patients with glioblastoma: Correlation with MGMT promoter methylation status. *Cancer, 115,* 3512–3518. doi:10.1002/cncr.24406

Central Brain Tumor Registry of the United States. (2010). *CBTRUS statistical report: Primary brain and central nervous system tumors diagnosed in the United States in 2004–2006.* Retrieved from http://www.cbtrus.org/2010-NPCR-SEER/CBTRUS-WEBREPORT-Final-3-2-10.pdf

Chamberlain, M.C., Glantz, M.J., & Fadul, C.E. (2007). Recurrent meningioma: Salvage therapy with long-acting somatostatin analogue. *Neurology, 69,* 969–973. doi:10.1212/01.wnl.0000271382.62776.b7

Chamberlain, M.C., & Raizer, J. (2009). Antiangiogenic therapy for high-grade glioma. *CNS and Neurological Disorders—Drug Targets, 8,* 184–194.

Elting, L., Rubenstein, E., Martin, C., Kurtin, D., Rodriguez, S., Laiho, E., ... Benjamin, R. (2001). Incidence, cost, and outcomes of bleeding and chemotherapy dose modification among solid tumor patients with chemotherapy-induced thrombocytopenia. *Journal of Clinical Oncology, 19,* 1137–1146.

Fred Hutchinson Cancer Research Center. (2009, April 14). Avastin effective at delaying brain tumor progression in recurrent disease. *Science Daily.* Retrieved from http://www.sciencedaily.com/releases/2009/04/090406151551.htm

Frenel, J.S., Botti, M., Loussouarn, D., & Campone, M. (2009). [Prognostic and predictive factors for gliomas in adults]. *Bulletin du Cancer, 96,* 357–367. doi:10.1684/bdc.2008.0776

Friedman, H.S., Prados, M.D., Wen, P.Y., Mikkelsen, T., Schiff, D., Abrey, L.E., ... Cloughesy, T. (2009). Bevacizumab alone and in combination with irinotecan in recurrent glioblastoma. *Journal of Clinical Oncology, 27,* 4733–4740. doi:10.1200/JCO.2008.19.8721

Goodman, E., Messinger, W., & White, J. (1946). Indications and results of surgery of the autonomic nervous system in Naval personnel. *Annals of Surgery, 124,* 204–217.

Gorlia, T., van den Bent, M.J., Hegi, M.E., Mirimanoff, M.O., Weller, M., Cairncross, J.C., ... Stupp, R. (2008). Nomograms for predicting survival of patients with newly diagnosed glioblastoma: Prognostic factor analysis of EORTC and NCIC trial 26981-22981/CE.3. *Lancet Oncology, 9,* 29–38. doi:10.1016/S1470-2045(07)70384-4

Hau, P., Stupp, R., & Hegi, M.E. (2007). MGMT methylation status: The advent of stratified treatment in glioblastoma. *Disease Markers, 23,* 97–104.

Hegi, M.E., Diserens, A.C., Godard, S., Dietrich, P.Y., Regli, L., Ostermann, S., ... Stupp, R. (2004). Clinical trial substantiates the predictive value of O-6-methylguanine-DNA methyltransferase promoter methylation in glioblastoma patients treated with temozolomide. *Clinical Cancer Research, 10,* 1871–1874. doi:10.1158/1078-0432.CCR-03-0384

Hirsch, J. (2006). An anniversary for cancer chemotherapy. *JAMA, 296,* 1518–1520. doi:10.1001/jama.296.12.1518

Kanamori, M., Kumabe, T., Sonoda, Y., Nishino, Y., Watanabe, M., & Tominaga, T. (2009). Predictive factors for overall and progression-free survival, and dissemination in oligodendroglial tumors. *Journal of Neuro-Oncology, 93,* 219–228. doi:10.1007/s11060-008-9762-7

Kesari, S., Schiff, D., Henson, J.W., Muzikansky, A., Gigas, D.C., Doherty, L., ... Wen, P.Y. (2008). Phase II study of temozolomide, thalidomide, and celecoxib for newly diagnosed glioblastoma in adults. *Neuro-Oncology, 10,* 300–308.

Khasraw, M., Bell, D., & Wheeler, H. (2009). Long term use of temozolomide: Could you use temozolomide safely for life in gliomas? *Journal of Clinical Neuroscience, 16,* 854–855. doi:10.1016/j.jocn.2008.09.005

Kim, L., & Glantz, M. (2006). Chemotherapeutic options for primary brain tumors. *Current Treatment Options in Oncology, 7,* 467–478.

Lin, S.H., & Kleinberg, L.R. (2008). Carmustine wafers: Localized delivery of chemotherapeutic agent in CNS malignancies. *Expert Reviews in Anticancer Therapies, 8,* 343–359. doi:10.1586/14737140.8.3.343

Marosi, C., Hassler, M., Rosessler, K., Reni, M., Sant, M., Mazza, E., & Vecht, C. (2008). Meningioma. *Critical Reviews in Oncology/Hematology, 67,* 153–171. doi:10.1016/j.critrevonc.2008.01.010

Nathoo, N., Ugokwe, K., Chang, A.S., Li, L., Ross, J., Suh, J.H., ... Barnett, G.H. (2007). The role of 111indium–octreotide brain scintigraphy in the diagnosis of cranial, dural-based meningioma. *Journal of Neuro-Oncology, 81,* 167–174. doi:10.1007/s11060-006-9210-5

National Cancer Institute Cancer Therapy Evaluation Program. (2009). *Common terminology criteria for adverse events* [v.4.02]. Retrieved from http://evs.nci.nih.gov/ftp1/CTCAE/CTCAE_4.02_2009-09-15_QuickReference_5x7.pdf

National Cancer Institute Surveillance, Epidemiology, and End Results. (2009, November). SEER stat fact sheets: Brain and other nervous system. Retrieved from http://seer.cancer.gov/statfacts/html/brain.html

National Comprehensive Cancer Network. (2010). *NCCN Clinical Practice Guidelines in Oncology™: Central nervous system cancers* [v.1.2010]. Retrieved from http://www.nccn.org/professionals/physician_gls/PDF/cns.pdf

Newton, H.B. (2007). Hydroxyurea chemotherapy in the treatment of meningiomas. *Neurosurgical Focus, 23,* E11. doi:10.3171/FOC-07/10/E11

Neyns, B., Tosoni, A., Hwu, W., & Reardon, D. (2010). Dose-dense temozolomide regimens: Antitumor activity, toxicity, and immunomodulatory effects. *Cancer, 116,* 2868–2877. doi:10.1002/cncr.25035

Nieder, C., Mehta, M.P., & Jalali, R. (2009). Combined radio- and chemotherapy of brain tumours in adult patients. *Clinical Oncology, 21,* 515–524. doi:10.1016/j.clon.2009.05.003

Norden, A.D., Drappatz, J., & Wen, P.Y. (2009). Advances in meningioma therapy. *Current Neurology and Neuroscience Reports, 9,* 231–240.

Piepmeier, J. (2009). Current concepts in the evaluation and management of WHO grade II gliomas. *Journal of Neuro-Oncology, 92,* 253–259. doi:10.1007/s11060-009-9870-z

Polovich, M., Whitford, J., & Olsen, M. (Eds.). (2009). *Chemotherapy and biotherapy guidelines and recommendations for practice* (3rd ed.). Pittsburgh, PA: Oncology Nursing Society.

Pritchard, J.B., Sweet, D.H., Miller, D.S., & Walden, R. (1999). Mechanism of organic anion transport across the apical membrane of choroid plexus. *Journal of Biological Chemistry, 274,* 33382–33387. doi:10.1074/jbc.274.47.33382

Rodriguez, D., Cheung, M., Housri, N., Quinones-Hinogosa, A., Camphasusen, K., & Koniaris, L. (2009). Outcomes of malignant CNS ependymomas: An examination of 2,408 cases through the Surveillance, Epidemiology, and End Results (SEER) database (1973–2005). *Journal of Surgical Research, 156,* 340–351. doi:10.1016/j.jss.2009.04.024

Rosenberg, L.A., Prayson, R.A., Lee, J., Reddy, C., Chao, S.T., Barnett, G.H., ... Suh, J.H. (2009). Long-term experience with WHO grade III meningiomas at a single institution. *International Journal of Radiation Oncology, Biology, Physics, 74,* 427–432. doi:10.1016/j.ijrobp.2008.08.018

Rudà, R., Gilbert, M., & Soffietti, R. (2008). Ependymomas of the adult: Molecular biology and treatment. *Current Opinion in Neurology, 21,* 754–761. doi:10.1097/WCO.0b013e328317efe8

Sarma, N. (2009). Stevens-Johnson syndrome and toxic epidermal necrolysis overlap due to oral temozolomide and cranial radiotherapy. *American Journal of Clinical Dermatology, 10,* 264–267. doi:10.2165/00128071-200910040-00007.

Scheie, D., Andresen, P., Cvancarova, M., Bo, A., Helseth, E., Skullerud, K., & Beiske, K. (2006). Fluorescence in situ hybridization (FISH) on touch preparations: A reliable method for detecting loss of heterozygosity at 1p and 19q in oligodendroglial tumors. *American Journal of Surgical Pathology, 30,* 828–837. doi:10.1097/01.pas.0000213250.44822.2e

Stupp, R., Hegi, M.E., Mason, W.P., van den Bent, M.J., Taphoorn, M.J., Janzer, R.C., ... Mirimanoff, R.O. (2009). Effects of radiotherapy with concomitant and adjuvant temozolomide versus radiotherapy alone on survival in glioblastoma in a randomised phase III study: 5-year analysis of the EORTC-NCIC trial. *Lancet Oncology, 10,* 459–466. doi:10.1016/S1470-2045(09)70025-7

Stupp, R., Mason, W.P., van den Bent, M.J., Weller, M., Fisher, B., Taphoorn, M., ... Mirimanoff, R.O. (2005). Radiotherapy plus concomitant and adjuvant temozolomide for glioblastoma. *New England Journal of Medicine, 352,* 987–1003.

Tatter, S.B. (2005). The new WHO classification of tumors affecting the central nervous system. Retrieved from http://neurosurgery.mgh.harvard.edu/newwhobt.htm

Tilleul, P., Brignone, M., Hassani, Y., Tailandier, L., Taillibert, S., Cartalat-Carel, S., ... Chinot, O. (2009). [Prescription guidebook for temozolomide usage in brain tumors]. *Bulletin du Cancer, 96,* 579–589. doi:10.1684/bdc.2009.0865

Tosoni, A., Franceschi, E., Ermani, M., Bertorelle, R., Bonaldi, L., Blatt, V., & Brandes, A.A. (2008). Temozolomide three weeks on and one week off as first line therapy for patients with recurrent or progressive low grade glioma. *Journal of Neuro-Oncology, 89,* 179–185. doi:10.1007/s11060-008-9600-y

Trinh, V., Patel, S., & Hwu, W. (2010). The safety of temozolomide in the treatment of malignancies. *Expert Opinion on Drug Safety, 8,* 493–499. doi:10.1517/14740330902918281

Vein, A. (2008). Scientist and fate: Lina Stern (1878–1969), a neurophysiologist and biochemist. *Journal of the History of the Neurosciences, 17,* 195–206. doi:10.1080/09647040601138478

Vitanovics, D., Balint, K., Hanzely, Z., Banczerowski, P., & Afra, D. (2010). Ependymoma in adults: Surgery, reoperation and radiotherapy for survival. *Pathology and Oncology Research, 16,* 93–99. doi:10.1007/s12253-00909104-5.

Vlassenbroeck, I., Califice, S., Diserens, A.C., Migliavacca, E., Straub, J., Di Stefano, I., ... Hegi, M.E. (2008). Validation of real-time methylation-specific PCR to determine O6-methylguanine-DNA methyltransferase gene promoter methylation in glioma. *Journal of Molecular Diagnostics, 10,* 332–337. doi:10.2353/jmoldx.2008.070169

Vredenburgh, J.J., Desjardins, A., Herndon, J.E., 2nd, Marcello, J., Reardon, D.A., Quinn, J.A., ... Friedman, H.S. (2007). Bevacizumab plus irinotecan in recurrent glioblastoma multiforme. *Journal of Clinical Oncology, 25,* 4722–4729. doi:10.1200/JCO.2007.12.2440

Wyss, M., Hofer, S., Bruehlmeier, M., Hefti, M., Uhlmann, C., Bärtschi, E., ... Roelcke, U. (2009). Early metabolic responses in temozolomide treated low-grade glioma patients. *Journal of Neuro-Oncology, 95*, 87–93. doi:10.1007/s11060-009-9896-2

Zhong, H. & Bowen, J.P. (2006). Antiangiogenesis drug design: Multiple pathways targeting tumor vasculature. *Current Medicinal Chemistry, 13*, 849–862.

CHAPTER 9

Treatment Modalities: Radiotherapy

Maurene A. McQuestion, RN, BScN, MSc, CON(C), and Maureen Daniels, BScN, RN

Introduction

Radiation therapy (RT) is a powerful and effective treatment for central nervous system (CNS) tumors. It is the treatment of choice in primary tumors when surgery or radiosurgery is not an option because of tumor type; inoperability of a tumor because of size, location, clinical status, or age of the patient; and when residual tumor remains following surgery. RT slows or halts the growth of these tumors for varying lengths of time. It also has a role in the management of benign tumors, recurrent malignant disease, and brain metastasis. New developments and improvements in the precision with which RT is delivered ensure that the targeted area of the brain receives maximal treatment while surrounding normal brain tissue is spared unnecessary exposure to radiation. RT works by targeting actively dividing cells, causing cell death through a process of DNA damage. Generally, patients tolerate a course of RT well, are able to receive their treatment on an outpatient basis, and are able to carry on with their usual activities with a few minor modifications to their daily routine.

Principles of Radiation Treatment

Several guiding principles of treatment relate to RT delivery to the brain or spinal cord. Controlling tumor growth for as long as possible is a primary goal of treatment. Of equal importance is maintaining the patient's quality of life by minimizing symptoms and side effects of treatment and the disease process. When a patient is facing a disease that has no cure, maintaining quality of life becomes of paramount importance in the overall treatment plan. RT for CNS tumors is often provided in conjunction with other treatment modalities such as surgery and chemotherapy. Although standard radiation dosage guidelines exist for several CNS tumor types, the treatment plan is always individualized to the patient, considering factors such as tumor biology, age of the patient, pre- and postoperative performance status, and the extent of the surgical resection. With ongoing advances in treatment and an evolving understanding of these tumors, the ability to tailor treatment plans to address the individual's tumor characteristics is improving. The hope is that this approach will lead to an improved patient quality of life and longer survival.

The goal of therapy is to deliver a dose of ionizing radiation to kill the tumor cells while minimizing the effects on normal tissue surrounding the tumor. Radiation damages cellular DNA and stops or reduces the cell's ability to divide and multiply. Damage can occur directly as a result of the ionizing effects of radiation on the DNA or indirectly through the interaction of radiation with intracellular water, causing the formation of free radicals that attack the DNA (Bruner, Haas, & Gosselin-Acomb, 2005). Radiation treatment can be delivered using a variety of technologies and techniques (see Figure 9-1).

Teletherapy, or external beam radiation, is the most common form of RT and uses high-energy x-rays, or electromagnetic waves, to accelerate electrons. The electrons then strike a target inside the linear accelerator (linac), producing photons, which emerge from the linac as a directed beam at the tumor target volume. Electromagnetic radiation can be produced through the decay of radioactive sources, such as cobalt 60 (Hancock & Burrow, 2004). Proton units may be used and produce extremely high energy from charged particles, but because of the Bragg peak (a sharp peak of energy delivered with a rapid dropoff of dose), a concentrated dose of radiation is delivered directly to the tumor with a rapid energy loss within a few millimeters of the target, thereby ensuring a high dose localized to the tumor while sparing more normal tissue (Bussière & Adams, 2003).

Primary Brain Tumors

Low-Grade Astrocytomas and Oligodendrogliomas

A wait-and-watch approach is often used with low-grade astrocytomas because the timing of radiation is not well de-

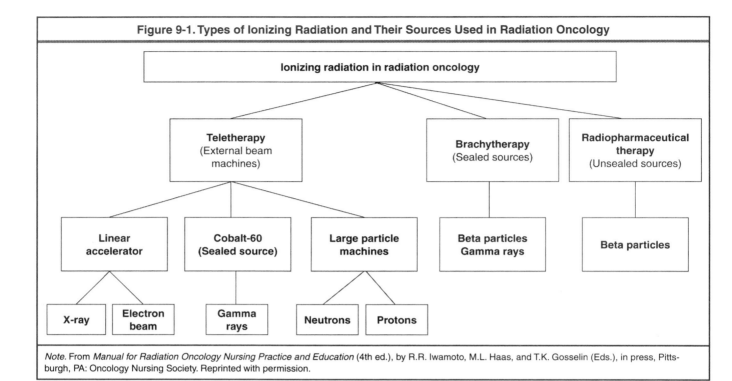

Figure 9-1. Types of Ionizing Radiation and Their Sources Used in Radiation Oncology

Note. From *Manual for Radiation Oncology Nursing Practice and Education* (4th ed.), by R.R. Iwamoto, M.L. Haas, and T.K. Gosselin (Eds.), in press, Pittsburgh, PA: Oncology Nursing Society. Reprinted with permission.

fined although most patients will eventually undergo radiation treatment at some point during the course of their illness. In the case of less-anaplastic tumors and a longer expected survival, radiation is delayed because of the cognitive effects from cranial irradiation. This approach is especially warranted in younger patients who are experiencing seizures but have no mass effect (mass or size of the tumor that can compress brain tissue and increase cranial pressure) or neurologic disability. Standard treatment for these patients is observation and anticonvulsant therapy (Karim et al., 2002). Karim et al. (2002) studied 311 patients comparing immediate postoperative radiation with delayed treatment. The five-year overall survival was 65% and 66%, respectively. Progression-free survival was 44% and 37%, respectively. Therefore, the watchful waiting includes careful monitoring with a magnetic resonance imaging (MRI) scan performed every three months with the time between scans increasing with prolonged stability of the tumor.

Patients presenting with mass effect, neurologic deficits, or enhancement on a computed tomography (CT) or MRI scan should be considered for upfront treatment, and observation is not usually offered in that situation. Genetic testing is performed on patients diagnosed with glial tumors. Molecular abnormalities include the loss of heterozygosity on chromosome 10q. In oligodendrogliomas, the loss of heterozygosity for 1p and 19q chromosomes is generally predictive of good prognosis and chemosensitivity (Behin, Hoang-Xuan, Carpentier, & Delattre, 2003; Kushen, Sonabend, & Lesniak, 2007).

In these cases, chemotherapy given prior to radiotherapy is a reasonable option to prolong the time before radiation is required. Tumors that do not have chromosome loss are associated with a less favorable prognosis and are less likely to be chemosensitive, so upfront radiotherapy is often advocated in this case.

Newly Diagnosed and Malignant Gliomas

Malignant gliomas include the following conditions: glioblastoma multiforme (GBM), malignant astrocytoma grades 3 and 4, anaplastic astrocytoma, anaplastic oligodendroglioma, anaplastic oligoastrocytoma, and anaplastic glioma. Many of these terms are overlapping and synonymous and can be divided into two categories: GBMs and anaplastic gliomas (Stupp et al., 2009). GBMs are the most common brain tumors but have a very poor overall prognosis.

External Beam Radiotherapy
External beam radiation has been shown in several early studies to significantly improve survival (Andersen, 1978; Kristiansen et al., 1981; Walker et al., 1978, 1980). With improvements in CT and MRI, clinicians have been moving away from using whole brain radiation therapy (WBRT) in favor of more focused treatments using regional fields and highly conformal RT planning. The high-dose tumor volume that is treated includes the radiologically enhanced tumor plus a 2 cm margin for the planned tumor volume (PTV)

(Buatti et al., 2008). This approach is used to prevent recurrence at the edge of the treatment field because the majority of recurrences occur at the original primary site (Hochberg & Pruitt, 1980; Wallner, Galicich, Krol, Arbit, & Malkin, 1989). Additionally, this approach has demonstrated similar survival when compared to WBRT for part or all of the scheduled treatment (Kita, Okawa, Tanaka, & Ikeda, 1989; Shapiro & Young, 1976). WBRT may be used in the presence of multifocal disease.

Following surgical resection, radiation is typically delivered to a dose of 60 Gy in 2 Gy fractions (#) given daily over six weeks (30#), along with concurrent temozolomide 75 mg/m^2 daily (Stupp et al., 2009). Concurrent treatment provides an improved mean survival from 12–15 months (Bleehen & Stenning, 1991; Buatti et al., 2008; Nelson et al., 1988). Stupp et al. (2005) observed a 16.1% increase in two-year survival, or 2.5-month median increased survival for patients receiving combined modality treatment with temozolomide as compared to radiation alone.

Many older patients do not tolerate radical RT, which can negatively affect quality of life. For patients older than 60 years, 60 Gy in 30# has been shown to be equivalent to 40 Gy in 15# (2.6 Gy per #) (Roa et al., 2004). Keime-Guibert et al. (2007) found that RT (50 Gy in 27# or 1.8 cGy per #) in addition to supportive care prolonged survival without reducing quality of life or cognitive function in patients older than 70, compared to supportive care alone. Therefore, patients older than 70 with a good performance status or those younger than 70 with a poor performance status may be recommended to undergo a shorter course of radiation treatments (Laperriere, Zuraw, Cairncross, & Cancer Care Ontario Practice Guidelines Initiative Neuro-Oncology Disease Site Group, 2002). Despite these study findings, the optimal dose of radiation for older patients has still not been determined. In patients with poor performance status, supportive care alone should be considered because of the poor treatment outcome in older patients following conventional radiation. Radiation is not recommended for patients who are confused or bedridden (Laperriere, Perry, Zuraw, & Cancer Care Ontario Practice Guidelines Initiative Neuro-Oncology Disease Site Group, 2005).

Hyperfractionated Radiation Therapy

Hyperfractionated RT is a modality for delivering more than one fraction per day with lower than standard doses per fraction, which results in a total higher dose delivered in the same overall time as compared to conventional radiation. However, hyperfractionated RT has not been shown to provide any survival benefit over conventional daily-fractionated RT (Buatti et al., 2008; Scott et al., 1998). Additionally, dose intensification or the use of radiation sensitizing agents, such as hypoxic cell sensitizers or halogenated pyrimidines, has not shown any added benefit or survival when compared to

standard therapy with doses of 50–60 Gy (Buatti et al., 2008; Horiot et al., 1988; Huncharek,1998; Werner-Wasik et al., 1996). As a result, neither of these approaches is recommended as standard therapy. Temozolomide has been the only drug that has shown improved survival with radiation treatment, but it is not clear if the drug acts as a radiosensitizer or if it has an adjuvant benefit (Athanassiou et al., 2005; Stupp et al., 2005).

Brachytherapy

Brachytherapy, also known as interstitial or implanted RT, uses a radioactive source such as iodine-125 (^{125}I) or iridium-192 (^{192}Ir) as a boost to conventional external beam radiation. It is an invasive procedure and has been associated with a high percentage of complications (Combs, Debus, & Schulz-Ertner, 2007; Laperriere et al., 1998). It has also been shown to increase dosage to normal surrounding tissue, increasing the risk of radiation damage in tumors larger than 6 cm (Suh & Barnett, 1999). Early studies evaluated the use of brachytherapy for recurrent tumors, leading to clinical trials incorporating brachytherapy with conventional external beam RT. To date, the evidence is insufficient to support its use for patients with newly diagnosed high-grade gliomas (Laperriere et al., 2002; McDermott et al., 2004). Other approaches using a radiolabeled antibody or radioactive colloid are under investigation.

Intraoperative GliaSite® Radiation Therapy System

The GliaSite® (Hologic, Inc.), an intraoperative form of brachytherapy, received U.S. Food and Drug Administration (FDA) approval in 2001 for the treatment of high-grade gliomas. An expandable balloon filled with radioactive ^{125}I that is connected to a subcutaneous reservoir is placed in the operative bed at the time of the initial debulking surgery (Strzelczyk & Safadi, 2004). Studies are ongoing to evaluate the use of GliaSite for recurrent as well as newly diagnosed gliomas (Kleinberg et al., 2009; Wernicke et al., 2010).

Anaplastic Gliomas

The standard management of anaplastic gliomas as a group is RT only, 60 Gy in 30# to a conformal volume as described previously for glioblastomas (Laperriere et al., 2005). Although the combination of radiotherapy and concurrent and adjuvant temozolomide has been shown to improve survival in GBM, no such data exist for anaplastic gliomas. International randomized trials looking at the possible benefit of temozolomide in this class of gliomas currently are just beginning to accrue patients. Despite this, while waiting for results from these recently undertaken studies, many centers offer patients with anaplastic gliomas the same treatment as for GBMs, namely radiation with concurrent and adjuvant temozolomide.

Recurrent Glioblastomas

Patients may be able to receive re-irradiation of a recurrent tumor if the volume of recurrence is small and the interval is significantly long (a few years) between the time of initial radiation treatment and the recurrence. Stereotactic radiosurgery (SRS) may be used to treat recurrent lesions. A recent pilot study evaluating the feasibility, risk, and effectiveness of stereotactic brachytherapy (SBT) using ^{125}I for small complex (smaller than 4 cm) recurrences determined that SBT is safe and minimally invasive (Schnell et al., 2008). With the implementation of high-precision treatments compared to conventional radiotherapy, further prospective studies are still required to evaluate the overall effectiveness and the role of SBT in combination with primary surgical resection and with recurrent disease. Patients may be provided with options that may include clinical trials of experimental treatments that use radiation and chemotherapy (Combs et al., 2007).

Ependymomas, Meningiomas, and Vestibular Schwannomas

Ependymomas develop in cells lining the ventricles and the spinal cord and can occur in both children and adults. They may spread from the brain to the spinal cord via the cerebrospinal fluid (CSF), thereby dictating the extent of treatment. RT is often given as adjuvant therapy following an incomplete surgical resection.

Meningiomas, arising within the layers lining the brain, are treated surgically if accessible. If surgery is not chosen for patients who are newly diagnosed and symptomatic, then radiation is the recommended treatment. For partially resected malignant meningiomas, radiation is given postoperatively to manage residual disease. Radiation is also warranted for recurrent disease. Stereotactic radiation is delivered for atypical, more infiltrative, recurrent, or malignant meningiomas, with excellent control rates (Elia, Shih, & Loeffler, 2007; Mirimanoff, 2004).

Vestibular schwannomas are often followed with imaging because of their slow growth. Surgery, radiosurgery, and fractionated stereotactic radiotherapy (SRT) all are acceptable treatment options; however, a recent study reported improved outcomes related to facial nerve and hearing with the use of GammaKnife® (Elekta) radiosurgery (Myresth, Møller, Pedersen, & Lund-Johansen, 2009).

Brain Metastases

Up to 30% of all brain tumors are brain metastases, most commonly having spread from the breast, lung, and kidney and from melanoma. Eighty percent of brain metastases occur in the cerebral hemispheres, with only one-third of the lesions being solitary lesions. Prognosis ranges from three to six months (Davey, 2002; Hoskin & Brada, 2001; Schaefer, Budzik, & Gonzalez, 1996).

Brain metastases are typically spherical lesions, often located at the junction of the gray-white matter, are associated with the presence of edema, and enhance on MRI scans (see Figure 9-2). Treatment of brain metastasis is always palliative with the primary goal being definitive local control. Treatment options may involve surgery plus WBRT, WBRT alone, or WBRT plus SRS depending on the treatment center, availability of technology, and patient factors. Patients who receive the most benefit from undergoing RT for brain metastasis are patients younger than 65 years with good performance status, those with primary disease control, and these with no other extracranial metastasis (Davey, 2002). Size and location of the metastatic lesions will determine treatment options.

Patients presenting with single-lesion brain metastasis, no evidence of extracranial disease, and good performance status should be considered for surgical resection followed by WBRT. This is based on the assumption that if one metastatic lesion is present, other lesions are likely to be present but are not visible on imaging. Postoperative WBRT is offered to reduce the risk of recurrence. Dose and fractionation schedules are typically 30 Gy in 10# or 20 Gy in 5#. Some centers prefer using 30 Gy/10# to reduce the fraction size because of concerns about long-term neurocognitive effects caused by a larger fraction size, but currently no evidence supports or refutes this practice (Mintz et al., 2006).

The addition of SRS with WBRT has been shown to improve median overall survival compared to WBRT alone for patients with single lesions compared to patients with multiple metastatic lesions (6.9 versus 4.9 months, $p = 0.04$) (Andrews et al., 2004). SRS with the addition of WBRT has not shown benefit in terms of overall median survival (7.5 versus 8 months, $p = 0.42$ for SRS and WBRT versus SRS alone), but patients treated with SRS alone had less local disease control, increased distal intracranial recurrence, and greater deterioration in cognitive function (Aoyama et al., 2006).

Patients with limited or controlled extracranial disease and a Karnofsky performance status score greater than 70 with one to three brain metastases smaller than 4 cm in maximal dimension can be considered for SRS as boost therapy in combination with WBRT (within six weeks of WBRT) or for SRS alone (McDermott & Sneed, 2005). Patients with recurrent brain metastasis may be treated with SRS (one to three metastases, smaller than 4 cm), surgery (single lesion with mass effect, or one to three metastases with one lesion causing significant mass effect and minimal extracranial disease), or repeat WBRT (minimum six months since prior WBRT) (Mintz et al., 2006). On occasion, patients with more than three recurrent brain metastases may also be treated with radiosurgery but generally not for more than five or six lesions.

Figure 9-2. Metastatic Brain Lesions From Lung Cancer

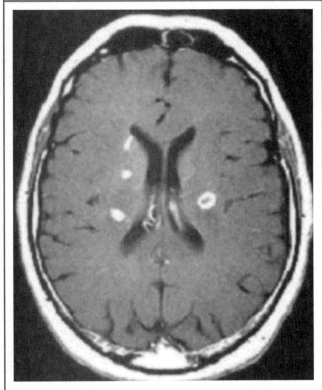

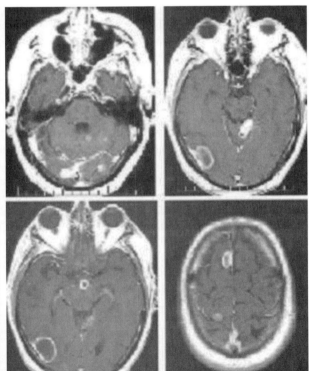

Note. Images courtesy of the Radiation Medicine Program, Princess Margaret Hospital, Toronto, Ontario, Canada. Used with permission.

Radiation Therapy Delivery Techniques

Intensity-Modulated Radiation Therapy

Older, conventional external beam RT uses a simple beam arrangement using a fluoroscopic simulator and results in larger treatment volumes and the potential for increased toxicity. Lead blocks are required to shield critical structures and protect normal tissue. Intensity-modulated RT (IMRT) provides a more advanced approach to three-dimensional (3-D) conformal RT through 3-D volumetric CT treatment planning with refinement of the dose configuration to deliver a highly conformal treatment target to the tumor, which limits as much exposure to normal tissue as possible and spares critical structures. Advanced imaging, computer software, and treatment machine design support the application of IMRT. A multileaf collimator inside the treatment gantry allows for individual movement of the leaves to shape to the tumor and vary the intensity of the dose in individual beams. The beams converge to deliver a higher dose of radiation to the tumor target while delivering a smaller dose to surrounding tissue. The use of IMRT for the treatment of CNS tumors has become a treatment modality of choice to improve precision and conformity of the target dose and reduce dose to normal tissue and organs at risk (e.g., optic chiasma, brain stem, cerebral cortex) (Chen et al., 2010). Studies to date comparing various IMRT protocols, including hypofractionated IMRT, standard fractionated IMRT, and IMRT boost following a non-IMRT treatment versus IMRT alone, have not shown an increased mean or overall survival benefit (Fuller et al., 2007). Acute toxicities across studies were similar. Benefits of IMRT may not have been observed as a result of the comparison of heterogeneous patient groups (Fuller et al., 2007; Voynov et al., 2002). The advantages of IMRT will definitely be more evident for children treated for brain tumor and adults with low-grade tumors (e.g., meningiomas, craniopharyngiomas) where long-term survival is the norm, and sparing normal brain tissue from the high-dose volume will be associated with less-prominent late effects, although this will always be a difficult end point to measure.

Image-Guided Radiotherapy

Image-guided RT (IGRT) uses in-room imaging modalities that support the merging of data from cone-beam CT images with the planning CT image, thereby allowing for real-time treatment adjustments to be made. The development of IGRT has supported changes in dose distributions, sparing of normal tissue, and changes in fractionation schedules (Greco & Ling, 2008).

Stereotactic Radiosurgery and Radiotherapy

SRS and SRT are the precise delivery of hypofractionated radiation. SRS is the use of a single high dose of radiation in one day, whereas SRT is a fractionated course of treatment provided over one to six weeks. Treatment planning involves highly conformal treatment planning with higher doses to the targeted tumor or cavity volumetric area and significantly smaller doses to surrounding tissue. This results in reduced toxicity, less time for immobilization to ensure reproducibility, and the prevention of movement during treatment delivery.

SRS is used for the treatment of benign or functional conditions (arteriovenous malformations, essential tremors, and trigeminal neuralgias), benign tumors (acoustic neuromas, meningiomas), primary brain tumors, and brain metastasis. SRS may be delivered as a primary therapy for a tumor that is surgically inaccessible, used to deliver a boost of radiation, or given as an adjuvant treatment for tumor recurrence. The tumor is shrunk at the rate of normal tumor growth by distorting the DNA in the tumor cells, causing the tumor to reduce in size over a period of time. SRS can be used to treat slow-growing tumors that are not life threatening or causing severe and debilitating side effects that need to be managed more rapidly. It may also be used in the presence of fast-growing tumors such as brain metastasis, as well as in patients who have already received WBRT or the maximum radiation dose (Gerosa, Nicolato, Foroni, Tomazzoli, & Bricolo, 2004; McDermott & Sneed, 2005).

Stereotactic Radiosurgery and Radiotherapy Treatment Delivery Systems

SRT (single treatment) and SRS (fractionated treatment) can be delivered using different technologies and equipment. They may be delivered using a cobalt-60 unit (GammaKnife, GammaKnife Perfexion™) or a linac (e.g., CyberKnife®, Accuray, Inc.; Synergy S®, Elekta). These various technologies are all able to provide single-fraction radiosurgery, but only the linac-based systems may be used for fractionated radiotherapy.

The GammaKnife has been used for more than 30 years. GammaKnife and Perfexion are used to treat smaller intracranial tumors (smaller than 3.5 cm; some centers smaller than 4 cm) and functional disorders of the brain (see Figure 9-3). They are also options in the management of brain metastases smaller than 4 cm, where surgical resection is not an option or the preferred treatment, and when SRS is technically advantageous over other approaches (Gerosa et al., 2004). The GammaKnife (cobalt source) is a stationary unit that uses 201 cobalt sources focused precisely on the tumor, whereas the Perfexion unit has 192 cobalt sources. The same principles apply to both units. Some centers will have either a GammaKnife or a Perfexion unit, but for centers that have both types of treatment units, they have the option of using the GammaKnife for functional and benign disorders and using the Perfexion unit for malignant disease, thereby maintaining separate oncology and non-oncology programs

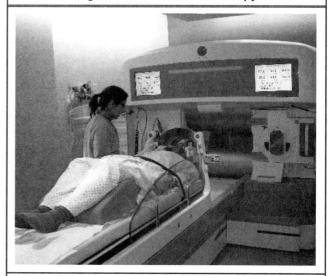

Figure 9-3. GammaKnife Therapy

Note. Photo courtesy of the Radiation Medicine Program, Princess Margaret Hospital, Toronto, Ontario, Canada. Used with permission.

within their institution. A stereotactic frame (e.g., Leksell® frame system, Elekta) is fixed to the skull with four screws or pins for stability.

The CyberKnife is a frameless IGRT system using a linac on a robotic arm (a mini linac) (see Figure 9-4). Fiducial markers are placed on the mask that is used for immobilization. Detectors in the robotic arm determine where the markers are located, determining treatment position. The robotic arm then delivers the radiation. The arm can adjust to correct for any movement by relocating the markers prior to delivering the dose of radiation (Fenwick, Tomé, Soisson, Mehta, & Mackie, 2006).

SRS with a linac uses a relocatable frame (e.g., Gill-Thomas-Cosman frame). The frame is the same as is used for fractionated treatments such as for pituitary tumors and meningiomas and is applied daily. The linac is used to treat larger intracranial tumors (larger than 3.5 cm), boosts to the nasopharynx, eye tumors, and treatments outside of the skull (spine and other tissues). Furthermore, the linac can use IMRT technology (see Figure 9-5). For fractionated (SRT) treatment of CNS tumors, the frame is not fixed to the skull but uses a mouth bite and straps, enabling multiple treatments with a less invasive device.

Particle Beam Proton Therapy

Proton therapy is a form of external beam radiation that uses protons rather than photons (x-rays). Only a few proton therapy units are located in the United States and Canada. Protons have a large mass (1,800 times greater than an electron) and are positively charged. The protons slow down as they pass through tissue and deliver a concentrated dose of radiation to the target volume at the end of their path, with little scatter. As a result, the dose of radiation to the surrounding normal tissue is lower than that delivered using IMRT because the dose drops off at the end of the beam

path (Bragg peak). Protons, unlike photons, do not continue to travel past the tumor target (Bussière & Adams, 2003).

Radiation Therapy Process

Consultation

The initial consultation for consideration of radiation for CNS tumor treatment involves a multidisciplinary team, including the radiation oncologist, radiation oncology nurse, social worker, and, depending on the treatment, a neurosurgeon. A full assessment is conducted, including a review of diagnostic tests, a physical and neurologic examination, evaluation of symptom presentation and experience, family and social support system evaluation, and assessment of the patient and family's understanding and expectations of the RT options and plan.

Simulation and Treatment Planning

RT simulation and planning involves additional members of the interdisciplinary team, including a medical physicist, dosimetrist, and medical radiation technologists (radiation therapists). Simulation includes the preparation or setup of any required mask or immobilization device that will be used during treatment (Hancock & Burrow, 2004). Simulation may be performed using a traditional simulator and two-dimensional planning or with 3-D CT simulation. CT simulation using axial, coronal, and sagittal images provides more accurate determination of the treatment volume for treatment planning. CT scans have good geometry, but tumors show up better with MRI. Computer software supports the fusing of MRI images with CT images to accurately delineate the tumor location and volume. This ensures that higher doses can be planned while ensuring accurate sparing of critical tissues (Hancock & Burrow, 2004).

Treatment planning includes defining the treatment volume. This includes the gross tumor volume (GTV), clinical tumor volume (CTV), and the PTV. For malignant tumors, the GTV includes the surgical cavity and any enhancement on imaging. The CTV would include an additional 0.5–1.5 cm margin for microscopic spread of tumor not visible on imaging. The PTV adds another 0.5 cm margin beyond the CTV and accounts for possible variation in positioning on a day-to-day basis (Laperriere et al., 2002). The radiation oncologist writes the treatment prescription, which includes the patient's name, medical record number, diagnosis, staging information, start date for treatment, total dose, daily dose, number of fractions, any planned boosts, treatment fields, and the energy that will be used during treatment delivery. The oncologist outlines or defines the tumor and normal structures. The dosimetrist then takes that information and creates a treatment plan based on the prescription, ensuring

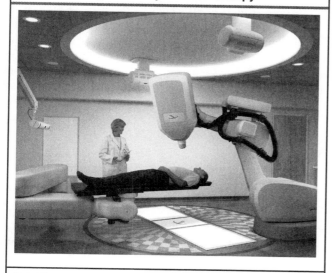

Figure 9-4. CyberKnife Therapy

Note. Photo courtesy of Accuray Incorporated. Used with permission.

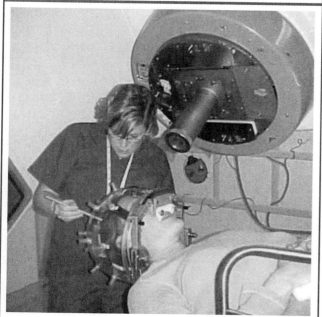

Figure 9-5. Traditional Linac Accelerator with Stereotactic Frame and Depth Helmet

Note. Photo courtesy of the Radiation Medicine Program, Princess Margaret Hospital, Toronto, Ontario, Canada. Used with permission.

precise dose distribution and field plan, which the oncologist will approve prior to treatment.

Planning systems are different for GammaKnife and the linac-based treatments, but RT planning systems are based on the same principles. They vary in how the beams are applied. The GammaKnife plan can conform very well to odd-shaped tumors, and because of the steep dose gradient, adjacent critical structures receive a much lower dose. Treatment can be close to the brain stem and optic nerves, ensuring a high dose to the tumor but sparing these critical structures. With a rapid falloff in dose (Bragg peak), less of the dose reaches the surrounding normal tissues. The drawback is the size of the tumor being treated, with recommendations to treat tumors 4 cm or smaller by GammaKnife (Mintz et al., 2006).

The main reason for choosing different technologies for treating patients relates to the tumor type (infiltrative tumors are not good cases for radiosurgery), tumor size (radiosurgery can only treat tumors 3 cm or smaller), and tumor location (tumors very near the optic nerves or chiasma can be more safely treated with fractionated radiation than with single-fraction radiosurgery) (Mintz et al., 2006).

Treatment Delivery

For fractionated treatments, the patient attends the treatment center daily (Monday through Friday) for the number of weeks required to deliver the fractions of treatment. The patient is also seen weekly in a review clinic to monitor for side effects and progress of treatment, provide ongoing support and education, and document the assessment and any changes to the treatment plan. In the case of SRS, the patient may be at the hospital or treatment center for the full day, which includes application of the treatment frame, CT simulation, and then waiting while the treatment plan is generated. Treatment is then delivered on the same day.

Follow-Up Care

Follow-up care varies with the type of tumor being treated. Patients with malignant gliomas are seen monthly for the adjuvant phase of their chemotherapy, whereas patients with low-grade gliomas are usually seen every three to six months following completion of their radiation. Serial MRI scans for baseline comparison review are performed every three months for at least one year. When tumor and clinical stability is prolonged, the time between MRIs may be extended. Although imaging provides valuable information about the radiologic state of the tumor, a full neurologic assessment by the radiation oncologist and an assessment by the radiation oncology nurse will ensure a global understanding of how the patient is managing following RT. Patients with meningiomas and schwannomas are usually seen every 6–12 months, whereas patients with brain metastases are usually reassessed every 3 months; however, this recommendation may vary among treatment centers.

Radiation Therapy Side Effects and Nursing Interventions

Patients undergoing RT to the brain may experience a number of potential acute side effects over the course of their treatment, as well as in the weeks, months, and years following completion of treatment. Nurses have a key role to play in the assessment, triage, and management of the RT side effects at all stages of the illness. Moreover, because a brain tumor diagnosis can result in the patient experiencing diminished cognitive functioning and physical impairment, nurses must ensure that the primary caregiver or caregivers receive supportive information and education that contributes to their understanding and ability to assist in managing these side effects. The RT side effects may be classified according to time of onset as acute, early delayed, and late delayed reactions (Abrey & Mason, 2003; Hancock & Burrow, 2004; Schultheiss, Kun, Ang, & Stephens, 1995) (see Table 9-1).

Acute Radiation Therapy Side Effects

Acute reactions will occur within hours to days of beginning treatment and are usually transient and not severe. These side effects include alopecia, scalp erythema, serous otitis media, and headache and may or may not be associated with neurologic deficit, nausea and vomiting, fatigue, and seizures (Hancock & Burrow, 2004). Although these side

Table 9-1. Common Side Effects of Radiation Therapy	
Timing During Therapy	Side Effect
Acute	• Alopecia • Scalp erythema • Serous otitis externa • Serous otitis media • Cerebral edema • Seizures • Headache • Nausea and vomiting • Neurologic deficits (motor, speech, vision, memory) • Fatigue
Early delayed	• Somnolence syndrome • Neurologic deficits (motor, speech, vision, memory) • Fatigue
Late	• Radiation necrosis • Dementia • Diminished higher cognitive functioning • Leukoencephalopathy • Decreased hormone production • New neoplasm • Fatigue

effects may appear quickly with the initiation of RT, some, such as fatigue and memory impairment, may persist well into the weeks and months following completion of radiation (Fox, Mitchell, & Booth-Jones, 2006; Schultheiss et al., 1995).

Treatment-related alopecia is an early and very visible side effect of RT that can be distressing for patients. Extent and timing of hair loss are dependent on the RT dose delivered and the size of the treatment field (Hancock & Burrow, 2004). For example, patients receiving focal radiation will experience patchy hair loss, whereas patients receiving WBRT will experience a total loss of hair on the scalp. During a course of fractionated RT, the hair loss typically occurs near the end of the third week of treatment. It may be three to six months following treatment before hair regrowth is seen, and it may continue for up to a year after treatment. Depending on the ultimate dose to the scalp, hair regrowth may be permanently quite thin. Hair color and texture may be altered as hair begins to regrow. Nursing interventions for managing treatment-related alopecia include educating the patient about the probability and timing of this side effect. Suggesting that patients acquire a wig or other suitable headwear prior to the onset of hair loss and referring them to an experienced hairstylist or wig boutique that specializes in assisting patients with cancer will ensure that they are prepared when the hair loss begins. After completion of RT, moisturizing the scalp with an unscented lotion or cream moisturizer will aid in promoting skin and follicle healing for hair regrowth (Bruner et al., 2005).

Erythema of the scalp is a common RT side effect where patients may experience something akin to sunburn. The scalp may become red and tender with some skin flaking. Although it is not usually severe, proper attention to this side effect will help to ameliorate the discomfort patients may experience. In this instance, nurses can provide guidance and expertise with respect to proper skin care and appropriate products that will soothe and assist in the healing of radiation dermatitis.

Serous otitis externa can develop in patients when the ear canal is within the RT field. Typical symptoms include dryness and pruritus of the ear canal. Assessing the degree to which patients are troubled by this side effect will help to determine what course of action, if any, is required. For more severe cases, anti-inflammatory medication and corticosteroid drops may be helpful. However, for most patients, reassurance that this is a common treatment side effect that will resolve on its own over time may be all that is required.

Serous otitis media can occur when the skull base and Eustachian tube are in the field. Typically patients experience a plugged ear sensation associated with decreased hearing, and onset is usually in the last two weeks of a four- to six-week course of RT. It is related to a fluid buildup within the middle ear. This situation typically resolves within two to three months of completing RT, and in rare instances tubes will need to be inserted into the eardrum (Hancock & Burrow, 2004).

With the initiation of RT, patients may experience acute side effects related to cerebral edema. These can include headache, nausea, vomiting, and a variety of neurologic deficits such as hemiparesis, problems with balance and movement, or speech deficits (Hancock & Burrow, 2004; Rabbitt & Page, 1998; Schultheiss et al., 1995). Rapid improvement within 24 hours of these symptoms is often observed with the institution of steroid therapy, most often dexamethasone (Rabbitt & Page, 1998). Steroids work by reducing the edema caused by the brain tumor, relieving the pressure in the brain and thus improving the symptoms. Because nurses have frequent, regular contact with patients throughout the course of their RT, they are well positioned to assess the severity or worsening of these types of neurologic deficits and provide guidance about steroid dosage. Although steroids are very useful in improving neurologic symptoms, they come with myriad side effects of their own, including insomnia, increased appetite and associated weight gain, emotional instability, aggressiveness, Cushingoid sequelae, steroid-induced diabetes, skin reactions, immunosuppression, and muscle atrophy (Batchelor & Byrne, 2006). Nurses need to ensure that patients receive information and teaching about these anticipated side effects so that they will understand when these sometimes puzzling and distressing symptoms appear and what can be done to moderate them. Finally, as a patient progresses through radiation treatment and neurologic symptoms begin to abate, weaning of the steroids is an optimal goal in order to minimize or alleviate the side effects associated with their administration (Rabbitt & Page, 1998). It is important to note that steroids should never be abruptly stopped, but rather, patients should be weaned off them in a planned way. There is no "one size fits all" approach to the weaning process. Factors such as current dosage, length of time on the steroids, amount of residual swelling, and the metabolism of the individual patient will influence how quickly a patient may be able to taper off steroids (Rabbitt & Page, 1998). Nurses can be very helpful by providing clear, written weaning schedules and education to patients and families about dosage adjustment should symptoms worsen during the weaning process. Often, because of the amount of residual tumor, patients may never be able to be completely weaned off steroids, but they should be tapered to the lowest dose possible (Bachelor & Byrne, 2006).

The incidence of seizures in patients with brain tumors is 20%–80% depending on the type of tumor, with low-grade tumors having a higher incidence of seizures than high-grade tumors (Abrey & Mason, 2003; Armstrong, Kanusky, & Gilbert, 2003). Seizure may be part of the initial presentation of the tumor or may occur later on in an individual's disease trajectory. It is important to note that although patients with a brain tumor are at a higher risk of experiencing seizures, RT does not cause the seizures and in fact may actually reduce seizure activity (Abrey & Mason, 2003). Seizures are most effectively treated with antiseizure medication. No set formula is available for prescribing these medications; many choices are available, and what works for one patient may not be effective at achieving reasonable seizure control in another patient. Phenytoin, carbamazepine, valproic acid, and levetiracetam are a few of the more commonly prescribed antiepileptic medications (Armstrong et al., 2003). Some patients may require more than one type of antiepileptic medication to achieve maximal seizure control.

The onset of seizure activity can be very distressing for both the patient and anyone who witnesses the event. Learning to cope with seizures may be part of accepting a new normal way of living. Education about first aid for seizures is crucial. Providing individual counseling to both the patient and caregivers about appropriate responses to seizure activity will help to limit the anxiety and fear surrounding a seizure and will ensure that the patient is safe and reassured during and after the event. Providing written educational material to reinforce this will provide a guide to refer to when necessary. The nurse should provide education to help patients understand the importance of taking their antiseizure medications and adhering to the prescribed treatment. In addition, nurses should ascertain that the patient's antiepileptic drug levels are being regularly monitored to ensure a therapeutic dose of the medication (Lovely, 2004).

Early Delayed Radiation Therapy Side Effects

Early delayed reactions develop within six weeks to six months of RT and are the result of transient demyelination caused by changes in capillary permeability or injury to oligodendrocytes from the radiation (Abrey & Mason, 2003). This condition may lead to a worsening of neurologic symptoms, which are impossible to differentiate from early tumor progression. However, they are reversible and can be effectively treated with steroids in much the same way as acute-onset neurologic side effects. At this time in the treatment trajectory, nurses should be assessing patients for exacerbation or worsening of neurologic symptoms. Providing education and information to patients and families that these changes may be an expected part of the recovery period after the completion of RT will be reassuring.

Radiation somnolence syndrome may be an early delayed reaction to RT. This syndrome is characterized by irritability, drowsiness, lethargy, and fatigue. Patients and caregivers may confuse this syndrome with symptoms associated with the flu (Faithfull & Brada, 1998). Although somnolence syndrome is typically self-limiting and abates over time, patients may feel overwhelmed and anxious with the severity of the symptoms they experience. These feelings of anxiety may be compounded as the somnolence syndrome develops at a phase in treatment where patients do not typically have daily contact with their healthcare team, and the symptoms may be

perceived as tumor progression. Nurses can help to prepare patients and caregivers by providing them with information and education about the possibility of early delayed effects prior to their onset. In addition, if and when these symptoms do occur, telephone support provided by nurses can reassure and guide patients.

Late Delayed Radiation Therapy Side Effects

Late delayed side effects of radiation typically develop months to years after completion of RT and can include radiation necrosis, dementia, effects on higher cognitive functioning, leukoencephalopathy, decreased hormone production, and in rare instances, development of a new neoplasm, usually within the radiation field (Abrey & Mason, 2003; Rabbitt & Page, 1998). Although the development of radionecrosis can occur six months to several years after the delivery of RT, the symptoms may vary in number and severity and include fatigue, memory impairment, personality changes, and dementia. The clinical and radiographic presentation of radionecrosis makes it impossible to distinguish from true tumor progression. Surgical intervention may be the only way to diagnose this unfortunate and potentially devastating side effect of RT to the brain. Treatment with steroids can be a temporizing approach, but in many instances surgery is not required (Abrey & Mason, 2003; Rabbitt & Page, 1998).

The incidence and severity of cognitive impairment following RT are still poorly understood. A variety of additional factors, including age, tumor type, radiation dosage, and exposure to additional treatments, make isolating the direct effect of RT on cognitive functioning difficult. The concept that RT may have a long-term negative impact on cognitive functioning is generally accepted, but the ability to predict who will be affected and to what degree is limited (Armstrong, Gyato, Awadalla, Lustig, & Tochner, 2004). Patients who completed their radiation treatment years prior may experience cognitive side effects ranging from mild to severe cognitive impairment and possible dementia with the loss of ability to care for oneself (Baumgartner, 2004; Fox et al., 2006).

Leukoencephalopathy results from the demyelination of brain lesions, multifocal coagulation of necrosis, and gliosis (Faithfull & Brada, 1998). It is characterized by personality changes, memory problems, disorientation, or dementia. These changes may be permanent. Regardless of the underlying cause or type of cognitive impairment, nursing interventions that address issues of cognitive impairment include encouragement to establish regular routines to cue memory, make and keep lists, or use a personal planner. In addition, reinforcing the benefit of proper rest, nutrition, and activity will help by ensuring that the cognitive challenges experienced by patients are not compounded by other factors such as fatigue, hunger, and boredom (Baumgartner, 2004).

Decreased hormone production can occur when patients have received radiation to the hypothalamic-pituitary axis. In children, the most sensitive hormone is growth hormone, followed by thyroid-stimulating hormone (TSH), and, far less frequently, the cortisol axis or the sex hormone axis. In adults, the most common hormone axis affected is thyroid hormone, which may be affected by lowering TSH by treatment to the brain or direct lowering of thyroid hormone by exit dose to the thyroid itself when craniospinal RT has been delivered (Chi, Béhin, & Delattre, 2008). In all cases, hormone replacement therapy can manage this development.

Finally, patients who have received radiation to the brain have a small risk for developing new neoplasms within the treatment field. This rare complication occurs in about 2%–3% of patients over the following 20 years (Abrey & Mason, 2003). Patients diagnosed with a tumor of the brain, regardless of tumor biology, will be followed closely and for the entire trajectory of their disease.

Nurses have a prominent role to play in the later stages of these diseases in terms of assessing new or worsening side effects and collaborating with the treating physician and members of the allied health team. Referral to community resources at appropriate times is an invaluable and necessary role of the nurse. These could include referrals to community-based nursing support, palliative care programs, support groups, and local or national brain tumor organizations (Laperriere et al., 2002; Leavitt, Lamb, & Voss, 1996). New or worsening symptoms and side effects can be both frightening and anxiety-provoking to patients and families. They present challenges to practical and functional aspects of everyday living. Nurses can provide empathic support and reassurance to contribute to improved quality of life (Leavitt et al., 1996).

Fatigue

Fatigue is a side effect of RT that patients may experience early in the course of RT and may be a lingering side effect months and years after the completion of the treatment. The fatigue that patients may experience may be multifactorial, related not only to their radiation treatment but also to the effects of the brain tumor plus other treatment modalities such as surgery, steroids, and chemotherapy and their associated side effects. It may also be related to the emotional distress of the disease itself (Lovely, 1998; Lovely, Miaskowski, & Dodd, 1999). Regardless of the cause, nurses can be instrumental throughout the disease trajectory with helping patients to live with and manage their fatigue. Increasing fatigue is associated with decreasing quality of life (Lovely et al., 1999). Suggestions for management strategies include energy conservation, pacing activities, adequate rest and relaxation, possibly including massage and healing touch, and engaging in appropriate types of exercise (Mitchell, Beck, Hood, Moore, & Tanner, 2009).

Summary

The diagnosis of a brain tumor is a terrifying and anxiety-provoking experience. For many patients, the diagnosis means a shortened life expectancy, grieving, and loss. For all patients diagnosed with a brain tumor, it is a life-changing experience that will influence the decisions they make and how they live life moving forward. Providing nursing care to patients undergoing RT to the brain for a CNS tumor and their families can be a very challenging but immensely rewarding experience. The diagnosis of a brain tumor brings with it objective symptoms such as headache, neurologic deficits, seizures, and a host of subjective symptoms, which include fatigue, personality changes, and depression.

In many treatment centers, nurses may be the most easily accessible members of the healthcare team, and patients and families will come to rely on nurses for advice and guidance as well as being a conduit for communication among team members. Throughout the RT process, nurses can provide practical, concrete information and advice about issues such as the correct way to take medication and side effect occurrence and management.

Nurses may be the first people to whom patients report new or concerning symptoms. Of equal importance is the provision of psychosocial support. Patients and families are frightened about what lies ahead, anxious about what they will have to experience, and desperately wanting hope and reassurance. CNS tumors affect not only the patients diagnosed with the tumor but also their loved ones. Physical and cognitive changes may make it difficult for the patients to perform the tasks within the family that they have traditionally carried out. Not only does this create a practical problem, but family members also find it emotionally and psychologically difficult to accept these very concrete changes in the person they knew. Referring both patients and caregivers to local community, psychoeducational, or psychotherapy support groups can help to connect them with others in similar circumstances (Honea et al., 2009). Knowledge about RT planning and delivery to the CNS, excellent assessment skills, and symptom management expertise are critical to support and guide patients during and following RT.

References

Abrey, L.E., & Mason, W.P. (2003). *Fast facts: Brain tumors*. Oxford, UK: Health Press Ltd.

Andersen, A.P. (1978). Postoperative irradiation of glioblastomas. Results in a randomized series. *Acta Radiologica: Oncology, Radiation, Physics, Biology, 17,* 475–484.

Andrews, D.W., Scott, C.B., Sperduto, P.W., Flanders, A.E., Gaspar, L.E., Schell, M.C., … Curran, W.J., Jr. (2004). Whole brain radiation therapy with or without stereotactic radiosurgery boost for patients with one to three brain metastases: Phase III results of the RTOG 9508 randomised trial. *Lancet, 363,* 1665–1672. doi:10.1016/S0140-6736(04)16250-8

Aoyama, H., Shirato, H., Tago, M., Nakagawa, K., Toyoda, T., Hatano, K., ... Kobashi, G. (2006). Stereotactic radiosurgery plus whole-brain radiation therapy vs. stereotactic radiosurgery alone for treatment of brain metastases: A randomized controlled trial. *JAMA, 295,* 2483–2491. doi:10.1001/jama.295.21.2483

Armstrong, C.L., Gyato, K., Awadalla, A.W., Lustig, R., & Tochner, Z.A. (2004). A critical review of the clinical effects of therapeutic irradiation damage to the brain: The roots of controversy. *Neuropsychology Review, 14,* 65–86.

Armstrong, T.S., Kanusky, J.T., & Gilbert, M.R. (2003). Seize the moment and learn about epilepsy in people with cancer. *Clinical Journal of Oncology Nursing, 7,* 163–169. doi:10.1188/03. CJON.163-169

Athanassiou, H., Synodinou, M., Maragoudakis, E., Paraskevaidis, M., Verigos, C., Misailidou, D., ... Karageorgis, P. (2005). Randomized phase II study of temozolomide and radiotherapy compared with radiotherapy alone in newly diagnosed glioblastoma multiforme. *Journal of Clinical Oncology, 23,* 2372–2377. doi:10.1200/JCO.2005.00.331

Batchelor, T.T., & Byrne, T.N. (2006). Supportive care of brain tumor patients. *Hematology/Oncology Clinics of North America, 20,* 1337–1361. doi:10.1016/j.hoc.2006.09.013

Baumgartner, K. (2004). Neurocognitive changes in cancer patients. *Seminars in Oncology Nursing, 20,* 284–290.

Behin, A., Hoang-Xuan, K., Carpentier, A.F., & Delattre, J. (2003). Primary brain tumours in adults. *Lancet, 361,* 323–331. doi:10.1016/S0140-6736(03)12328-8

Bleehen, N.M., & Stenning, S.P. (1991). A Medical Research Council trial of two radiotherapy doses in the treatment of grades 3 and 4 astrocytoma. The Medical Research Council Brain Tumour Working Party. *British Journal of Cancer, 64,* 769–774. Retrieved from http://www.ncbi.nlm.nih.gov/pmc/articles/PMC1977696/pdf/brjcancer00074-0171.pdf

Bruner, D.W., Haas, M.L., & Gosselin-Acomb, T.K. (Eds.) (2005). *Manual for radiation oncology nursing practice and education* (3rd ed.). Pittsburgh, PA: Oncology Nursing Society.

Buatti, J., Ryken, T.C., Olson, J.J., Smith, M.C., Sneed, P., Suh, J.H., & Mehta, M. (2008). New treatment guidelines for newly diagnosed glioblastoma issued by American Association of Neurological Surgeons/Congress of Neurological Surgeons. *Oncology Times, 30*(19), 30–32. doi:10.1097/01.COT.0000340746.00671.e9

Bussière, M.R., & Adams, J.A. (2003). Treatment planning for conformal proton radiation therapy. *Technology in Cancer Research and Treatment, 2,* 389–399.

Chen, M.J., Santos Ada, S., Sakuraba, R.K., Lopes, C.P., Gonçalves, V.D., Weltman, E., ... Cruz, J.C. (2010). Intensity-modulated and 3D-conformal radiotherapy for whole-ventricular irradiation as compared with conventional whole-brain irradiation in the management of localized central nervous system germ cell tumors. *International Journal of Radiation Oncology, Biology, Physics, 76,* 608–614. doi:10.1016/j.ijrobp.2009.06.028

Chi, D., Béhin, A., & Delattre, J. (2008). Neurologic complications of radiation therapy. In D. Schiff, S. Kesari, & P.Y. Wen (Eds.), *Cancer neurology in clinical practice: Neurologic complications of cancer and its treatment* (2nd ed., pp. 259–286). Totowa, NJ: Humana Press.

Combs, S.E., Debus, J., & Schulz-Ertner, D. (2007). Radiotherapeutic alternatives for previously irradiated recurrent gliomas. *BMC Cancer, 7,* 167. doi:10.1186/1471-2407-7-167

Davey, P. (2002). Brain metastasis: Treatment options to improve outcomes. *CNS Drugs, 16,* 325–338.

Elia, A.E., Shih, H.A., & Loeffler, J.S. (2007). Stereotactic radiation treatment for benign meningiomas. *Neurosurgical Focus, 23,* E5. doi:10.3171/FOC-07/10/E5

Faithfull, S., & Brada, M. (1998). Somnolence syndrome in adults following cranial irradiation for primary brain tumours. *Clinical Oncology, 10,* 250–254. doi:10.1016/S0936-6555(98)80011-3

Fenwick, J.D., Tomé, W.A., Soisson, E.T., Mehta, M.P., & Mackie, T.R. (2006). Tomotherapy and other innovative IMRT delivery systems. *Seminars in Radiation Oncology, 16,* 199–208. doi:10.1016/j.semradonc.2006.04.002

Fox, S.W., Mitchell, S.A., & Booth-Jones, M. (2006). Cognitive impairment in patients with brain tumors: Assessment and intervention in the clinic setting. *Clinical Journal of Oncology Nursing, 10,* 169–176.

Fuller, C.D., Choi, M., Forthuber, B., Wang, S.J., Rajagiriyil, N., Salter, B.J., & Fuss, M. (2007). Standard fractionation intensity modulated radiation therapy (IMRT) of primary and recurrent glioblastoma multiforme. *Radiation Oncology, 2,* 26. doi:10.1186/1748-717X-2-26

Gerosa, M., Nicolato, A., Foroni, R., Tomazzoli, L., & Bricolo, A. (2004). Regional treatment of metastasis: Role of radiosurgery in brain metastasis—gamma knife radiosurgery. *Annals of Oncology, 15*(Suppl. 4), iv113–iv117. doi:10.1093/annonc/mdh914

Greco, C., & Ling, C.C. (2008). Broadening the scope of image-guided radiotherapy (IGRT). *Acta Oncologica, 47,* 1193–1200. doi:10.1080/02841860802241956

Hancock, C.M., & Burrow, M.A. (2004). The role of radiation therapy in the treatment of central nervous system tumors. *Seminars in Oncology Nursing, 20,* 253–259. doi:10.1016/j.soncn.2004.07.005

Hochberg, F.H., & Pruitt, A. (1980). Assumptions in the radiotherapy of glioblastoma. *Neurology, 30,* 907–911.

Honea, N.J., Sherwood, P.R., Northouse, L.L., Brintnall, R.A., Colao, D.B., Somers, S.C., & Given, B.A. (2009). ONS PEP resource: Caregiver strain and burden. In L.H. Eaton & J.M. Tipton (Eds.), *Putting evidence into practice: Improving oncology patient outcomes* (pp. 57–62). Pittsburgh, PA: Oncology Nursing Society.

Horiot, J.C., van den Bogaert, W., Ang, K.K., Van der Schueren, E., Bartelink, H., Gonzalez, D., ... Blabbeke, M. (1988). European Organization for Research and Treatment of Cancer trials using radiotherapy with multiple fractions per day: A 1978–1987 survey. *Frontiers in Radiation Therapy and Oncology, 22,* 149–161.

Hoskin, P.J., & Brada, M. (2001). Radiotherapy for brain metastasis: Second Workshop on Palliative Radiotherapy and Symptom Control. *Clinical Oncology, 13,* 91–94.

Huncharek, M. (1998). Meta-analytic re-evaluation of misonidazole in the treatment of high grade glioma. *Anticancer Research, 18,* 1935–1939.

Karim, A.B.M.F., Afra, D., Cornu, P., Bleehan, N., Schraub, S., De Witte, O., ... Van Glabbeke, M. (2002). Randomized trial on the efficacy of radiotherapy for cerebral low-grade glioma in the adult: European Organization for Research and Treatment of Cancer Study 22845 with the Medical Research Council study BRO4: An interim analysis. *International Journal of Radiation Oncology, Biology, Physics, 52,* 316–324.

Keime-Guibert, F., Chinot, O., Taillandier, L., Cartalat-Carel, S., Frenay, M., Kantor, G., ... Delattre, J.Y. (2007). Radiotherapy for glioblastoma in the elderly. *New England Journal of Medicine, 356,* 1527–1535. doi:10.1056/NEJMoa065901

Kita, M., Okawa, T., Tanaka, M., & Ikeda, M. (1989). Radiotherapy of malignant glioma—prospective randomized clinical study of whole brain vs. local irradiation. *Gan No Rinsh, 35,* 1289–1294.

Kleinberg, L., Yoon, G., Weingart, J.D., Parisi, M., Olivi, A., Detorie, N., & Chan, T.A. (2009). Imaging after GliaSite brachytherapy: Prognostic MRI indicators of disease control and recurrence. *International Journal of Radiation Oncology, Biology, Physics, 75,* 1385–1391. doi:10.1016/j.ijrobp.2008.12.074

Kristiansen, K., Hagen, S., Kollevold, T., Torvik, A., Holme, I., Nesbakken, R., ... Elgen, K. (1981). Combined modality therapy of operated astrocytomas grade III and IV. Confirmation of the value of postoperative irradiation and lack of potentiation of bleomycin on survival time: A prospective multicenter trial of the Scandinavian Glioblastoma Study Group. *Cancer, 47,* 649–652.

Kushen, M.C., Sonabend, A.M., & Lesniak, M.S. (2007). Current immunotherapeutic strategies for central nervous system tumors. *Surgical Oncology Clinics of North America, 16,* 987–1004. doi:10.1016/j.soc.2007.07.003

Laperriere, N., Perry, J., Zuraw, L., & Cancer Care Ontario Practice Guidelines Initiative Neuro-Oncology Disease Site Group. (2005). *Radiotherapy for newly diagnosed malignant glioma in adults: A clinical practice guideline.* Retrieved from http://www.cancercare. on.ca/common/pages/UserFile.aspx?fileId=14234

Laperriere, N.J., Leung, P.M., McKenzie, S., Milosevic, M., Wong, S., Glen, J., ... Bernstein, M. (1998). Randomized study of brachytherapy in the initial management of patients with malignant astrocytoma. *International Journal of Radiation Oncology, Biology, Physics, 41,* 1005–1011.

Laperriere, N.J., Zuraw, L., Cairncross, G., & Cancer Care Ontario Practice Guidelines Initiative Neuro-Oncology Disease Site Group. (2002). Radiotherapy for newly diagnosed malignant glioma in adults: A systematic review. *Radiotherapy and Oncology, 64,* 259–273.

Leavitt, M.B., Lamb, S.A., & Voss, B.S. (1996). Brain tumor support group: Content themes and mechanisms of support. *Oncology Nursing Forum, 23,* 1247–1256.

Lovely, M.P. (1998). Quality of life of brain tumor patients. *Seminars in Oncology Nursing, 14,* 73–80.

Lovely, M.P. (2004). Symptom management of brain tumor patients. *Seminars in Oncology Nursing, 20,* 273–283.

Lovely, M.P., Miaskowski, C., & Dodd, M. (1999). Relationship between fatigue and quality of life in patient with glioblastoma multiforme. *Oncology Nursing Forum, 26,* 921–925.

McDermott, M.W., Berger, M.S., Kunwar, S., Parsa, A.T., Sneed, P.K., & Larson, D.A. (2004). Stereotactic radiosurgery and interstitial brachytherapy for glial neoplasms. *Journal of Neuro-Oncology, 69,* 83–100. doi:10.1023/B:NEON.0000041873.42938.13

McDermott, M.W., & Sneed, P.K. (2005). Radiosurgery in metastatic brain cancer. *Neurosurgery, 57*(Suppl. 5), S45–S53.

Mintz, A.P., Perry, J., Laperriere, N., Cairncross, G., Chambers, A., Spithoff, K., & the Neuro-Oncology Disease Site Group. (2006, August). *Management of single brain metastasis: A clinical practice guideline.* Retrieved from http://www.cancercare.on.ca/ common/pages/UserFile.aspx?fileId=14226

Mirimanoff, R.O. (2004). New radiotherapy technologies for meningiomas: 3D conformal radiotherapy? Radiosurgery? Stereotactic radiotherapy? Intensity-modulated radiotherapy? Proton beam radiotherapy? Spot scanning proton radiation therapy ... or nothing at all? *Radiotherapy and Oncology, 71,* 247–249. doi:10.1016/j.radonc.2004.05.002

Mitchell, S.A., Beck, S.L., Hood, L.E., Moore, K., & Tanner, E.R. (2009). ONS PEP resource: Fatigue. In L.H. Eaton & J.M. Tipton (Eds.), *Putting evidence into practice: Improving oncology patient outcomes* (pp. 155–174). Pittsburgh, PA: Oncology Nursing Society.

Myresth, E., Møller, P., Pedersen, P.H., & Lund-Johansen, M. (2009). Vestibular schwannoma: Surgery or gamma knife radiosurgery? A prospective, nonrandomized study. *Neurosurgery, 64,* 654–671. doi:10.1227/01.NEU.0000340684.60443.55

Nelson, D.F., Diener-West, M., Horton, J., Chang, C.H., Schoenfeld, D., & Nelson, J.S. (1988). Combined modality approach to treatment of malignant gliomas—re-evaluation of RTOG 7401/ ECOG 1374 with long-term follow-up: A joint study of the Radiation Therapy Oncology Group and the Eastern Cooperative Oncology Group. *Journal of the National Cancer Institute Monographs, 6,* 279–284.

Rabbitt, J.E., & Page, M.S. (1998). Selected complications in neuro-oncology patients. *Seminars in Oncology Nursing, 14,* 53–60. doi:10.1016/S0749-2081(98)80043-0

Roa, W., Brasher, P.M.A., Bauman, G., Anthes, M., Bruera, E., Chan, B., ... Forsyth, P. (2004). Abbreviated course of radiation therapy in older patients with glioblastoma multiforme: A prospective randomized clinical trial. *Journal of Clinical Oncology, 22,* 1583–1588. doi:10.1200/JCO.2004.06.082

Schaefer, P.W., Budzik, R.F., Jr., & Gonzalez, R.G. (1996). Imaging of cerebral metastasis. *Neurosurgery Clinics of North America, 7,* 393–423.

Schnell, O., Schöller, K., Ruge, M., Siefert, A., Tonn, J.C., & Kreth, F.W. (2008). Surgical resection plus stereotactic ^{125}I brachytherapy in adult patients with eloquently located supratentorial WHO grade II glioma—Feasibility and outcome of a combined local treatment concept. *Journal of Neurology, 255,* 1495–1502. doi:10.1007/ s00415-008-0948-x

Schultheiss, T.E., Kun, L.E., Ang, K.K., & Stephens, L.C. (1995). Radiation response of the central nervous system. *International Journal of Radiation Oncology, Biology, Physics, 31,* 1093–1112.

Scott, C.B., Curran, W.J., Yung, W.K., Scarantino, C., Urtasun, R., Movsas, B., ... Nelson, J. (1998). Long-term results of RTOG 9006: A randomized study of hyperfractionated radiotherapy (RT) to 72.0 Gy and carmustine vs. standard RT for malignant glioma patients with emphasis on anaplastic astrocytoma (AA) patients [Abstract]. *Proceedings of the Annual Meeting of the American Society of Clinical Oncology, 17,* 401a.

Shapiro, W.R., & Young, D.F. (1976). Treatment of malignant glioma. A controlled study of chemotherapy and irradiation. *Archives in Neurology, 33,* 494–500.

Strzelczyk, J., & Safadi, R. (2004). Radiation safety considerations in GliaSite ^{125}I brain implant procedures. *Health Physics, 86*(Suppl. 2), S120–S123.

Stupp, R., Hegi, M.E., Mason, W.P., van den Bent, M.J., Taphoorn, M.J., Janzer, R.C., ... Mirimanoff, R.O. (2009). Effects of radiotherapy with concomitant and adjuvant temozolomide versus radiotherapy alone on survival in glioblastoma in a randomised phase III study: 5-year analysis of the EORTC-NCIC trial. *Lancet Oncology, 10,* 459–466. doi:10.1016/S1470-2045(09)70025-7

Stupp, R., Mason, W.P., van den Bent, M.J., Weller, M., Fisher, B., Taphoorn, M.J.B., ... Mirimanoff, R.O. (2005). Radiotherapy plus concomitant and adjuvant temozolomide for glioblastoma. *New England Journal of Medicine, 352,* 987–996. doi:10.1056/ NEJMoa043330

Suh, J.H., & Barnett, G.H. (1999). Brachytherapy for brain tumors. *Hematology/Oncology Clinics of North America, 13,* 635–650.

Voynov, G., Kaufman, S., Hong, T., Pinkerton, A., Simon, R., & Dowsett, R. (2002). Treatment of recurrent malignant gliomas with stereotactic intensity modulated radiation therapy. *American Journal of Clinical Oncology, 25,* 606–611.

Walker, M.D., Alexander, E., Jr., Hunt, W.E., MacCarty, C.S., Mahaley, M.T., Jr., Mealey, J., Jr., ... Strike, T.A. (1978). Evaluation of BCNU and/or radiotherapy in the treatment of anaplastic gliomas: A cooperative clinical trial. *Journal of Neurosurgery, 49,* 333–343. doi:10.3171/jns.1978.49.3.0333

Walker, M.D., Green, S.B., Byar, D.P., Alexander, E., Jr., Batzdorf, U., Brooks, W.H., ... Strike, T.A. (1980). Randomized comparisons of radiotherapy and nitrosoureas for the treatment of malignant glioma after surgery. *New England Journal of Medicine, 303,* 1323–1329.

Wallner, K.E., Galicich, J.H., Krol, G., Arbit, E., & Malkin, M.G. (1989). Patterns of failure following treatment for glioblastoma multiforme and anaplastic astrocytoma. *International Journal of Radiation Oncology, Biology, Physics, 16,* 1405–1409. doi:10.1016/0360-3016(89)90941-3

Werner-Wasik, M., Scott, C.B., Nelson, D.F., Gaspar, L.E., Murray, K.J., Fischbach, J.A., ... Curran, W.J., Jr. (1996). Final report of a phase I/II trial of hyperfractionated and accelerated hyperfractionated radiation therapy with carmustine for adults with supratentorial malignant gliomas. Radiation Therapy Oncology Group Study 83-02. *Cancer, 77,* 1535–1543.

doi:10.1002/(SICI)1097-0142(19960415)77:8<1535::AID-CNCR17>3.0.CO;2-0

Wernicke, A.G., Sherr, D.L., Schwartz, T.H., Pannullo, S.C., Stieg, P.E., Boockvar, J.A., ... Nori, D. (2010). The role of dose escalation with intracavitary brachytherapy in the treatment of localized CNS malignancies: Outcomes and toxicities of a prospective study. *Brachytherapy, 9,* 91–99. doi:10.1016/j.brachy.2009.06.005

CHAPTER 10

Special Considerations: Pediatric Therapeutic Modalities

Corrine Hoeppner, MSN, ARNP

Introduction

The diagnosis of a brain tumor in a child carries with it myriad considerations specific to the pediatric population. Brain development starts in utero, continues rapidly from birth, and reaches mature levels of nerve fiber tracts and a high level of gray matter development by four years old. From birth through adolescence alone, brain volume increases fourfold (Johnson, 2001). Because of the vulnerability of the location of central nervous system (CNS) tumors, as well as the morbidity of the current treatments, these tumors can present a potentially devastating prognosis. However, advances over the past two decades in imaging modalities, ongoing research, advances in current treatments, and the judicious use of effective chemotherapy agents have made for increased survival rates in the population with pediatric tumors. Multidisciplinary teams are vital in the ongoing care of children with CNS tumors, with nurses and advanced practice nurses participating as a valuable part of this team.

Brain tumors are the most common solid tumor diagnosed in childhood, and even brain tumors that are histologically considered benign can create troublesome to potentially life-threatening symptoms. Approximately 3,750 children were diagnosed with a brain tumor in 2007, and of those, 2,820 were younger than 15 years old. The highest incidence of brain tumors occurs in children from birth to four years old. The survival rate is 72.1% for individuals younger than 19 years old who are diagnosed with primary brain and CNS tumors (Central Brain Tumor Registry of the United States, 2010). With so many different subtypes of tumors, the number of children with each type of tumor will be small, especially in comparison to adult numbers. As opposed to adult brain tumors, which are most often in the cerebrum, approximately 60% of all pediatric brain tumors are located in the posterior fossa, consisting of the brain stem and cerebellum (see Chapter 2, Figures 2-3 and 2-6) (von Koch, Schmidt, & Perry, 2004). The symptom management of children with CNS tumors is very different than from the adult population, particularly in children younger than six years old

who are still undergoing neuronal development and are much more vulnerable to treatment morbidities. Over the past decades, all three of the treatment modalities—surgery, radiation, and chemotherapy—for pediatric CNS tumors have improved. One outcome of increased survivorship is that clinicians now realize that long-term effects of having and surviving a brain tumor can be complex and life altering.

Surgical Considerations in Pediatric Patients

Surgical resection of a brain tumor is the frontline treatment of a tumor, with few exceptions. Intrinsic brain stem tumors are not resected because of their infiltrative qualities into the brain stem, which would make for unacceptable morbidities. Pineal region and deep, centrally located tumors that are difficult to access without potential harm to the patient but could be highly responsive to chemotherapy and radiation are often biopsied and not fully resected. These include germ cell tumors and pineoblastomas (Miller, 2001).

Surgery is most often the primary treatment modality in pediatric CNS tumors and for some histologically benign tumors can sometimes be the only treatment, along with close postsurgical follow-up. A complete surgical resection is prognostic of a favorable outcome in malignant tumors. If less than a gross total resection of the tumor, a second surgery is warranted, often after chemotherapy courses are used to potentially shrink the tumor (Abdullah, Qaddoumi, & Bouffet, 2008). The extent of the care of these patients is determined by the age of the child, the location of the tumor, the patient's preoperative or postoperative clinical status, and the extent of the surgery.

More aggressive surgeries can be performed with less damage to the child through advances in computer-guided stereotaxis, laser dissection of the tumor, and intraoperative physiologic monitoring that can inform the surgeon of potential damage to vital brain structures (Ahn & Goumnerova, 2010). In addition, improved surgical techniques have changed the recovery period of children after removal of CNS tumors. The use of endoscopy and intraoperative guidance systems have shortened the recovery period for children postoperatively. Preoperatively, the use of new imaging modalities, such as functional magnetic resonance imaging (fMRI), have reduced postoperative morbidity. fMRI is a specialized MRI scan that measures the hemodynamic response of a neural stimulus in the brain. This means that when an area responsible for some type of language or motor function is utilized by an awake patient undergoing fMRI, this neural area of the brain will be identified through color coding on the fMRI (Vézina, 2008). This helps the surgeon to map out important areas of function prior to surgery. Given that a near-complete surgical resection greatly improves outcomes in children with malignant tumors, these recent surgical advances leading to more aggressive surgeries with less morbidity have contributed greatly to the ongoing improved survival in children with CNS tumors (Vézina, 2008).

Most children with CNS tumors present with increased intracranial pressure (Miller, 2001), and surgical removal of the tumor is often the first step in decreasing intracranial pressure. Postoperatively, most patients with infratentorial tumors will have in place an external drain to remove excess cerebrospinal fluid (CSF). Steroids, most often dexamethasone, are almost universally used postoperatively for craniotomies. Although very effective as anti-inflammatory agents, they have short- and long-term side effects that take their toll on the pediatric patient. The short-term side effects include increased appetite, weight gain, susceptibility to infection, potentially severe irritability, and sleep difficulties (Taketomo, Hodding, & Kraus, 2009). In an already stressful postoperative period, many of these side effects are intolerable. Steroids should be tapered as quickly as possible and increased again in the postoperative period only if the patient experiences a sudden loss of neurologic function, with the goal being to preserve long-term overall ability.

Increased intracranial pressure and the presence of a supratentorial tumor can put the pediatric patient at risk for a seizure before tumor detection, during the surgery, and after the removal of the tumor. Multiple opinions exist regarding the use of anticonvulsant therapy postoperatively, but it is generally thought to be judicious to use some type of antiseizure medication, for a period of six weeks to six months if used prophylactically or potentially for the patient's lifetime if a seizure disorder occurs as a result of the tumor or surgery (Khan, Boop, Onar, & Sanford, 2006). Electrocorticography is helpful in the identification of true seizure activity in the cerebral cortex. Seizures can look very different from what is perceived, ranging from subtle eye movements in infants to grand mal, tonic/clonic activity. Adding to this complexity in children is their inability to report symptoms in a way that would lead quickly to a diagnosis of a seizure. Teaching points for families include identifying normal neurologic behavior in children, such as

"jerking" movements during sleep, and encouraging families to be aware of and to report other suspicious symptoms (Wilson & Bryant, 2007).

In the postoperative period, clinical changes in the pediatric patient can happen quickly and can be potentially life threatening. A loss of neurologic function in patients with a CNS tumor could be permanent; therefore, close monitoring requiring a postoperative stay in the pediatric intensive care unit is warranted. Immediate postoperative nursing considerations for patients with a CNS tumor include support for the family at a very critical time and identification and possible notification of the multidisciplinary brain tumor team. This team often consists of a pediatric oncologist that specializes in neuro-oncology and a specialized neuro-oncology nurse or advanced practice nurse. Early intervention of support through child life specialists and social workers can also help, as the family is likely facing the beginning of a long treatment process, and early identification of stressful procedural situations for the child could help for long-term coping (Wilson & Bryant, 2007).

Posterior fossa syndrome, also called cerebellar mutism, is a symptom complex including decreased or absent speech, irritability, hypotonia (low muscle tone), ataxia (unsteadiness and deceased coordination), and the inability to coordinate voluntary movements. It is seen after surgery for tumors in the posterior fossa region of the brain (see Figure 10-1) and affects about 25% of patients with cerebellar

Figure 10-1. Posterior Fossa Syndrome

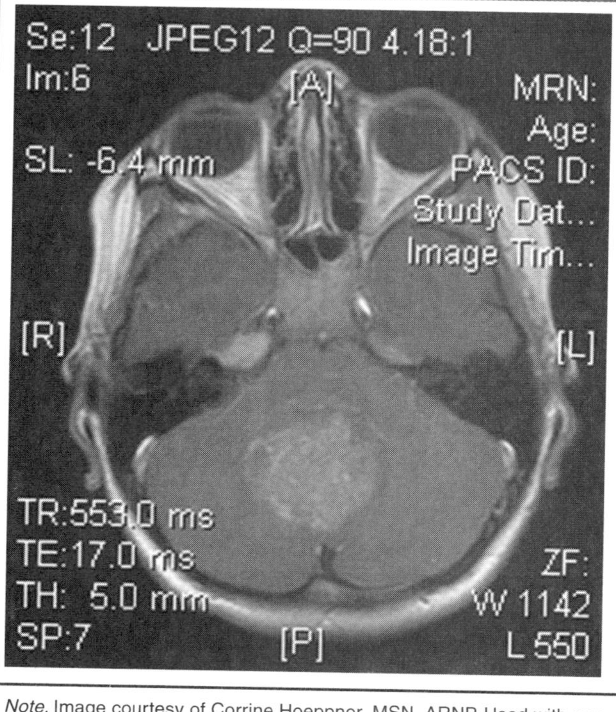

Note. Image courtesy of Corrine Hoeppner, MSN, ARNP. Used with permission.

tumors, most commonly medulloblastomas, astrocytomas, and ependymomas (Taylor & Rutka, 2008). It is reported in adults but is most commonly seen in pediatrics. The exact cause of posterior fossa syndrome is unknown, but it has been associated with more midline tumors and was thought to be caused by the splitting of the vermis, the thick layer of tissue that separates the lobes of the cerebellum. However, recent theories suggest that it may be caused by injury to both sets of dentatothalamocortical outflow tracks from the cerebellum to the cerebral cortex. These tracts are the nerve fibers that arise from the vermis and communicate out to the lobes of the cerebellum. The children who are affected often wake up postoperatively able to talk, but their speech is often atonal and with a flat affect. Within 24–48 hours, the child stops talking, may develop generalized weakness, and can develop severe emotional irritability. The syndrome presents as a spectrum, and deficits range from mild to incapacitating. Mutism has been reported to last as few as six days and as many as 52 months (Kirk, Howard, & Scott, 1995). No cases have been reported where a child with cerebellar mutism did not regain functional speech; however, the quality of this speech is often changed, becoming slower, higher pitched, and atonal. Nursing care of a child with posterior fossa syndrome is extremely challenging, as the families are experiencing a completely altered child postoperatively, with no good answers as to when the child will recover. Agents such as risperidone and lorazepam show some limited ability to help with the irritability caused by the syndrome (Charalambides, Dinopoulos, & Sgouros, 2009). Intensive rehabilitation, especially speech therapy, is required for these children but may not be immediately effective if the syndrome is severe. Speech therapy is effective in providing children who cannot verbally communicate with an alternative communication means, such as hand signals, sign language, and communication boards (De Smet et al., 2009).

Radiation Therapy

Radiation therapy remains one of the core modalities of treatment for pediatric brain tumors despite the risk of long-term radiation exposure (Radiation Therapy Oncology Group [RTOG], 2009). Nursing considerations differ for infants compared to older children but for all ages include education, treatment coordination, and management of side effects. Radiation advances over the past few decades have limited the field of exposure of healthy tissue to radiation beams, but treatment requires strict immobilization. This includes the children having a tight mask fitted over their face to keep them still during delivery of radiation. The mask is a mesh-like material that is bolted to the radiation table. For older children, this often requires a skilled team that ideally includes child life therapists to help these children deal

with this process, which usually lasts an average of 25–35 sessions. For younger children, those who are cognitively delayed, and sometimes for children with severe postoperative posterior fossa syndrome, immobilization can only be achieved through anesthesia. Ideally, these children should be scheduled early in the morning because they will not be allowed to eat anything for a time prior to undergoing anesthesia.

Radiation Side Effects

Radiation side effects depend mostly on the area of the tumor, although full craniospinal radiation is common in the treatment of malignant tumors, especially in children older than three years old (Duffner et al., 1993). Radiation should be delayed until a child is at least 12 months old, and focal radiation should be used as much as possible, especially in children younger than three years old. Younger children, especially infants, are much more vulnerable to the long-term effects of radiation because their brains remain in critical stages of development (RTOG, 2009). Generally, acute radiation side effects include nausea and vomiting, fatigue, hair loss that may be permanent, and loss of appetite. The acute side effects are often from swelling in the area of the radiation field and can be managed by steroids. Ideally, a short and higher dose burst of steroids should be used and then rapidly tapered as the swelling decreases, which will be apparent by the decrease in symptoms. The acute effect period is defined as side effects that occur during the course of treatment and two to four months after radiation.

Especially challenging are brain stem tumors, which in children are often large in this critical area. Not only do symptoms related to critical structures occur, but even mild swelling in this area can cause the blockage of CSF flow, resulting in hydrocephalus. This may warrant high doses of steroids and symptom management that may be too complex for outpatient management. Cerebellar tumor symptoms include a possible exacerbation of posterior fossa syndrome symptoms, ataxia, and visual changes. Radiation to the area of the hypothalamus results in decreased appetite, acute endocrine dysfunction, and possible sudden-onset vision changes. Supratentorial radiation side effects can also result in decreased appetite, as well as personality changes, increased impairment to speech and motor function, and seizures. Full craniospinal radiation is more likely to cause a decrease in blood counts resulting in immune suppression because of the direct effect of radiation bone marrow suppression in a large volume of the skull and spinal bones (CureSearch.org Medical Editorial Board, 2006).

Fatigue is another acute radiation side effect, which can be mild to severe. Somnolence syndrome is experienced more in children than in adults and is a period of extreme sleepiness along with symptoms of headache, loss of appetite, irritability, and nausea that occurs around one to six months after radiation. It will spontaneously resolve within days to weeks, but symptoms can be reduced by a short course of steroids (RTOG, 2009). Adequate nutrition during radiation can be very challenging because of both appetite suppression and the possibility of these children being on food and liquid restriction for the procedure. Radiation is often administered postoperatively and prior to a potentially long course of chemotherapy, when it may also be difficult to continue to maintain adequate nutrition. Nurses can be essential advocates when nutrition begins to be an issue by including a nutritionist in the care plan, as well as educating and assisting the family with decisions regarding enteral feeding to prevent severe malnourishment (Wilson & Bryant, 2007).

Long-term side effects have been reduced over the past two decades by the introduction of new radiation techniques, developed when it became clear that pediatric patients who became long-term survivors had considerable challenges after their CNS tumor treatment. The pathophysiology of long-term effects is based on both the direct effects of radiation on glial cells and the effect of radiation on the vasculature of the brain (RTOG, 2009). The predominant long-term side effects are a potential for severe decreased cognitive ability, problems with short-term memory, hearing loss, and hormonal deficiencies, including growth failure and precocious puberty.

Many of the technologic advances in radiation therapy over the past 20 years have been in the arena of delivery, as photons and protons continue to be the radiation sources used. High-resolution imaging has made it easier to determine tumor targets. Immobilization techniques, especially of the very young, have improved. Technologically advanced radiation software has allowed for three-dimensional conformal radiation to be developed. This has enabled radiation oncologists to substantially decrease the size of the field needed to cover the tumor, the standard being the target plus a margin. Through blocking and beam arrangements, critical normal tissue can be spared. Intensity-modulated radiation therapy is a recent innovation that uses multiple non-uniform beams to configure the radiation dose in a precise manner around a normal structure (Yock & Tarbell, 2004).

Proton Beam Radiation

Technologic advances in radiation therapy over the past 20 years have sought to improve both short-term and long-term side effects in patients with CNS tumors. The goal is to adequately treat the tumor while trying to avoid untargeted, normal brain structures (Yock & Tarbell, 2004). Photon beams are the radiation energy source used at most cancer centers. High-energy photons are x-rays that are produced by a linear accelerator. As the photon beam enters the patient, energy in the path initially increases and then exponentially decreases as the beam exits the patient. This means that normal tissue will be exposed to radiation, albeit in lower doses than the target area.

An alternative source of radiation is the proton. Proton beams are produced by a cyclotron and have a very different size and mass compared to photons. The energy produced along the path of the beam is low, increases as the beam deposits energy at the target, and produces no exit dose. Limiting radiation exposure to healthy tissue in this way will hopefully decrease long-term side effects (Kirsch & Tarbell, 2004). When comparing both modalities, the radiation dose delivered to normal tissue through proton beam therapy is approximately one-half of the exposure that photon beam therapy creates (Yock & Tarbell, 2004). The long-term effects of proton beam therapy continue to be studied, with the hope that the long-term side effects of radiation on children with CNS tumors can be ameliorated, especially in cognition and learning difficulties. To date, only a small number of proton beam centers around the world are capable of treating children with CNS tumors.

Chemotherapy

The use of chemotherapy in the treatment of pediatric brain tumors has changed significantly over the past 30 years. In the past decade it has come to include new categories of chemotherapy agents, including biologic therapy and antiangiogenesis agents, which will be discussed in the following section. Chemotherapy for use in brain tumors must be very specific, as many agents do not cross the blood-brain barrier and are therefore toxic to the host without being toxic to the tumor. Because of this, it is very important that pediatric patients with brain tumors are treated in a standard way, with agents that have been researched, tested, and known to be effective. Because each geographic area in any region would have a small number of pediatric patients diagnosed each year, cooperative groups started forming in the 1970s to provide national and international research on pediatric patients, with the goal to treat all pediatric patients with cancer using standardized regimens. Studies within groups such as the Children's Oncology Group have been responsible for increasing progression-free survival of patients with CNS tumors.

The goal of chemotherapy agents is to interfere with or destroy the tumor cells in a variety of ways that prevents them from proliferating. The ultimate goal is to make the tumors both go away and stay away. Chemotherapy is most often administered as combination therapy, either with other chemotherapy agents or in combination with radiation in an attempt to increase the effectiveness of the radiation. Table 10-1 gives an overview of agents specifically used with CNS tumors (Wilson & Bryant, 2007).

Overview of Biologic Agents Used in Pediatrics

A more recent development in chemotherapy agents is the use of biologic agents. As opposed to conventional

Table 10-1. Overview of Agents Used in the Treatment of Pediatric Brain Tumors		
Type of Chemotherapy	Name of Drug	Common Side Effects
Alkylating agents	Busulfan Lomustine Carboplatin Cisplatin Cyclophospha- mide Ifosfamide Temozolomide Procarbazine	Immune suppression Nausea and vomiting (can be delayed) Alopecia Hearing loss (cispla- tin, less common with carboplatin) Hemorrhagic cystitis (ifosfamide and cy- clophosphamide)
Antimetabolites	Methotrexate	Mouth sores Immunosuppression Rashes and skin sensitivity
Plant alkaloids	Vincristine Vinblastine Irinotecan	Peripheral neurop- athies Constipation Diarrhea Alopecia
Antiangiogenesis agents	Thalidomide Lenalidomide Bevacizumab	Interferes with wound healing Peripheral neurop- athy Potential for bleeding at surgical sites

Note. Based on information from Kline, 2004.

chemotherapy, which works on weakened and rapidly dividing tumor cells, biologic agents work by supporting or affecting the host's immune system in various ways to make one's own immune system destroy the cancer cells (National Cancer Institute, 2004). These include making cancer cells more recognizable by the immune system, boosting the destructive power of the immune system to attack abnormal cells, and interfering with the process that changes normal cells into cancer cells. Biologic agents, also called biologic response modifier therapy, includes vaccines, interferons, interleukins, colony-stimulating factors, monoclonal antibodies, and cytokine therapy. Many of these agents are in clinical trials and are showing some promise in the treatment of pediatric CNS tumors. Some of these agents are at the phase one level of clinical research in pediatrics, which measures toxicities from new agents or new combinations of agents. Common side effects of biologic agents are flu-like symptoms, fevers, chills, nausea, and fatigue (National Cancer Institute, 2004). Because they are different from conventional chemotherapy agents, it is the ongoing hope that these agents will be effective against pediatric CNS tumors while being less toxic to

patients in both short- and long-term effects (Wilson & Bryant, 2007).

Symptom Management

Acute Endocrine Effects

Endocrine dysfunction in newly diagnosed pediatric patients with CNS cancer can be complex and life threatening, and the likelihood and severity of the issues are often contingent on the location of the tumor. Pediatric patients with brain tumors can have widely varied electrolyte issues postoperatively that can be more acute and more difficult to manage than their adult counterparts, which is a reason many pediatric patients are placed in the intensive care unit for 24–48 hours postoperatively (Shiminski-Maher, 2007). Diabetes insipidus (DI) can develop in patients who have pineal region, pituitary tumors, or tumors in the hypothalamic regions. Water balance is controlled by the release of vasopressin from the posterior pituitary gland and controlled by the hypothalamus. If the tumor has injured this primary area or if the pituitary stalk is injured by the tumor or surgery, then the syndrome of inappropriate secretion of antidiuretic hormone (SIADH) can occur. Vasopressin controls the amount of water that the kidney retains or excretes and helps to keep electrolytes such as sodium in balance. If DI occurs, and large volumes of fluid are retained, then sodium levels can drop to critically low levels, and seizures can occur. These symptoms can be well controlled with close monitoring of fluid intake and output and the use of desmopressin acetate (DDAVP®, sanofi-aventis), which is exogenous vasopressin taken orally or intranasally (Shiminski-Maher, 2007).

Cerebral salt wasting can also occur postoperatively. It is different from SIADH in that patients with cerebral salt wasting are hypovolemic, and patients with SIADH are normal to hypervolemic. Cerebral salt wasting involves centrally mediated renal sodium wasting and is treated by sodium supplementation. It almost always resolves within weeks to months of the removal of the tumor, and until sodium levels return to normal, close follow-up of serum sodium levels and ongoing supplementation are necessary (Shiminski-Maher, 2007).

Late Endocrine Effects

Survivors of pediatric brain tumors are at high risk for long-term endocrine issues. In a survey of pediatric cancer survivors who have survived cancer for five or more years, the Childhood Cancer Survivor Study, medical records, and self-reports from more than 1,600 pediatric patients with a brain tumor showed that 43% reported one or more long-term endocrine condition (Packer et al., 2003). These endocrine late effects can present a much higher risk for morbidity in the pediatric population than in their adult counterparts.

Unique to children is the long-term deficit of growth hormone. Human growth hormone is responsible not only for linear growth but also for muscle development, including cardiac muscles. Studies have shown a significant decrease in lean body mass, increased fat mass, and decreased bone density two years after cessation of linear growth of adolescents with childhood-onset growth hormone deficiency. This puts an extra burden of increased cardiac risk factors on these adolescents as they age into adulthood (Boot, van der Sluis, Krenning, & de Muinck Keizer-Schrama, 2009). Currently, growth hormone can only be administered via a subcutaneous injection daily, something that is often not well tolerated by children and is prohibitively expensive. Even if covered by insurance, the co-pay for this treatment may be burdensome for a family to cover monthly over years. Both of these factors can contribute to noncompliance. The study also reported that 104 of 1,066 of survivors needed hormones to either stop or induce puberty, and 255 of 1,066 had hypothyroidism (Gurney et al., 2003). These deficits over time can affect metabolism and body mass and could contribute to both male and female issues with future fertility and childbearing. Also, cardiac issues could occur, which could be further complicated by the potential for central obesity in patients with long-term steroid use.

Nursing considerations for these patients include educating the families that lifelong endocrinopathy screening is crucial for the ongoing health maintenance of pediatric CNS tumor survivors, especially those who have had any type of radiation that may have directly affected the pituitary or thyroid glands. The basic health teachings of maintaining a healthy weight and exercising would also be of benefit (Boot et al., 2009).

Hydrocephalus

Most brain tumors in adults are located in the supratentorium, or upper part of the brain. In children, approximately 60% of tumors are in the infratentorium, composed of the brain stem, the cerebellum, and the fourth ventricle (Taylor & Rutka, 2008). Hydrocephalus is a common occurrence with these types of tumors, and it is often the symptom of increased intracranial pressure that brings children with brain tumors to medical attention. The hydrocephalus may be obstructive and require immediate medical attention, or could occur again postoperatively from postsurgical scarring or blood and debris after tumor resection.

Approximately 50% of children with brain tumors will require either the placement of a permanent shunt or an endoscopic third ventriculostomy (ETV) (Shiminski-Maher, 2007). ETV is a surgical procedure using an endoscope through a burr hole that diverts the flow of CSF through the floor of the third ventricle and returns it to normal subarachnoid space. ETV procedures have been performed more frequently over the past 10 years with the advent of better surgical endoscopy

techniques and have a success rate around 75% (Ray et al., 2005). If the surgical team has not deemed an ETV to be appropriate, then an internalized shunt is placed, most often a ventriculoperitoneal, or VP, shunt. Factors that increase the likelihood of a shunt include age younger than 10 years, midline tumor, infection, persistent fluid collections, and incomplete tumor resection (Shiminski-Maher, 2007).

The placement of a permanent shunt in a child comes with the potential for many challenges, including the fact that this static device will be placed in a patient that will continue growing; thus, the ventricular anatomy of the child must be known (see Figure 10-2). Other considerations include the placement of a foreign device long-term in patients and issues around infection. This is complicated by the fact that many patients with a brain tumor go on to adjuvant therapies that will render their immune systems compromised, leaving the patients with a shunt susceptible to meningitis. Patients with shunts that present with even vague symptoms of increased intracranial pressure should be assessed quickly because of the high likelihood of shunt malfunction. These symptoms include change in mental status, lethargy, and early morning vomiting with no concomitant nausea. A noncontrast head computed tomography scan, with no sedation or need for IV contrast, is a quick way to determine if the patient has hydrocephalus. Although it is not ideal to expose children to scans with high radiation content, hydrocephalus is a life-threatening condition, and morbid increased intracranial pressure can occur in less than 24 hours (Ray et al., 2005).

Cognitive and Neuropsychological Issues

Neurocognitive changes happen to all children diagnosed and treated with a brain tumor, from a combination of the direct impact of the destruction of normal brain from the tumor and the subsequent therapy used to treat the tumor if needed (Zebrack et al., 2004). The treatment modality most often cited for causing the biggest cognitive impact is radiation (Packer et al., 2003). Radiation damage can be divided into either effects on the vasculature of the brain or direct effects on the glial cells of the white matter and their precursors. Radiation-induced inflammation and possible necrosis can also directly cause cellular damage (RTOG, 2009).

The most severe deficits occur in children younger than five years old and children who receive full craniospinal irradiation. Additionally, the severity of effects is dose dependent, with higher doses of radiation causing more severe deficits. Neurocognitive decline begins within one to two years of radiation treatment and is progressive in nature. This progressive nature reflects more the inability of the child to acquire new skills than the ongoing loss of skills (Packer et al., 2003).

The areas most affected are those of short-term memory, attention span, expressive and receptive language skills, and mathematics. In comparison to age- and sex-matched siblings, it has been found that brain tumor survivors utilize special

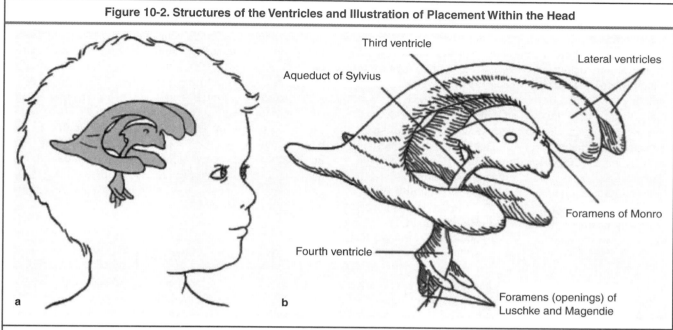

Figure 10-2. Structures of the Ventricles and Illustration of Placement Within the Head

Note. From "Hydrocephalus" (p. 33), by N. Nielsen, K. Pearce, E. Limbacher, and D. Wallace in C.C. Cartwright and D.C. Wallace (Eds.), *Nursing Care of the Pediatric Neurosurgery Patient*, 2007, New York, NY: Springer. Copyright 2007 by Springer. Reprinted with permission.

education services at a much higher rate (Landier & Bhatia, 2008). Nurses and school nurses can help by advocating for early intervention of special educational services, use of a proper school environment for sensory deficits, and aid in the class to help remember even simple tasks, such as lists for homework.

The Childhood Cancer Survivor Study uses a large cohort of cancer survivors, more than 20,000 pediatric cancer survivors across the United States and Canada, to obtain information through questionnaires on various survivor issues, including psychological and health-related quality of life (Zebrack et al., 2004; Zeltzer et al., 2009). It was found that brain tumor survivors report higher levels of impaired health compared to other cancer survivors, which leads to lower expectations of future life satisfaction. CNS tumor survivors also report more depression, somatization, and an overall lower health-related quality of life.

Sensory Issues: Ototoxicity

Hearing loss in patients with CNS tumors results from the treatment modalities with platinum-based chemotherapy and from long-term effects of radiation (Geyer et al., 2005; Wilson & Bryant, 2007). Cisplatin chemotherapy alone can be responsible for hearing loss and synergistically with radiation can cause long-term hearing loss. The hearing loss from radiation and cisplatin is sensorineural and initially affects high frequencies. With cisplatin, the villi

of the sound conduction system of the auditory canal are directly affected. The damage to the villi is dose dependent, and frequent systematic monitoring is vital to prevention of complete damage to hearing. Once an audiology examination determines that chemotherapy is affecting the patient's ability to hear high frequencies, it is crucial that the team is aware of the potentially progressive nature of the damage and makes decisions for dose reduction of cisplatin at this point (Geyer et al., 2005). Amplification devices and hearing aids can benefit children a great deal, especially younger children who will need all sounds for language development. Hearing aids are especially helpful in school, where background noise can greatly diminish the child's ability to hear. Given the popularity of portable music devices such as mp3 players, another good teaching point for families and young adults is the ongoing protection of damaged hearing by keeping the volume down on listening devices to prevent further physical sensorineural damage and the judicious use of ear plugs if the child has frequent exposure to loud noise levels (Geyer et al., 2005).

Infants

In the area of CNS tumors, infants require their own subset of special considerations. In CNS tumor classification for the purpose of research studies, infants are defined as children younger than three years old, and this group is frequently categorized and evaluated separately from children older than three years old. Infant tumors are histologically more aggressive and include atypical teratoid rhabdoid tumors, primitive neuroectodermal tumors, ependymomas, and the choroid plexus tumors. Along with the tumors being more aggressive, the treatments can potentially greatly affect the infant's rapidly developing brain (Fouladi et al., 2005; Geyer et al., 2005). Surgical removal remains the primary intervention. Radiation should be delayed to one year of age at the earliest, and chemotherapy can be used to treat malignant tumors until the child is older than one year (Geyer et al., 2005). Ideally, radiation should be delayed as long as possible, especially full craniospinal radiation, but this may put the child with a malignant tumor at greater risk for recurrence (Geyer et al., 2005). The morbidity of radiation is primarily neurocognitive, with studies showing that many children who have radiation prior to three years old have IQ scores of less than 70, putting them in the severely disabled classification (Fouladi et al., 2005). Input and availability of the neuropsychology team can be beneficial in assisting the treatment team and family through the decision-making process for treatment of infants with aggressive tumors. At this juncture, nurses can be advocates for the families, ensuring that good communication and education happens prior to the decisions for aggressive treatment. Families need to have all the facts for potential long-term outcomes before initiation of aggressive treatment of infants in order to understand the impact of these treatments when making these very difficult decisions. Nurses are instrumental in pulling together all key members of the team to provide these facts, as well as supporting the family in this difficult time.

Supporting the Family

Supporting a child diagnosed with a CNS tumor means supporting the family as a unit. Evidence-based medicine shows that interventions during critical time periods in areas such as procedural pain, realization of long-term effects, stress at diagnosis, and the importance of relationships can help in the overall support of families at this stressful time. Conservative estimates show that post-traumatic stress symptoms have been found in 20% of survivors of childhood cancer and 25% of their parents (Kazak, 2005). The developmental stages of children in coping with a cancer diagnosis must be taken into consideration when referring patients and their families to community, psychoeducational, or psychotherapeutic support groups (Honea et al., 2009) or providing physical rehabilitation.

Pediatric Palliative Care

Special considerations for the palliative care of a pediatric patient could be covered in an entire separate textbook;

however, a few key points can be made in the context of this chapter. The palliative care of a child is much less linear and much more complex than for an adult. Decision making along the way takes in the entire family unit and must consider all family members, including siblings. The decision-making process for a dying child is inherently difficult and fraught with devastating emotional impact. Given the emotional issues along this process, the early intervention of a palliative care or hospice team is imperative to start difficult conversations earlier as opposed to when the family is in full crisis mode. Nurses are crucial in their role in this process and can help with decisions that can affect a family in their grieving process, with the potential for aiding and supporting a more positive grief experience.

Summary

CNS tumors in children create challenges unique to this population. Treatment decisions need to take into consideration the quality-of-life issues of the child along with the long-term issues that will present along the life span of the person living with the side effects of that treatment. This is a balance between making decisions that will not just improve survivorship but will do so with looking toward a functional future for the brain tumor survivor. Working with this vulnerable population in the context of a family requires specialized multidisciplinary care. But similar to most neurologic conditions, the outcomes can be variable, and the opportunity to intervene and support these families can result in outcomes that are rewarding for all involved.

References

Abdullah, S., Qaddoumi, I., & Bouffet, E. (2008). Advances in the management of pediatric central nervous system tumors. *Annals of the New York Academy of Sciences, 1138,* 22–31. doi:10.1196/annals.1414.005

Ahn, E.S., & Goumnerova, L. (2010). Endoscopic biopsy of brain tumors in children: Diagnostic success and utility in guiding treatment strategies. *Journal of Neurosurgery: Pediatrics, 5,* 255–262. doi:10.3171/2009.10.PEDS09172

Boot, A.M., van der Sluis, I.M., Krenning, E.P., & de Muinck Keizer-Schrama, S.M. (2009). Bone mineral density and body composition in adolescents with childhood-onset growth hormone deficiency. *Hormone Research, 71,* 364–371.

Central Brain Tumor Registry of the United States. (2010). *CBTRUS statistical report: Primary brain and central nervous system tumors diagnosed in the United States in 2004–2006.* Retrieved from http://www.cbtrus.org/2010-NPCR-SEER/CBTRUS-WEBREPORT-Final-3-2-10.pdf

Charalambides, C., Dinopoulos, A., & Sgouros, S. (2009). Neuropsychological sequelae and quality of life following treatment of posterior fossa ependymomas in children. *Child's Nervous System, 25,* 1313–1320. doi:10.1007/s00381-009-0927-2

CureSearch.org Medical Editorial Board. (2006, October). Radiation therapy side effects. Retrieved from http://www.curesearch.org/for_parents_and_families/intreatment/medical/article.aspx?ArticleId=3866&StageId=3&TopicId=71&Level=1

De Smet, H.J., Baillieux, H., Wackenier, P., De Praeter, M., Engelborghs, S., Paquier, P.F., ... Mariën, P. (2009). Long-term cognitive deficits following posterior fossa tumor resection: A neuropsychological and functional neuroimaging follow-up study. *Neuropsychology, 23*, 694–704. doi:10.1037/a0016106

Duffner, P.K., Horowitz, M.E., Krischer, J.P., Friedman, H.S., Burger, P.C., Cohen, M.E., ... Kun, L.E. (1993). Postoperative chemotherapy and delayed radiation in children less than three years of age with malignant brain tumors. *New England Journal of Medicine, 328*, 1725–1731.

Fouladi, M., Gilger, E., Kocak, M., Wallace, D., Buchanan, G., Reeves, C., ... Mulhern, R. (2005). Intellectual and functional outcome of children 3 years old or younger who have CNS malignancies. *Journal of Clinical Oncology, 23*, 7152–7160. doi:10.1200/JCO.2005.01.214

Geyer, J.R., Sposto, R., Jennings, M., Boyett, J.M., Axtell, R.A., Breiger, D., ... Shiminski-Maher, T. (2005). Multiagent chemotherapy and deferred radiotherapy in infants with malignant brain tumors: A report from the Children's Cancer Group. *Journal of Clinical Oncology, 23*, 7621–7631. doi:10.1200/JCO.2005.09.095

Gurney, J.C., Kadan-Lottick, N.S., Packer, R.J., Neglia, J.P., Sklar, C.A., Punyko, J.A., ... Robison, L.L. (2003). Endocrine and cardiovascular late effects among adult survivors of childhood brain tumors: Childhood Cancer Survivor Study. *Cancer, 97*, 663–673. doi:10.1002/cncr.11095

Honea, N.J., Sherwood, P.R., Northouse, L.L., Brintnall, R.A., Colao, D.B., Somers, S.C., & Given, B. (2009). ONS PEP resource: Caregiver strain and burden. In L.H. Eaton & J.M. Tipton (Eds.), *Putting evidence into practice: Improving oncology patient outcomes* (pp. 57–62). Pittsburgh, PA: Oncology Nursing Society.

Johnson, M.H. (2001). Functional brain development in humans. *Nature Reviews Neuroscience, 2*, 475–483. doi:10.1038/35081509

Kazak, A.E. (2005). Evidence-based interventions for survivors of childhood cancer and their families. *Journal of Pediatric Psychology, 30*, 29–39. doi:10.1093/jpepsy/jsi013

Khan, R.B., Boop, F.A., Onar, A., & Sanford, R.A. (2006). Seizures in children with low-grade tumors: Outcome after tumor resection and risk factors for uncontrolled seizures. *Journal of Neurosurgery, 104*(Suppl. 6), 377–382. doi:10.3171/ped.2006.104.6.377

Kirk, E.A., Howard, V.C., & Scott, C.A. (1995). Description of posterior fossa syndrome in children after posterior fossa brain tumor surgery. *Journal of Pediatric Oncology Nursing, 12*, 181–187. doi:10.1177/104345429501200402

Kirsch, D.G., & Tarbell, N.J. (2004). New technologies in radiation therapy for pediatric brain tumors: The rationale for proton radiation therapy. *Pediatric Blood Cancer, 42*, 461–464. doi:10.1002/pbc.10471

Kline, N. (Ed.). (2004). *The pediatric chemotherapy and biotherapy curriculum.* Glenview, IL: Association of Pediatric Hematology/Oncology Nurses.

Landier, W., & Bhatia, S. (2008). Cancer survivorship: A pediatric perspective. *Oncologist, 13*, 1181–1192. doi:10.1634/theoncologist.2008-0104

Miller, D.C. (2001). Surgical neuropathology. In R.F. Keating, J.T. Goodrich, & R.J. Packer (Eds.), *Tumors of the pediatric central nervous system* (pp. 44–102). New York, NY: Thieme.

National Cancer Institute. (2004, December 29). Biological therapy. Retrieved from http://www.cancer.gov/cancertopics/biologicaltherapy

Packer, R.J., Gurney, J.G., Punyko, J.A., Donaldson, S.S., Inskip, P.D., Stovall, M., ... Robison, L.L. (2003). Long-term neurologic and neurosensory sequelae in adult survivors of a childhood brain tumor: Childhood Cancer Survivor Study. *Journal of Clinical Oncology, 21*, 3255–3261. doi:10.1200/JCO.2003.01.202

Radiation Therapy Oncology Group. (2009). RTOG acute radiation morbidity scoring criteria. Retrieved from www.rtog.org/members/toxicity/acute.html

Ray, P., Jallo, G., Kim, R.Y., Kim, B.S., Wilson, S., Kothbauer, S., & Abbott, R. (2005). Endoscopic third ventriculostomy for tumor-related hydrocephalus in a pediatric population. *Neurosurgical Focus, 19*, 1–4.

Shiminski-Maher, T. (2007). Tumors of the central nervous system. In C.C. Cartwright & D.C. Wallace (Eds.), *Nursing care of the pediatric neurosurgery patient* (pp. 119–148). New York, NY, Springer.

Taketomo, C., Hodding, J.H., & Kraus, D.M. (2009). *Lexi-Comp's pediatric dosage handbook: Including neonatal dosing, drug administration, and extemporaneous preparations* (16th ed.). Hudson, OH: Lexi-Comp and American Pharmacists Association.

Taylor, M.D., & Rutka, J.T. (2008). Pediatric posterior fossa tumors. In M. Bernstein & M. Berger (Eds.), *Neuro-oncology: The essentials* (2nd ed., pp. 287–298). New York, NY: Thieme.

Vézina, L.G. (2008). Imaging of central nervous system tumors in children: Advances and limitations. *Journal of Child Neurology, 23*, 1128–1135. doi:10.1177/0883073808320753

von Koch, C.S., Schmidt, M.H., & Perry, V. (2004). Neuronal tumors. In N. Gupta, A. Banerjee, & D. Haas-Krogan (Eds.), *Pediatric CNS tumors* (pp. 143–156). New York, NY: Springer.

Wilson, K., & Bryant, R. (Eds.). (2007). *APHON's foundation of pediatric hematology nursing: A comprehensive orientation and review course.* Glenview, IL: Association of Pediatric Hematology/Oncology Nurses.

Yock, T.I., & Tarbell, N.J. (2004). Technology insight: Proton beam radiotherapy for treatment in pediatric brain tumors. *Nature Clinical Practice: Oncology, 1*, 97–103. doi:10.1038/ncponc0090

Zebrack, B.J., Gurney, J.G., Oeffinger, K., Whitton, J., Packer, R.J., Mertens, A., ... Zeltzer, L.K. (2004). Psychological outcomes in long-term survivors of childhood brain cancer: A report from the Childhood Cancer Survivor Study. *Journal of Clinical Oncology, 22*, 999–1006. doi:10.1200/JCO.2004.06.148

Zeltzer, L.K., Recklitis, C., Buchbinder, D., Zebrack, B., Casillas, J., Tsao, J.C., ... Krull, K. (2009). Psychological status in childhood cancer survivors: A report from the Childhood Cancer Survivor Study. *Journal of Clinical Oncology, 27*, 2396–2404. doi:10.1200/JCO.2008.21.1433

CHAPTER 11

Symptom Management and Psychological Issues

Paula R. Sherwood, RN, PhD, CNRN, and Mary Beth Baer, BS

Introduction

Because of a multitude of factors, data on symptom management in neuro-oncology are sparse in comparison with that of other cancers. As previous chapters have illustrated, central nervous system (CNS) tumors occur much less frequently than other primary sites, yet mortality and morbidity rates are extremely high. Considering these factors along with the difficulty of delivering antineoplastic medication to the CNS, the majority of research in neuro-oncology has focused on new chemotherapeutic and radiation regimens as well as alternative surgical approaches. Symptom management research in neuro-oncology, then, has been primarily limited to reporting frequencies of side effects associated with new treatment regimens. In turn, even fewer intervention studies have been implemented that are aimed at symptom management. In the following sections, available data on the most prevalent symptoms in neuro-oncology are presented. For each symptom, incidence, associated factors, and nursing care are presented.

Surgical Complications

Complications following CNS tumor surgery are closely linked to the location and grade of the tumor, length of surgery, and the patient's comorbid conditions. In people with a brain tumor, postoperative complications have been categorized as neurologic, regional, or systemic (Sawaya et al., 1998) (see Table 11-1).

Incidence and Associated Factors

Sawaya et al. (1998) performed one of the largest studies of postoperative complications in patients undergoing surgery for a glioma or metastatic tumor. Tumor grade was the only variable that approached significance as a predictor of major neurologic complications (e.g., motor/sensory deficit,

Table 11-1. Postoperative Complications in Patients Following Brain Tumor Resection	
Category	**Complication**
Neurologic	Aphasia/dysphasia Motor or sensory deficit Visual field deficit
Regional	Cerebrospinal fluid leak Hematoma Hydrocephalus Meningitis Pneumocephalus Seizure Wound infection
Systemic	Central line infection Deep vein thrombosis Esophageal candidiasis Gastritis Hyponatremia Pneumothorax Psychosis Pulmonary embolism Pulmonary infection Sepsis Urinary tract infection

Note. Based on information from Sawaya et al., 1998.

aphasia/dysphasia). Higher tumor grades were associated with increased incidence of neurologic complications (Taylor & Bernstein, 1999). Regarding regional complications (seizure, hematoma, and cerebrospinal fluid [CSF] leak), higher numbers of complications were found in patients who were older, had worse preoperative physical function, and had infratentorial tumors than in other patients with CNS cancer. Finally, older patients, those with a higher tumor grade, and those with an anaplastic glioma were more likely to have systemic complications (e.g., pulmonary infection, urinary tract infection) than others with CNS cancer.

In a descriptive study of 93 people with a glioma, Yeh et al. (2005) found that 26% of patients reported somnolence five years following diagnosis, and 17% reported memory impairments. Yeh et al. also reported that receiving postoperative radiation was associated with reports of memory impairment. Other variables associated with postoperative complications in people with a brain tumor have included the caseload of the hospital and surgeon (Barker, Klibanski, & Swearingen, 2003) and the degree of preoperative neurologic deficit (Khan et al., 2006).

Little research has reported about postoperative complications following surgery for a spinal cord tumor. In a large retrospective study, Patil, Patil, Lad, and Boakye (2008) found the most common complications during the inpatient postoperative period were urinary and renal complications, hemorrhage or hematoma, and pulmonary complications. The authors also reported that African Americans and patients with multiple comorbid conditions were more likely to have postoperative complications. In turn, having a poor surgical outcome was more likely in those who had postoperative complications, those older than 64 years of age, and those who had multiple comorbid conditions.

Nursing Care

In the past, surgical complications have been the primary focus for nurses in the inpatient setting. However, because of advances in surgical techniques coupled with decreased insurance reimbursement, many patients now undergo a limited length of stay following resection. For some patients, tumor resection is an outpatient procedure. Assessment of surgical complications, then, often becomes the responsibility of the outpatient clinic and family caregivers. Several texts are available that serve as excellent references for postoperative care of patients undergoing tumor resection in the brain and spine, such as *The Clinical Practice of Neurological and Neurosurgical Nursing* (Hickey, 2009) and *Neuroscience Nursing: A Spectrum of Care* (Barker, 2008). In addition, clinical practice guidelines for caring for patients undergoing craniotomy for a brain tumor and patients undergoing cervical and lumbar spinal surgery are available from the American Association of Neuroscience Nurses Web site, www.aann.org (AANN, 2006, 2007). Highlights of the guidelines are presented in Tables 11-2 and 11-3.

A primary goal of controlling postoperative complications in people undergoing surgery for a CNS tumor is control of edema. Tissue in the CNS swells in response to insult (e.g., resection), peaking approximately 48–72 hours after surgery (Hickey, 2009). Although postoperative edema is a common complication for any tumor resection, the fact that CNS tissue is enclosed within a rigid structure, such as the cranium or spinal column, makes this complication a potentially life-threatening condition. Corticosteroids are the principal therapy for controlling postoperative edema and should be accompanied with patient education for continuing steroid therapy in the home. Patients also require education regarding the side effects of corticosteroids, which are detailed in a later section. Other postoperative nursing care goals include assessing for and preventing hemorrhage and systemic postoperative complications. Regular and complete neurologic examinations are key to quickly identifying postoperative complications and should be particularly targeted toward the location of the tumor. For example, in a patient with a tumor at the fourth and fifth lumbar vertebrae, particular attention should be paid during assessment to the neurologic function controlled by the spinal column three to four levels above and below the surgical site. If edema or hemorrhage occurs, the spine swells vertically (enclosed within the vertebral column) and the patient can have ascending or descending edema resulting in further loss of neurologic function (Hickey, 2009). In patients with a brain tumor, edema can cause site-specific complications, such as memory loss in patients with a frontal lobe tumor, or more generalized symptoms, such as lethargy and decreased level of consciousness. Regular assessment and good communication with the healthcare team are vital in decreasing the incidence and lowering the severity of complications.

Fatigue

Fatigue is one of the most commonly reported symptoms associated with a tumor in the CNS (particularly with brain tumors), and patients have reported that the incidence and severity of fatigue are important factors to consider when determining the value of continuing with treatment (Butt et al., 2008). In addition, fatigue has been closely linked with patient reports of quality of life (Gustafsson, Edvardsson, & Ahlström, 2006) although it is often underdiagnosed (Fox, Lyon, & Farace, 2007). Patients have described feelings of fatigue as excessive exhaustion and tiredness, which can result as a direct effect of the tumor, as a side effect of medical treatments, or because of psychological or existential issues associated with the diagnosis (Faithfull & Brada, 1998; Pelletier, Verhoef, Khatri, & Hagen, 2002). Because of this multitude of causal factors, it can be difficult for clinicians to implement interventions to lower its severity.

Incidence and Associated Factors

Levels of fatigue in patients with a brain tumor have been shown to be comparable to those in patients with other types of cancer (Osoba, Brada, Prados, & Yung, 2000). In patients with higher-grade tumors, 89%–94% of patients report feeling fatigued (Osoba et al., 2000); a slightly lower rate (77%) has been reported in patients with lower-grade tumors (Gustafsson et al., 2006). In addition, high levels of fatigue have

Table 11-2. Postoperative Nursing Considerations for Patients Following Craniotomy for Brain Tumor

Potential Problem	Causes	Nursing Considerations
Generalized Care and Monitoring		
Neurologic and vital signs	Disrupted brain tissue and structures from surgical procedure Increased intracranial pressure Brain stem lesion	Confer with neurosurgeon to identify expected deficits. Monitor patient closely for new or worsening deficits. Monitor patient per institution guidelines/physician's orders. Compare with baseline. Maintain ordered parameters. Assess for respiratory depression if brain stem lesion; monitor oxygen saturation and rate per physician's orders.
Pain	Surgery	Assess patient's pain using institution's preferred pain scale. Administer analgesics as ordered; assess patient response. Assist patient with complementary pain management techniques.
Seizures	Frontal, temporal, and parietal lobe tumors (40% occurrence rate with these tumor types) Occipital tumors (14% occurrence rate) History of seizures (Patients with a positive preoperative seizure history have an increased risk of seizures in the first 24 hours after surgery.)	Monitor patient for seizures. Keep patient safe if seizure observed; call physician. Monitor anticonvulsant therapy level. Maintain anticonvulsant level in therapeutic range as ordered.
Venothromboembolism: Deep vein thrombosis	Brain tumor resection (Incidence for postcraniotomy for brain tumor resection is 1.6%–4%.)	Enforce bed rest for patient and keep legs elevated. Assist patient with compression stockings. Administer anticoagulant therapy as ordered. Prepare patient for insertion of vena cava filter if indicated.
Identification and Monitoring of Postoperative Procedures		
Cerebrospinal fluid (CSF) leak	Posterior fossa craniotomy with dural opening (Patients have an increased risk of CSF leak after this type of surgery.)	Monitor patient for clear fluid escaping from nose, ears, or operative site. Assess patient for salty-sweet taste in mouth. Keep patient on bed rest with the head of the bed elevated unless patient has a posterior fossa CSF leak. Administer stool softeners/laxatives regularly to prevent straining with bowel movements. Administer acetazolamide as ordered to decrease CSF production. If necessary, prepare patient for insertion of lumbar drain or surgical repair of dural defect.
Increased intracranial pressure	Hemorrhage Cerebral edema Retraction of brain tissue during surgery Interference of venous drainage Cerebral infarction Pain Fever or infection	Assist with management of underlying cause. Raise the head of the bed to a 30°–45° angle. Administer osmotic diuretics with mannitol as ordered. Keep patient cool; avoid hyperthermia. Instruct patient to hyperventilate once daily to promote vasoconstriction. Infuse hypertonic saline as ordered. Monitor ventricular catheter drainage for amount, color, and consistency.
Hemorrhage	Subdural, epidural, intraparenchymal, or intraventricular bleeding	Correct coagulopathy levels if indicated and as ordered. Prepare patient for immediate surgery as indicated.
Hydrocephalus	Buildup of intracranial fluid	Prepare patient for ventriculostomy (drain inserted into ventricle). Monitor drain. Measure color and amount of CSF drained.

(Continued on next page)

Table 11-2. Postoperative Nursing Considerations for Patients Following Craniotomy for Brain Tumor *(Continued)*

Potential Problem	Causes	Nursing Considerations
Identification and Monitoring of Postoperative Procedures *(cont.)*		
Peritumoral edema	Blood-brain barrier breakdown	Administer dexamethasone 4–10 mg IV or orally every six hours or as ordered. Do not discontinue dexamethasone abruptly; taper dose over 7–10 days as ordered.
Pneumocephalus (air in subdural, epidural, subarachnoid, intraparenchymal, or intraventricular spaces)	Postprocedure: lumbar puncture or surgery	May occur 24 hours to 7 days postoperatively. Usually resolves without treatment in one to three days. Monitor neurologic signs. Administer 100% oxygen (unless patient has received previous bleomycin) to encourage air absorption.
Risk for Infection		
Wound	Bacteria Fungi Viruses Parasites Myelosuppression	Assess head dressing for drainage; record drainage amount and characteristics. Outline drainage edge directly on dressing immediately postoperatively and monitor for changes. Remove head dressing 24 hours after surgery. Monitor incision for erythema and drainage. Keep staples and stitches dry.
Meningitis	Bacteria Viruses Fungi Parasites Myelosuppression	Perform lumbar puncture to confirm diagnosis **ONLY AFTER** a computed tomography scan. Monitor vital signs, neurologic signs, and mental status. Assess for photophobia or petechial rash. Monitor for seizures. Administer antibiotics and corticosteroids as ordered. Prepare patient for surgical intervention if indicated.
Risk for Alterations in Electrolyte Balance		
Diabetes insipidus	Develops almost exclusively when area around posterior lobe of pituitary gland is disturbed Insufficient antidiuretic hormone (ADH)	Usually resolves within 36 hours. Monitor postoperative blood sugar before meals and before sleep. Monitor patient for increased thirst, increased urine output, decreased specific gravity, increased serum sodium, and increased serum osmolality. Replace oral and IV fluids as ordered to prevent dehydration. Administer desmopressin acetate or aqueous vasopressin, as ordered.
Syndrome of inappropriate ADH	Increased ADH Water intoxication (water from kidney tubules continuously reabsorbed into system)	Monitor intake and output. Restrict daily fluid intake to less than 1 liter. Monitor serum sodium; replace accordingly.
Cerebral salt wasting	Loss of sodium by kidneys	Monitor for the following signs and symptoms: hypovolemia, decreased sodium, decreased weight, increased blood urea nitrogen, increased hematocrit, confusion, lethargy, and seizures. Replace urine with isotonic saline cc-for-cc. Administer sodium orally. Administer fludrocortisone acetate 0.2 mg/day IV or orally, as ordered.

Note. Based on information from American Association of Neuroscience Nurses, 2006.

Table 11-3. Nursing Care for Patients Following Cervical Spine Surgery for Cancer

Factor	Nursing Considerations
Postoperative neurologic examination	• Monitor and compare to baseline: – Neurologic status – Extremity strength and sensation. • Postoperative swelling may occur if nerve roots were extensively handled during surgery and manifests as neurologic deficits. – Assess patient for signs of edema (neurologic deficits) three to four levels above and below the level of the cervical surgery. – Administer corticosteroids 24–28 hours postoperatively as ordered. • Administer oral antibiotics for 24 hours after surgery if ordered.
Incision care: Generalized and specific	• General care – Assess site for swelling, hematoma, or infection. – Monitor site for bleeding, hemorrhage, dehiscence, or cerebrospinal fluid leak. – Change dressing and cleanse as ordered. Notify physician if drainage characteristics change. • For anterior procedure – Assess patient for sore throat or raspy, hoarse voice. – Monitor patient for excessive phlegm production and ability to speak and swallow. • For posterior procedure – Assess and document length of incision, usually five to six inches. – Assess cervical collar for fit and comfort. Teach patient rationale for collar and expected length of use.
Mobility	• Variable according to preoperative ambulation, diagnosis, and surgery performed. • Immediately after surgery, assist patient to roll to one side, keeping his or her head and neck still, explaining the process as it occurs. • Depending on procedure performed, the patient may be able to ambulate within two hours of surgery. • Refer the patient to physical therapy for a walker or gait training as needed. • Refer the patient to occupational therapy as indicated.
Pain	• Posterior procedures cause muscle spasms and significantly more pain than anterior procedures. • Assess patient for pain and administer IV analgesics (hydromorphone or morphine sulfate) as ordered immediately after surgery. • Assess patient for pain and administer oral opioids with or without a nonsteroidal anti-inflammatory drug when patient is able to swallow. • Assess patient for muscle spasms and administer antispasmodics as ordered. Apply warm packs to areas of muscle spasms.
Constipation	• Monitor intake and output. • Assess patient for dehydration or abdominal pain and cramping. • Encourage and assist patient to increase ambulation as ordered. • Palpate abdomen and perform rectal examination if appropriate. (Never perform a rectal examination on immunocompromised patients.) • Administer stool softeners or bulk-forming laxatives as ordered. • Increase patient's fluid and fiber intake.
Urination	• Assess patient for temporary postoperative urinary hesitancy. • Monitor intake and output. • Assess bladder for adequate emptying.
Patient education	• Keep incision dry at all times. Assess incision daily for redness, swelling, drainage, or infection. If any signs are present, check temperature and notify physician. • Contact physician immediately for – Temperature higher than 101.5°F – Neck swelling – Drainage that is excessive or foul-smelling – Increased upper extremity weakness or numbness – Increased pain.

(Continued on next page)

Table 11-3. Nursing Care for Patients Following Cervical Spine Surgery for Cancer *(Continued)*	
Factor	**Nursing Considerations**

Patient education *(cont.)*	• Limited motion postprocedure as specified by the physician.
	  – Advise the patient to not lift anything heavier than a gallon of milk for a minimum of 4 weeks.
	  – Tell the patient to avoid working or lifting over head.
	  – Instruct the patient to avoid flexing, bending, or twisting the neck at any time.
	• Instruct the patient to wear cervical collar at all times unless the physician specifies otherwise.
	  – The patient should not move the head while cleaning the collar.
	  – The patient should hold the neck still while facing a mirror to clean pads and change collar.
	  – One part of the collar should remain intact and in place at all times during cleaning procedure.
	• The patient should not drive while taking opioids or wearing a cervical collar.
	• Instruct the patient to slowly resume his or her preoperative daily schedule of activities.
	  – The patient should ask family, neighbors, or community members for assistance with household chores.
	  – Return to work is dependent upon occupational physical requirements, sedentary versus active.

Note. Based on information from American Association of Neuroscience Nurses, 2007.

been shown to continue for months following diagnosis. Both Pelletier et al. (2002) and Struik et al. (2009) reported fatigue in long-term brain tumor survivors, 42% of the sample and 39% of the sample, respectively.

As with other cancers, fatigue rarely occurs in isolation. Fox et al. (2007) found that patients with a brain tumor commonly developed two clusters of symptoms, and fatigue played a role in both clusters. The cluster of fatigue, sleep disturbance, depression, and cognitive impairment had a significant impact on quality of life. The second cluster of symptoms (depression, fatigue, sleep disturbance, cognitive impairment, and pain) significantly affected the patient's functional status.

Fatigue has been related to the location of the tumor and treatment modalities. Brown, Ballman, et al. (2006) reported higher levels of fatigue in patients with tumors on the right side of the brain, but these data have not been replicated to date. Chemotherapeutic agents that have been associated with fatigue are temozolomide, carboplatin, tamoxifen, and erlotinib (Cohen, Johnson, & Pazdur, 2005; Prados et al., 2006; Tang et al., 2006). Data also suggest that the combination of chemotherapy and radiation places the patient at particular risk for fatigue, such as concomitantly administering temozolomide and radiotherapy (Cohen et al., 2005; Prados et al., 2006; Tang et al., 2006). Taphoorn et al. (2007) found higher levels of fatigue in patients receiving both radiation and chemotherapy compared to those receiving radiation only, although significant differences were found only at the onset of treatment, and no significant differences were observed when chemotherapy treatment ended.

In general, patients who receive radiotherapy report high levels of fatigue, which are cyclical in nature and correspond to radiation treatment cycles (Brown, Clark, et al., 2006; Faithfull & Brada, 1998). When radiation is delivered in high doses, somnolence syndrome may occur, a condition marked by extreme fatigue, drowsiness, flu-like symptoms, and lethargy (Faithfull & Brada, 1998). Somnolence syndrome has

been associated with the level of fractionation during radiation and has been reported to hinder both physical and mental functioning. Table 11-4 delineates the factors associated with fatigue in patients with CNS cancers.

Fatigue affects multiple aspects of patients' lives, including their ability to resume prediagnosis activities (Pelletier et al., 2002). Struik et al. (2009) found that severe fatigue was significantly associated with reduced motivation and problems concentrating. Postdiagnosis employment status (specifically the inability to return to work) has been linked to fatigue (Butt et al., 2008; Pelletier et al., 2002), and patients with fatigue have been shown to be less likely to be employed and experience more work limitations for years following diagnosis (Feuerstein, Hansen, Calvio, Johnson, & Ronquillo, 2007). As such, fatigue can significantly affect health-related and overall quality of life and potentially survival (Brown, Ballman, et al., 2006; Butt et al., 2008).

Nursing Care

The first step in fatigue management for patients with a CNS tumor is routine assessment. The subjective nature of each person's experience with fatigue makes patient self-report the best form of assessment (Eaton, 2009). Several tools to measure fatigue have been validated in patients with cancer, and although few are specifically targeted toward patients with a CNS tumor, the following have been used in this population. The Multidimensional Fatigue Symptom Inventory–Short Form measures general fatigue, physical fatigue, emotional fatigue, mental fatigue, and vigor using a 30-item scale (Stein, Jacobsen, Blanchard, & Thors, 2004). The Checklist of Individual Strength measures four aspects of fatigue: severity, concentration problems, reduced motivation, and reduced activity; a score of more than 35 indicates severe fatigue (Struik et al., 2009; Vercoulen et al., 1994). The Brief Fatigue Inventory (nine items) can be useful as a screening tool for fatigue, measuring the severity of fatigue and its resulting distress (Mendoza et al., 1999). Other tools are available that are not specifically targeted toward measuring fatigue but include either specific questions related to fatigue or have been used to indicate fatigue. The Symptom Distress Scale and the Functional Assessment of Cancer Therapy–Brain (often referred to as FACT-BR) both contain items related to fatigue (McCorkle & Quint-Benoliel, 1983; Weitzner et al., 1995). Fatigue has been assessed using general quality-of-life questionnaires such as the European Organisation for Research and Treatment of Cancer QLQ-C30 (+3) and the Brain Cancer Module 20 (Osoba et al., 1996). Although all of these tools have been proved valid and reliable in patients with cancer, nurses need to consider clinical implications such as the length of the tool and measurement of a single dimension, such as the Oncology Nursing Society's numeric rating fatigue scale (Eaton, 2009), versus multiple dimensions of fatigue. Regardless of the tool chosen, most researchers suggest that the patient's level of fatigue, along with its affect on multiple aspects of the patient's life, should be routinely monitored both during active treatment and into cancer survivorship.

Few interventions have been aimed at decreasing fatigue specifically in patients with a CNS tumor. Drug treatment with a CNS stimulant, methylphenidate, is currently under investigation with inconsistent results. Meyers, Weitzner, Valentine, and Levin (1998) studied 30 patients with primary brain tumors who received methylphenidate twice a day and reported improvements in cognition, motor function, and mood. However, these results were not replicated by Butler et al. (2007). Modafinil has also been evalu-

ated in the treatment of fatigue. Blackhall, Petroni, Shu, Baum, and Farace (2009) showed a reduction in fatigue, depression, and anxiety and improved quality of life in the weeks following administration, yet how representative the sample was of those with a CNS tumor is unclear. An abstract of a paper presented at the 2006 annual meeting of the American Society of Clinical Oncology reported that in a pilot study of patients with brain tumors, modafinil was associated with improvements in mood, fatigue, and cognitive function. Common side effects were headache (42%), insomnia (26%), dizziness (23%), and dry mouth (23%) (Kaleita et al., 2006).

Brown evaluated a structured, multidisciplinary intervention to decrease fatigue in patients with a CNS tumor (Brown, Ballman, et al., 2006; Brown, Clark, et al., 2006). The intervention consisted of eight 90-minute sessions over two weeks. Each session began with physical exercise, provided educational information, cognitive-behavioral strategies, discussion, and support, and ended with guided relaxation. Both the control and intervention groups reported significant levels of fatigue at baseline, and no significant differences in levels of fatigue postintervention were reported. Until more research is done specifically testing interventions for fatigue in patients with a CNS tumor, fatigue management strategies may be based upon general oncology guidelines, such as those provided by the National Comprehensive Cancer Network (2010) and the Oncology Nursing Society (Mitchell, Beck, Hood, Moore, & Tanner, 2009). Current nursing interventions to combat fatigue should be tailored to each person and situation and include exercise, education interventions, energy conservation and activity management,

Table 11-4. Factors Associated With Fatigue in Patients With Central Nervous System Cancer	
Factor	**Comment**
Brain tumor	Symptom clusters • Fatigue, sleep disturbance, depression, and cognitive impairment • Fatigue, sleep disturbance, depression, cognitive impairment, and pain
Grade of brain tumor	Direct correlation with level of fatigue • High grade = high fatigue. • Low grade = low fatigue.
Location of brain tumor	Tumor in right side of brain = high fatigue.
Treatment modalities • Chemotherapy and radiation therapy	• Patients at high risk for fatigue • Fatigue is high at onset of treatment in patients receiving concomitant therapy.
• Cytotoxic agents	• Temozolomide, carboplatin, tamoxifen, and erlotinib have fatigue as a side effect.
• Radiation therapy	• Patients experience a high level of fatigue that occurs with treatment cycles. • High-dose radiation therapy associated with somnolence syndrome: extreme fatigue, drowsiness, flu-like symptoms, and lethargy.

Note. Based on information from Brown, Clark, et al., 2006; Cohen et al., 2005; Faithfull & Brada, 1998; Fox et al., 2007; Gustafsson et al., 2006; Osoba et al., 2000; Prados et al., 2006; Tang et al., 2006; Taphoorn et al., 2007.

measures to optimize sleep quality, and relaxation (Mitchell et al., 2009).

Nausea and Vomiting

Incidence and Associated Factors

Nausea and vomiting have been associated with high levels of anxiety and depression as well as lower levels of satisfaction with daily living in patients with a CNS tumor (Enblom, Axelsson, Steineck, Hammar, & Börjeson, 2009). Although they are not as prevalent as fatigue, nausea and vomiting are common side effects for patients with a CNS tumor, particularly as they are going through active treatment. Approximately 26%–45% of patients with a CNS tumor report nausea and vomiting, which can be related to a multitude of factors (Enblom et al., 2009; Italian Group for Antiemetic Research in Radiotherapy, 1999; Prados et al., 2006) (see Table 11-5). Tumor location and size may cause nausea, which may be one of the initial symptoms that can lead to the diagnosis. Large tumors or tumors that grow quickly (such as high-grade tumors) can cause nausea and vomiting by increasing intracranial pressure. Patients with high-grade, infratentorial tumors that grow into the fourth ventricle are at high risk for nausea and vomiting, and intractable vomiting in particular (Cohen, Hassenbusch, Maor, Pfeffer, & Ram, 2002; Fujimura et al., 2004). Glioblastoma multiforme with poor differentiation, for

example, tends to shed tumor cells and seed the CSF more vigorously than tumors that are more differentiated (Cohen et al., 2002). Fujimara et al. (2004) suggested that intractable vomiting may result from CSF seeding into the fourth ventricle and may serve as an early warning sign of tumor progression.

The type of anesthesia used during surgery to remove a CNS tumor can also affect the presence and severity of nausea and vomiting. Manninen and Tan (2002) compared nausea and vomiting between patients who received an "awake" craniotomy (intermittent boluses of midazolam and fentanyl, an infusion of remifentanil, and/or a bolus or infusion of propofol) versus those who received general anesthesia (receiving some combination of thiopental or propofol, nitrous oxide, isoflurane or desflurane, and/or fentanyl). The authors reported that patients undergoing an awake craniotomy had less nausea (4% versus 23%) and vomiting (0% versus 11%) during the first four hours after surgery compared with those who underwent general anesthesia.

Common chemotherapeutic agents used with CNS tumors are moderate emetogenic agents, such as temozolomide, and the highly emetogenic agents of nimustine hydrochloride, lomustine, and carmustine (Grunberg et al., 2005; Yano et al., 2004). Nausea and vomiting are less strongly associated with radiation therapy than chemotherapy, and several authors have described the risk for nausea and vomiting following radiation therapy as low (Enblom et al., 2009; Kris et al., 2006). When receiving radiation alone, approximately 6%–15% of patients are at risk for vomiting and 16%–33% are at risk for nausea

Table 11-5. Factors Associated With Nausea and Vomiting in Patients With Central Nervous System Cancer

Factor	Comment
Anxiety	High level associated with nausea and vomiting
Depression	High level associated with nausea and vomiting
Satisfaction with daily living	Low level associated with nausea and vomiting
Tumor location and size	Large or rapidly growing tumor can cause increased intracranial pressure and nausea and vomiting. High-grade, infratentorial tumor in fourth ventricle can cause intractable vomiting.
Tumor type	Poorly differentiated glioblastoma multiforme tumor sheds cells that seed the cerebrospinal fluid, which can cause nausea and vomiting.
Anesthesia	Lower risk of nausea and vomiting with awake craniotomy Higher risk of nausea and vomiting with general anesthesia
Prior chemotherapy	Higher risk of nausea and vomiting during radiation therapy
Chemotherapy	Moderately emetogenic agents currently used to treat central nervous system tumors
Radiation therapy	Risk for nausea slightly higher than low risk for vomiting
Chemotherapy and radiation therapy	Incidence of nausea is higher compared to incidence of vomiting for radiation and temozolomide.

Note. Based on information from Cohen et al., 2002; Cohen et al., 2005; Enblom et al., 2009; Fujimura et al., 2004; Italian Group for Antiemetic Research in Radiotherapy, 1999; Manninen & Tan, 2002.

(Cohen et al., 2005; Italian Group for Antiemetic Research in Radiotherapy, 1999). However, when patients are undergoing concomitant chemotherapy and radiation (the standard of care for a large number of CNS tumors), rates are much higher. Cohen et al. (2005) reported that the percentage of patients receiving radiation therapy who reported nausea rose from 16% for those receiving radiation alone to 36% for those receiving radiation and temozolomide and 49% for those receiving a maintenance dose of temozolomide. Similarly, percentages of patients reporting vomiting increased from 6% in those receiving radiation alone to 20% in those receiving radiation and temozolomide and 29% in those receiving the maintenance dose of temozolomide. These data are supported by other researchers who have shown that when patients have a previous experience with chemotherapy, rates of nausea and vomiting increase during radiation (Italian Group for Antiemetic Research in Radiotherapy, 1999).

Nursing Care

Assessment of nausea and vomiting typically varies, and few tools with established reliability and validity address these symptoms alone. Measurement has included hospital observations of frequency of emesis and occurrences of nausea, as well as participants' diaries of their emesis occurrence and gradation of nausea according to cause and effect on normal daily life (Enblom et al., 2009; National Cancer Institute Cancer Therapy Evaluation Program [NCI CTEP], 2009; Italian Group for Antiemetic Research in Radiotherapy, 1999; Yano et al., 2004).

Despite the availability of multiple treatment modalities for nausea and vomiting, research has suggested that approximately one-third of patients undergoing treatment for a CNS tumor experience nausea and would like better symptom management (Enblom et al., 2009). Several pharmacologic agents are available for nausea and vomiting, the majority of which are 5-HT$_3$ receptor antagonists. They gain their antiemetic effects from selectively binding to 5-HT$_3$ receptors on peripheral vagal nerve terminals and centrally in the chemoreceptor zone. Ondansetron is commonly prescribed during radiation therapy, and ramosetron and granisetron have both been shown specifically to relieve nausea and vomiting during most chemotherapy administrations in patients with a CNS tumor (Grunberg et al., 2005; Yano et al., 2004).

No research to date has evaluated nonpharmacologic interventions to control nausea and vomiting in patients with a CNS tumor. Similar to fatigue, guidelines for the general management of nausea and vomiting are available from the National Comprehensive Cancer Network and for the management of chemotherapy-induced nausea and vomiting from the Oncology Nursing Society (Friend et al., 2009), among others. National CNS tumor support groups also offer advice. The American Brain Tumor Association (2008), for example, advises patients to use relaxation or diversion techniques, like playing games or watching videos, before or during treatment to manage nausea and vomiting. It also recommends that patients avoid eating before chemotherapy treatment, and when eating, pick plain and bland foods rather than spicy, fatty, or strong-smelling foods.

Changes in Cognition

Incidence and Associated Factors

Cognitive dysfunction is an extremely common symptom in patients with a CNS tumor, primarily for brain tumors. Noting the significant impact of cognitive function on patients' ability to resume previously held roles, multiple studies have reported cognitive deficits in patients with a brain tumor (Davies, Clarke, & Hopkins, 1996; Kaleita et al., 2004; Marciniak, Sliwa, Heinemann, & Semik, 2001; Yeh et al., 2005). The majority of work in this area is aimed at determining the effect of radiation therapy on cognitive function; few studies have evaluated changes in cognitive function over time following surgery. In general, impairments in cognitive function have been linked to tumor location, tumor type, tumor volume, and undergoing radiation treatment (Correa et al., 2007; Gregor et al., 1996; Hahn et al., 2003; Kaleita et al., 2004; Marciniak et al., 2001).

Correa et al. (2007) reported that psychomotor skills and nonverbal memory were worse in patients undergoing radiation therapy, and patients on antiepileptic polytherapy had decreased psychomotor skills. In addition, patients with increased white-matter changes on magnetic resonance imaging demonstrated lower scores on executive functioning. Age also appears to affect cognitive status. Kaleita et al. (2004) found that older patients had lower scores in multiple domains of cognitive function, with the exception of attention. The authors also suggested that measures of attention and concentration were the most sensitive measures of neurocognition.

Nursing Care

Assessment of cognitive dysfunction is a challenge. Valid and reliable measure of cognitive function requires the administration of a lengthy battery of tools by a well-trained clinician. Tests from multiple domains of cognition are required in order to identify specific deficits and target interventions appropriately. Referral to a neuropsychologist can provide this assessment and recommendations for treatment. In the absence of a complete assessment, screening of cognitive function can be performed using a brief screening tool such as the Mini-Mental Status Examination or the Neuro-Psychological Inventory. It is crucial, however, that if deficits on these tests are identified, the patient is referred to a neuropsychologist for more complete assessment.

Resolution of cognitive deficits is largely dependent upon their cause. If cerebral edema, pressure from the tumor itself, or radiation necrosis is causing a temporary loss of function, corticosteroid therapy or tumor debulking may improve function. If, however, the loss of function is related to irreversible tissue damage, interventions are aimed at helping patients compensate for loss of function and assisting family caregivers to deal with symptoms as they arise.

Donepezil, an acetylcholinesterase inhibitor, was originally created to treat dementia associated with Alzheimer disease but has recently been used to help with memory loss after brain damage. Morey, Cilo, Berry, and Cusick (2003) reported significant improvements in immediate and delayed memory when donepezil was administered to patients who had persistent memory disorder following traumatic brain injury; these results have been supported by Zhang, Plotkin, Wang, Sandel, and Lee (2004). Other authors have failed to find significant improvements following the administration of donepezil although this may be related to limitations in study design (e.g., use of a global, rather than specific, measure of cognitive dysfunction) (Walker et al., 2004). No studies to date have reported the effects of donepezil on patients with a brain tumor.

Methylphenidate therapy, a stimulant used predominantly for managing the symptom of fatigue during or after completion of cancer treatments, has undergone some limited study for improving cognition. Specific areas of cognitive function that may be positively affected by methylphenidate therapy are those of attention, psychomotor speed, and executive control (Meyers et al., 1998; Wen et al., 2006). Although most clinical trials have involved pediatric survivors (Conklin et al., 2007; Mulhern et al., 2004), the results are mixed regarding the effects on cognitive function (Meyers et al., 1998); therefore, results are mixed regarding their quality of life (Butler et al., 2007).

Cognitive rehabilitation programs that teach adults various techniques to practice their cognitive abilities as well as compensatory strategies have shown some limited benefits (Gehring et al., 2009; Locke et al., 2008). In one randomized controlled trial with 140 adults with primary brain tumors, computerized cognitive retraining sessions over six weeks with trained neuropsychologists and an additional six psychoeducational sessions focused on compensatory strategy training showed improvements in attention and memory, but not in executive control, at a six-month follow-up evaluation (Gehring et al., 2009). Most intervention subjects reported continued use of compensatory strategies after six months as well as perceptions of improved cognitive functioning and everyday function. In a feasibility study for delivering cognitive rehabilitation sessions and psychoeducational sessions on compensatory strategies involving dyads (the patient and the caregiver), most participants and caregivers continued to report use of their training and compensatory strategies over time (Locke

et al., 2008). As this was an intervention feasibility study, they did not observe statistical improvements in cognitive function most likely because of the small sample size (12 dyads completing the study) and participants had only mild cognitive impairment at baseline.

The biologic mechanisms for the cognitive impairments observed over time in patients with primary brain tumors and metastatic disease during and after completion of treatment are not fully understood. Rapid, easy to use and interpret, and sensitive measures for determining cognitive impairment and change over time are still developing. As the International Cognition and Cancer Task Force (2010) pursues its objective of examining the comprehensive issues affecting cognition and cancer, sustainable interventions for improving or preventing cognitive dysfunction that may be useful in this population are on the horizon.

Side Effects of Biotherapy and Chemotherapy

Incidence and Associated Factors

This section will first focus on bevacizumab, a new and exciting treatment for primary malignant brain tumors, and then will discuss more common treatment regimens. Bevacizumab, commonly taken in conjunction with chemotherapy, is a humanized immunoglobulin G1 monoclonal antibody that interacts with vascular endothelial growth factor receptors to inhibit activity. Few studies have reported side effects of bevacizumab in patients with a brain tumor. Vredenburgh et al. (2007) found that in 35 patients with glioblastoma multiforme, 11 patients discontinued therapy because of various toxicities (NCI Common Terminology Criteria for Adverse Events [CTCAE]): grade 2 proteinuria, thromboembolic complications, grade 3 gastrointestinal symptoms, and fatigue (NCI CTEP, 2006). Narayana et al. (2009) reported a lower incidence of toxicity following treatment with bevacizumab. Complications within their sample of 61 patients with a high-grade glioma included deep vein thrombosis (with or without subsequent pulmonary embolism), extreme fatigue, intracerebral hemorrhage, and bone marrow toxicity. Finally, from a retrospective chart audit of patients receiving bevacizumab with conventional chemotherapy, Norden et al. (2008) found that bone marrow suppression, fatigue, and nausea were common, although this may have been attributed to the patient's chemotherapeutic agent. Of 55 patients, 9 had documentation of hemorrhage (epistaxis or other mucosal bleeding), 2 developed asymptomatic brain hemorrhage, and 5 had CTCAE grade 3 or 4 thromboembolic complications.

Side effects of common chemotherapeutic agents often include fatigue, nausea, and vomiting. Besides these, patients often experience several other symptoms. Temozolomide, common in treating CNS tumors, has been linked to anorexia, headache, constipation, and rash (Cohen et al., 2005). When combined with bischloroethylnitrosourea (BCNU), temozolomide has been associated with grade 3–4 thrombocytopenia, granulocytopenia, and anemia (Chang et al., 2004). When given in combination with Gliadel® Wafers (Eisai, Inc.), temozolomide has been linked with myelosuppression (McGirt et al., 2009). A chemotherapy regimen of carboplatin and tamoxifen has been associated with headaches, thrombocytopenia, anemia, and anorexia, and a combination of cisplatin and BCNU has been linked with neutropenia, thrombocytopenia, and nausea and vomiting (Silvani et al., 2009; Tang et al., 2006). High rates of myelosuppression have also been associated with procarbazine-lomustine-vincristine (commonly known as PCV) (Buckner et al., 2003).

Several biotherapeutic agents are used in the treatment of CNS tumors. Unfortunately, research related to side effects is scarce. Pegylated interferon is a form of interferon alpha and has been used to treat some primary malignant brain tumors. Dickinson, Barr, Hiscock, and Meyers (2009) failed to find any significant decline in quality of life or cognition following treatment; however, patients whose tumor showed positive growth during the study were excluded, resulting in a biased sample. In a small sample of patients who received BCNU-impregnated biodegradable wafers during tumor resection and follow-up therapy with interferon alfa-2b, therapy was associated with fatigue, a decline in cognition, myalgia, and arthralgia (Olson et al., 2008). Interferon beta-1a has been associated with nausea and vomiting, leukopenia, and CNS effects (Colman et al., 2006). Adoptive immunotherapy has also been evaluated in the literature in patients with CNS tumors and in one small sample was associated with induration at the site of vaccination, low-grade fever, chills, and muscle spasms (Sloan et al., 2000).

Nursing Care

A small number of studies have evaluated biotherapies and immune targeted therapies; thus, a limited amount of information is known regarding symptom management during these treatment regimens. In addition, research that exists often used very small sample sizes (generally less than 20 participants), which precludes generalizability. As a result, neuro-oncology clinicians need to be aware that a multitude of side effects and symptoms may occur, which requires a consistent, multiple symptom assessment and interventions as needed.

Corticosteroids

Incidence and Associated Factors

Corticosteroids are common in the treatment of cerebral and spinal edema during the postoperative period, radiation

therapy, and in the case of tumor recurrence or CNS metastases (Sturdza et al., 2008). These drugs, however, increase the patient's risk for hyperglycemia and steroid-induced psychosis (Hempen, Weiss, & Hess, 2002; Sinha, Bastin, Wardlaw, Armitage, & Whittle, 2004). Steroid-related hyperglycemia can occur as a result of intraoperative administration of corticosteroids (Pasternak, McGregor, & Lanier, 2004), with one study suggesting that higher levels are found when intraoperative corticosteroids are given to patients with no history of taking the medication and in patients who have longer surgical procedures (Lukins & Manninen, 2005). In turn, hyperglycemia has been associated with increased mortality in patients with an astrocytoma (Derr et al., 2009; McGirt et al., 2008).

Corticosteroids may cause patients to experience psychiatric symptoms, which can induce a mood disorder or even a psychotic disorder. Steroid psychosis can present with a wide array of symptoms ranging from depression to mania. In a review of the literature, Lewis and Smith (1983) reported that steroid psychosis occurs in approximately 5% of patients taking steroids; a much lower percentage (0.87%) has been suggested in other studies (Wada et al., 2001). Why corticosteroid use induced steroid psychosis is unclear, but it may be related to increased dosages or resumption of use.

Nursing Care

Nursing care for patients on corticosteroids is centered on monitoring for hyperglycemia and preparing patients for the physical and cognitive side effects that may occur. Increased appetite, weight gain, insomnia, gastrointestinal problems, muscle weakness, irritability, and personality changes have all been associated with corticosteroid therapy and can have a large impact on quality of life (Sturdza et al., 2008). Serum glucose levels should be routinely monitored both during corticosteroid therapy and in the period after therapy has been discontinued. Patients should be carefully monitored for psychiatric symptoms or changes in cognitive status during the first two weeks of therapy and when receiving high doses (Brown, Khan, & Nejtek, 1999). Patients are commonly prescribed corticosteroids for six months during treatment or, in the case of metastases or advanced disease, until the end of life (Hempen et al., 2002). Assessment of potential complications should be routine and continue while the therapy continues.

Psychological Issues

Psychological issues studied in patients with a CNS tumor are typically depression and depressive symptoms. Depressive symptoms include sadness, lack of energy, and lack of interest in daily activities. Controversy exists regarding whether depression is a result of physiologic processes or a situational response. Regardless of the cause, depression has been associated with increased mortality in patients with several different types of cancer, including CNS cancers.

Incidence and Associated Factors

Rates of depressive symptoms in cross-sectional studies have been found to vary from 28% to 50% in patients with CNS tumors (Davies et al., 1996; Wellisch, Kaleita, Freeman, Cloughesy, & Goldman, 2002), and data have suggested that patients with a brain tumor are greater than nine times more likely to have a major depressive disorder than the general population. In a study of 21 men diagnosed with a glioma, Davies et al. (1996) found that moderate or severe depression, anxiety, irritability, or fatigue was present in more than half of the subjects who were classified as "inactive" (those with poor physical function). Depression was associated with life changes and hopelessness, which can be expected given the amount of physical and cognitive dysfunction that can occur following diagnosis of a glioma and the potential for a short, terminal trajectory.

Research has shown that depressive symptoms have been linked to gender, tumor type, employment status, tumor location, corticosteroid and interferon therapy, and a family history of psychiatric illness (American Psychiatric Association [APA], 2000; Mainio, Hakko, Niemelä, Koivukangas, & Räsänen, 2005; Pelletier et al., 2002; Wellisch et al., 2002). Subsequently, increased levels of depression have been linked to mortality. In patients with a low-grade glioma, Mainio et al. (2006) found that depressive symptoms significantly affected survival, but they did not find this relationship in patients with high-grade gliomas or those with benign tumors. They found that in patients with a low-grade glioma, those with depressive symptoms had a survival time of 3.3–5.8 years, compared with 10–11.7 years in those who did not report depressive symptoms (Mainio et al., 2006). The relationship between depressive symptoms and survival in patients with a CNS tumor has been replicated in several studies (Gathinji et al., 2009; Litofsky et al., 2004; Litofsky & Resnick, 2009).

Nursing Care

Because of the frequency of depressive symptoms in patients with a CNS tumor and the significant impact of depressive symptoms on not only the quality but potentially the quantity of life, assessment and intervention are of primary concern. Unfortunately, practitioner and patient assessment of depressive symptoms may be incongruent. Litofsky et al. (2004) found that in a sample of patients with brain tumors, more than 90% reported symptoms consistent with depression, whereas only 15% of the patients' practitioners reported depression. The gold standard for diagnosing a major depressive episode is the *Diagnostic and Statistical Manual of Mental Disorders* (*DSM-IV-TR*) (APA, 2000). *DSM-IV-TR* criteria require patients to have at least five of the following symptoms nearly every day during the same two-week period that are a change from previous functioning and are in the absence of drug or alcohol abuse or bereavement: (a) depressed mood most of the day, (b) diminished interest or pleasure in activities, (c) significant weight loss or weight gain, (d) insomnia or hypersomnia, (e) psychomotor agitation or retardation, (f) fatigue, (g) feelings of worthlessness or inappropriate guilt, (h) diminished ability to think or concentrate, and (i) recurrent thoughts of death or suicidal ideation.

Because several of these criteria are likely to be a result of the disease process or treatment (e.g., fatigue, insomnia, weight loss), controversy exists regarding the utility of the *DSM-IV-TR* criteria in evaluating depression in patients with cancer. Administering these criteria requires the use of a psychiatrist or psychologist to both make the official diagnosis and to differentiate somatic symptoms from the disease versus a psychological state. Because of these issues, many oncology practices use shortened screening forms to identify patients at risk for depression. These forms are less time intensive, can often be self-administered, and are short enough to prove clinically useful. Forms such as the Beck Depression Inventory and the Center for Epidemiologic Studies–Depression use a Likert-type scale to ask respondents to indicate the degree to which they agree with statements. Responses have a numeric value and items are summed to provide a total score of depressive symptoms. Common depressive symptom measures have established cutoff scores to indicate those patients at risk for major depression disorder.

Patients should be monitored for depressive symptoms at routine intervals throughout the disease trajectory with particular attention to any changes in disease status (see Table 11-6). No studies to date have reported the effectiveness of interventions to alleviate depressive symptoms in patients with a CNS tumor. However, the standard of care in treating depressive symptoms in patients with other types of tumors is the concomitant use of antidepressants with counseling or therapy (Fulcher, Badger, Gunter, Marrs, & Reese, 2009).

Complementary and Alternative Therapies

Incidence and Associated Factors

Over the past decade, use of complementary and alternative therapies has become more common (Armstrong et al., 2006; Fox, Laws, Anderson, & Farace, 2006). Types of complementary and alternative therapies are typically grouped into the following five domains.
- Alternative medical systems (acupuncture, Chinese medicine)
- Mind-body modalities (meditation and prayer)

- Biologically based modalities (neoplastics, herbs, hydrazine sulfate, macrobiotic diet, shark cartilage, and vitamins)
- Manipulative and body-based therapies (massage and yoga)
- Energy-based modalities (faith healing, therapeutic touch)

Fox et al. (2006) found that in a sample of patients with a high-grade glioma, 32% reported having used some form of complementary therapy. The most frequently used therapies included meditation (31%), vitamins (23%), herbs (22%), and shark cartilage (12%). Although those who used complementary therapies reported a higher level of quality of life, no statistically significant difference was reported between those who did and did not use the therapies.

Verhoef, Hagen, Pelletier, and Forsyth (1999) also studied alternative therapies in people with CNS tumors. At the time of diagnosis, almost one-half of the sample was familiar with more than two alternative therapies, the majority being herbal therapies (69%), mind-body practices (40%), and animal/vegetable-derived therapies (36%). Although only one-fourth of the sample used alternative therapies, the majority of those who used alternative therapies perceived positive effects; 35% of patients attributed lack of tumor regrowth or tumor shrinkage to the therapy. The most commonly reported benefits were improved mental or physical well-being and increased energy. Only 37% of participants reported the costs of their alternative therapy, but the median reported cost was $55, with 90% of participants or their families paying all of the costs (Verhoef et al., 1999). Armstrong et al. (2006) reported similar results but with a higher percentage of patients using therapies (34%). In addition, Armstrong et al. found significant relationships between complementary therapy use and both physical function and quality of life.

Nursing Care

Both Armstrong et al. (2006) and Fox et al. (2006) found that the use of alternative therapies helped participants feel more in control of their treatment. However, Verhoef et al. (1999) and Armstrong et al. reported that only 45%–74% of patients indicated that their physicians were aware of their use of alternative therapies. These data underscore the necessity for doing a complete assessment with each clinic visit, as the number and variety of therapies may change rapidly during the course of the disease. In turn, because studies in

Table 11-6. Depression Assessment Guide		
Assessment	**Yes**	**No**
Physical Symptoms		
• Changes in appetite, weight, sleep, and psychomotor activity		
• Decreased energy		
Psychosocial Symptoms		
• Feelings of worthlessness or guilt		
• Recurrent thoughts of death or suicidal ideation, plans, or attempts		
Cognitive Changes		
• Difficulty thinking, concentrating, or making decisions		
• Flat affect		
Risk and Contributing Factors		
• Medications		
• Family history		
• Medical conditions (e.g., endocrine disorders, cardiovascular conditions, neurologic conditions, immune disorders)		
• History of substance abuse		

Note. Based on information from Albright & Valente, 2006; Dahlin, 2006.

From "Depression" (p. 106), by L.H. Eaton in L.H. Eaton and J.M. Tipton (Eds.), *Putting Evidence Into Practice: Improving Oncology Patient Outcomes*, 2009, Pittsburgh, PA: Oncology Nursing Society. Copyright 2009 by the Oncology Nursing Society. Reprinted with permission.

this area have been descriptive in nature, neuro-oncology practitioners have very little information regarding potential interactions and side effects. Some Web sites, such as Memorial Sloan-Kettering Cancer Center (www.mskcc.org), offer information about side effects of herbal supplements. However, in addition to performing adequate assessments at each visit, practitioners need to be cautious of potential interactions of complementary and alternative therapies with mainstream therapy.

Family Caregiver Distress

Incidence and Associated Factors

It has been estimated that 31% of the adult population has provided care for a family member; the number of family caregivers in the United States is likely to rise and continue to be the largest source of long-term care (U.S. Department of Health and Human Services, 1998). Noting the expected increase in the number of family caregivers, the reduction in reimbursable healthcare services, and the risk for negative outcomes for caregivers, it is vital to maintain family caregiver health. Providing adequate support to family caregivers not only improves their health but may also improve the care they provide to the patient with a CNS tumor.

Despite decades of research underscoring the negative emotional and physical responses that can occur as a result of providing care to someone with a chronic illness, little of this work has been done in neuro-oncology. In oncology and dementia research, family caregivers have been shown to be at high risk for depression, anxiety, burden, altered sleep patterns, poor self-care behaviors, altered cytokine production, high blood pressure, and increased overall mortality (Beach, Schulz, Yee, & Jackson, 2000; Carter, 2002; Pinquart & Sörensen, 2003; Vitaliano, Zhang, & Scanlan, 2003). Caregiver distress (so named to encompass caregiver burden, depression, anxiety, and other negative emotional responses) has been consistently linked to behavior problems and cognitive impairment in the care recipient (the patient). Poor physical health in the care recipient has also been associated with caregiver distress although its impact is typically considered secondary to that of behavioral and cognitive dysfunction (Pinquart & Sörensen, 2004). Other factors that may lead to poor outcomes in family caregivers include providing care for an extended time, being a younger caregiver, being a spouse of the care recipient, and being female. In addition, poor outcomes have been associated with caregivers who have higher levels of neuroticism and those who have lower levels of self-efficacy, marital satisfaction, and social support (Gallant & Connell, 2003; Jang, Clay, Roth, Haley, & Mittelman, 2004; Nijboer, Tempelaar, Triemstra, van den Bos, & Sanderman, 2001).

Nursing Care

Several researchers have reported neuro-oncology caregivers' difficulty in communicating with healthcare practitioners (Sherwood, Given, Doorenbos, & Given, 2004; Strang, Strang, & Ternestedt, 2001; Wideheim, Edvardsson, Påhlson, & Ahlström, 2002). As such, nurses' primary responsibility is to establish a trusting relationship with the caregiver-care recipient dyad. Information should be given orally and backed up with written material and should target the dyad's needs. For example, caregivers have reported having difficulty accessing information on end of life and have reported the need to understand what to expect with disease progression (Lipsman, Skanda, Kimmelman, & Bernstein, 2007; Sherwood et al., 2004). In turn, unmet needs in neuro-oncology caregivers have been linked to depression and lower reports of quality of life. Janda and colleagues reported that caregivers needed help adjusting to changes in the care recipient's mental and thinking ability, managing difficult care recipient behaviors, feeling less alone in providing care, and finding appropriate rehabilitation services (Janda, Eakin, Bailey, Walker, & Troy, 2006; Janda et al., 2007, 2008).

Screening caregivers for emotional distress and intervening to alleviate those symptoms is challenging. Caregiver distress measures that are multidimensional in nature allow for more accurate screening, yet these tools are often lengthy, which limits their clinical utility. Caregiver distress measures that are shorter tend to be less sensitive to identifying those in need. Examples of measurement tools for caregiver strain and burden include (Sherwood & Given, 2008)

- Caregiver Strain Index (13 items)
- Zarit Burden Inventory (22 items)
- Caregiver Reaction Assessment (24 items).

Caregivers experiencing strain often benefit from cognitive-behavioral interventions such as focusing on time management, developing problem-solving abilities, or reengaging in pleasant activities, to cite a few (Sörensen, Pinquart, & Duberstein, 2002). Nurses can help to improve caregiver outcomes, and thus patient outcomes, by incorporating cognitive-behavioral interventions into their practice (Honea et al., 2009).

Ultimately, caregivers who are distressed should be referred appropriately (e.g., counseling, therapy, or to their primary care practitioner for follow-up). It is important to remember that caregivers often forgo their own health needs to meet the demands of the care situation; adequate follow-up measures should be in place to ensure caregivers receive the care they need.

Summary

As the previous sections have illustrated, the science of symptom management in neuro-oncology is just beginning.

The data available have started to describe the incidence and associated factors involved in several common symptoms in patients with a CNS tumor. Very little work has been done to identify therapeutic interventions to alleviate symptom distress. In addition, family reports of difficulty in communicating with healthcare providers and patient reports of not fully informing physicians of treatments underscore the necessity of opening lines of communication between practitioners and patients. When therapeutic communication occurs, symptom management becomes a cooperative effort and a realistic goal.

References

Albright, A.V., & Valente, S.M. (2006). Depression and suicide. In R.M. Carroll-Johnson, L.M. Gorman, & N.J. Bush (Eds.), *Psychosocial nursing care along the cancer continuum* (2nd ed., pp. 241–260). Pittsburgh, PA: Oncology Nursing Society.

American Association of Neuroscience Nurses. (2006). *Guide to the care of the patient with craniotomy post-brain tumor resection.* Retrieved from http://www.aann.org/pdf/cpg/aanncraniotomy.pdf

American Association of Neuroscience Nurses. (2007). *Cervical spine surgery: A guide to preoperative and postoperative care.* Retrieved from http://www.aann.org/pubs/cpg/cervicalspine.pdf

American Brain Tumor Association. (2008). Help with side effects—Chemotherapy. Retrieved from http://www.abta.org/index.cfm?contentid=144

American Psychiatric Association. (2000). *Diagnostic and statistical manual of mental disorders* (4th ed., text revision). Washington, DC: American Psychiatric Publishing.

Armstrong, T., Cohen, M.Z., Hess, K.R., Manning, R., Lee, E.L., Tamayo, G., ... Gilbert, M. (2006). Complementary and alternative medicine use and quality of life in patients with primary brain tumors. *Journal of Pain and Symptom Management, 32,* 148–154. doi:10.1016/j.jpainsymman.2006.02.015

Barker, E. (Ed.). (2008). *Neuroscience nursing: A spectrum of care* (3rd ed.). St. Louis, MO: Elsevier Mosby.

Barker, F.G., II, Klibanski, A., & Swearingen, B. (2003). Transsphenoidal surgery for pituitary tumors in the United States, 1996–2000: Mortality, morbidity, and the effects of hospital and surgeon volume. *Journal of Clinical Endocrinology and Metabolism, 88,* 4709–4719. doi:10.1210/jc.2003-030461

Beach, S.R., Schulz, R., Yee, J.L., & Jackson, S. (2000). Negative and positive health effects of caring for a disabled spouse: Longitudinal findings from the caregiver health effects study. *Psychology and Aging, 15,* 259–271. doi:10.1037/0882-7974.15.2.259

Blackhall, L., Petroni, G., Shu, J., Baum, L., & Farace, E. (2009). A pilot study evaluating the safety and efficacy of modafinil for cancer-related fatigue. *Journal of Palliative Medicine, 12,* 433–439. doi:10.1089/jpm.2008.0230

Brown, E.S., Khan, D.A., & Nejtek, V.A. (1999). The psychiatric side effects of corticosteroids. *Annals of Allergy, Asthma, and Immunology, 83*(6, Pt. 1), 495–503.

Brown, P., Clark, M.M., Atherton, P., Huschka, M., Sloan, J.A., Gamble, G., ... Rummans, T.A. (2006). Will improvement in quality of life (QOL) impact fatigue in patients receiving radiation therapy for advanced cancer? *American Journal of Clinical Oncology, 29,* 52–58. doi:10.1097/01.coc.0000190459.14841.55

Brown, P.D., Ballman, K.V., Rummans, T.A., Maurer, M.J., Sloan, J.A., Boeve, B.F., ... Buckner, J.C. (2006). Prospective study of quality of life in adults with newly diagnosed high-grade gliomas.

Journal of Neuro-Oncology, 76, 283–291. doi:10.1007/s11060-005-7020-9

Buckner, J.C., Gesme, D., Jr., O'Fallon, J.R., Hammack, J.E., Stafford, S., Brown, P.D., ... Jenkins, R. (2003). Phase II trial of procarbazine, lomustine, and vincristine as initial therapy for patients with low-grade oligodendroglioma or oligoastrocytoma: Efficacy and associations with chromosomal abnormalities. *Journal of Clinical Oncology, 21,* 251–255. doi:10.1200/JCO.2003.06.023

Butler, J.M., Jr., Case, L.D., Atkins, J., Frizzell, B., Sanders, G., Griffin, P., ... Shaw, E.G. (2007). A phase III, double-blind, placebo-controlled prospective randomized clinical trial of d-threo-methylphenidate HCl in brain tumor patients receiving radiation therapy. *International Journal of Radiation Oncology, Biology, Physics, 69,* 1496–1501. doi:10.1016/j.ijrobp.2007.05.076

Butt, Z., Rosenbloom, S.K., Abernethy, A.P., Beaumont, J.L., Paul, D., Hampton, D., ... Cella, D. (2008). Fatigue is the most important symptom for advanced cancer patients who have had chemotherapy. *Journal of the National Comprehensive Cancer Network, 6,* 448–455. Retrieved from http://www.jnccn.org/content/6/5/448.full.pdf+html

Carter, P.A. (2002). Caregivers' descriptions of sleep changes and depressive symptoms. *Oncology Nursing Forum, 29,* 1277–1283. doi:10.1188/02.ONF.1277-1283

Chang, S.M., Prados, M.D., Yung, W.K., Fine, H., Junck, L., Greenberg, H., ... Schold, C. (2004). Phase II study of neoadjuvant 1, 3-bis (2-chloroethyl)-1-nitrosourea and temozolomide for newly diagnosed anaplastic glioma: A North American Brain Tumor Consortium trial. *Cancer, 100,* 1712–1716. doi:10.1002/cncr.20157

Cohen, M.H., Johnson, J.R., & Pazdur, R. (2005). Food and Drug Administration drug approval summary: Temozolomide plus radiation therapy for the treatment of newly diagnosed glioblastoma multiforme. *Clinical Cancer Research, 11*(19, Pt. 1), 6767–6771. doi:10.1158/1078-0432.CCR-05-0722

Cohen, Z.R., Hassenbusch, S.J., Maor, M.H., Pfeffer, R.M., & Ram, Z. (2002). Intractable vomiting from glioblastoma metastatic to the fourth ventricle: Three case studies. *Neuro-Oncology, 4,* 129–133.

Colman, H., Berkey, B.A., Maor, M.H., Groves, M.D., Schultz, C.J., Vermeulen, S., ... Yung, W.K.A. (2006). Phase II Radiation Therapy Oncology Group trial of conventional radiation therapy followed by treatment with recombinant interferon-beta for supratentorial glioblastoma: Results of RTOG 9710. *International Journal of Radiation Oncology, Biology, Physics, 66,* 818–824. doi:10.1016/j.ijrobp.2006.05.021

Conklin, H.M., Khan, R., Reddick, W.E., Helton, S., Brown, R., Howard, S.C., ... Mulhern, R.K. (2007). Acute neurocognitive response to methylphenidate among survivors of childhood cancer: A randomized, double-blind, cross-over trial. *Journal of Pediatric Psychology, 32,* 1127–1139. doi:10.1093/jpepsy/jsm045

Correa, D.D., DeAngelis, L.M., Shi, W., Thaler, H.T., Lin, M., & Abrey, L.E. (2007). Cognitive functions in low-grade gliomas: Disease and treatment effects. *Journal of Neuro-Oncology, 81,* 175–184. doi:10.1007/s11060-006-9212-3

Dahlin, C. (2006). Depression. In D. Camp-Sorrell & R.A. Hawkins (Eds.), *Clinical manual for the oncology advanced practice nurse* (2nd ed., pp. 1119–1125). Pittsburgh, PA: Oncology Nursing Society.

Davies, E., Clarke, C., & Hopkins, A. (1996). Malignant cerebral glioma-I: Survival, disability, and morbidity after radiotherapy. *BMJ, 313,* 1507–1512. Retrieved from http://www.bmj.com/cgi/content/full/313/7071/1507?view=long&pmid=8978224

Derr, R.L., Ye, X., Islas, M.U., Desideri, S., Saudek, C.D., & Grossman, S.A. (2009). Association between hyperglycemia and survival in patients with newly diagnosed glioblastoma.

Journal of Clinical Oncology, 27, 1082–1086. doi:10.1200/JCO.2008.19.1098

Dickinson, M.D., Barr, C.D., Hiscock, M., & Meyers, C.A. (2009). Cognitive effects of pegylated interferon in individuals with primary brain tumors. *Journal of Neuro-Oncology, 95,* 231–237. doi:10.1007/s11060-009-9920-6

Eaton, L.H. (2009). Fatigue. In L.H. Eaton & J.M. Tipton (Eds.), *Putting evidence into practice: Improving oncology patient outcomes* (pp. 149–154). Pittsburgh, PA: Oncology Nursing Society.

Enblom, A., Axelsson, B.B., Steineck, G., Hammar, M., & Börjeson, S. (2009). One third of patients with radiotherapy-induced nausea consider their antiemetic treatment insufficient. *Supportive Care in Cancer, 17,* 23–32. doi:10.1007/s00520-008-0445-x

Faithfull, S., & Brada, M. (1998). Somnolence syndrome in adults following cranial irradiation for primary brain tumours. *Clinical Oncology, 10,* 250–254.

Feuerstein, M., Hansen, J.A., Calvio, L.C., Johnson, L., & Ronquillo, J.G. (2007). Work productivity in brain tumor survivors. *Journal of Occupational and Environmental Medicine, 49,* 803–811. doi:10.1097/JOM.0b013e318095a458

Fox, S., Laws, E.R., Jr., Anderson, F., Jr., & Farace, E. (2006). Complementary therapy use and quality of life in persons with high-grade gliomas. *Journal of Neuroscience Nursing, 38,* 212–220.

Fox, S.W., Lyon, D., & Farace, E. (2007). Symptom clusters in patients with high-grade glioma. *Journal of Nursing Scholarship, 39,* 61–67. doi:10.1111/j.1547-5069.2007.00144.x

Friend, P.J., Johnston, M.P., Tipton, J.M., McDaniel, R.W., Barbour, L.A., Star, P., ... Ripple, M.L. (2009). ONS PEP resource: chemotherapy-induced nausea and vomiting. In L.H. Eaton & J.M. Tipton (Eds.), *Putting evidence into practice: Improving oncology patient outcomes* (pp. 71–83). Pittsburgh, PA: Oncology Nursing Society.

Fujimura, M., Kumabe, T., Jokura, H., Shirane, R., Yoshimoto, T., & Tominaga, T. (2004). Intractable vomiting as an early clinical symptom of cerebrospinal fluid seeding to the fourth ventricle in patients with high-grade astrocytoma. *Journal of Neuro-Oncology, 66,* 209–216. doi:10.1023/B:NEON.0000013487.71148.5d

Fulcher, C.D., Badger, T.A., Gunter, A.K., Marrs, J.A., & Reese, J.M. (2009). ONS PEP resource: Depression. In L.H. Eaton & J.M. Tipton (Eds.), *Putting evidence into practice: Improving oncology patient outcomes* (pp. 111–118). Pittsburgh, PA: Oncology Nursing Society.

Gallant, M.P., & Connell, C.M. (2003). Neuroticism and depressive symptoms among spouse caregivers: Do health behaviors mediate this relationship? *Psychology and Aging, 18,* 587–592. doi:10.1037/0882-7974.18.3.587

Gathinji, M., McGirt, M.J., Attenello, F.J., Chaichana, K.L., Than, K., Olivi, A., ... Quinones-Hinojosa, A. (2009). Association of preoperative depression and survival after resection of malignant brain astrocytoma. *Surgical Neurology, 71,* 299–303. doi:10.1016/j.surneu.2008.07.016

Gehring, K., Sitskoorn, M.M., Gundy, C.M., Sikkes, S.A., Klein, M., Postma, T.J., ... Aaronson, N.K. (2009). Cognitive rehabilitation in patients with gliomas: A randomized, controlled trial. *Journal of Clinical Oncology, 27,* 3712–3722. doi:10.1200/JCO.2008.20.5765

Gregor, A., Cull, A., Traynor, E., Stewart, M., Lander, F., & Love, S. (1996). Neuropsychometric evaluation of long-term survivors of adult brain tumours: Relationship with tumour and treatment parameters. *Radiotherapy and Oncology, 41,* 55–59.

Grunberg, S.M., Osoba, D., Hesketh, P.J., Gralla, R.J., Borjeson, S., Rapoport, B.L., ... Tonato, M. (2005). Evaluation of new antiemetic agents and definition of antineoplastic agent emetogenicity—An update. *Supportive Care in Cancer, 13,* 80–84. doi:10.1007/s00520-004-0718-y

Gustafsson, M., Edvardsson, T., & Ahlström, G. (2006). The relationship between function, quality of life and coping in patients with low-grade gliomas. *Supportive Care in Cancer, 14,* 1205–1212. doi:10.1007/s00520-006-0080-3

Hahn, C.A., Dunn, R.H., Logue, P.E., King, J.H., Edwards, C.L., & Halperin, E.C. (2003). Prospective study of neuropsychological testing and quality-of-life assessment of adults with primary malignant brain tumors. *International Journal of Radiation Oncology, Biology, Physics, 55,* 992–999. doi:10.1016/S0360-3016(02)04205-0

Hempen, C., Weiss, E., & Hess, C.F. (2002). Dexamethasone treatment in patients with brain metastases and primary brain tumors: Do the benefits outweigh the side-effects? *Supportive Care in Cancer, 10,* 322–328. doi:10.1007/s00520-001-0333-0

Hickey, J.V. (2009). Neurological assessment. In J.V. Hickey (Ed.), *The clinical practice of neurological and neurosurgical nursing* (6th ed., pp. 154–180). Philadelphia, PA: Wolters Kluwer/Lippincott Williams & Wilkins.

Honea, N.J., Sherwood, P.R., Northouse, L.L., Brintnall, R.A., Colao, D.B., Somers, S.C., ... Given, B.A. (2009). ONS PEP resource: Caregiver strain and burden. In L.H. Eaton & J.M. Tipton (Eds.), *Putting evidence into practice: Improving oncology patient outcomes* (pp. 57–62). Pittsburgh, PA: Oncology Nursing Society.

International Cognition and Cancer Task Force. (2010). Mission statement. Retrieved from http://www.icctf.com/index.php?3

Italian Group for Antiemetic Research in Radiotherapy. (1999). Radiation-induced emesis: A prospective observational multicenter Italian trial. *International Journal of Radiation Oncology, Biology, Physics, 44,* 619–625.

Janda, M., Eakin, E.G., Bailey, L., Walker, D., & Troy, K. (2006). Supportive care needs of people with brain tumours and their carers. *Supportive Care in Cancer, 14,* 1094–1103. doi:10.1007/s00520-006-0074-1

Janda, M., Steginga, S., Dunn, J., Langbecker, D., Walker, D., & Eakin, E. (2008). Unmet supportive care needs and interest in services among patients with a brain tumour and their carers. *Patient Education and Counseling, 71,* 251–258. doi:10.1016/j.pec.2008.01.020

Janda, M., Steginga, S., Langbecker, D., Dunn, J., Walker, D., & Eakin, E. (2007). Quality of life among patients with a brain tumor and their carers. *Journal of Psychosomatic Research, 63,* 617–623. doi:10.1016/j.jpsychores.2007.06.018

Jang, Y., Clay, O.J., Roth, D.L., Haley, W.E., & Mittelman, M.S. (2004). Neuroticism and longitudinal change in caregiver depression: Impact of a spouse-caregiver intervention program. *Gerontologist, 44,* 311–317.

Kaleita, T.A., Wellisch, D.K., Cloughesy, T.F., Ford, J.M., Freeman, D., Belin, T.R., & Goldman, J. (2004). Prediction of neurocognitive outcome in adult brain tumor patients. *Journal of Neuro-Oncology, 67,* 245–253. doi:10.1023/B:NEON.0000021900.29176.58

Kaleita, T.A., Wellisch, D.K., Graham, C.A., Steh, B., Nghiemphu, P., Ford, J.M., ... Cloughesy, T.F. (2006). Pilot study of modafinil for treatment of neurobehavioral dysfunction and fatigue in adult patients with brain tumors [Abstract]. *Journal of Clinical Oncology, 24*(Suppl. 18), Abstract No. 1503. Retrieved from http://meeting.ascopubs.org/cgi/content/abstract/24/18_suppl/1503

Khan, R.B., Gutin, P.H., Rai, S.N., Zhang, L., Krol, G., & DeAngelis, L.M. (2006). Use of diffusion weighted magnetic resonance imaging in predicting early postoperative outcome of new neurological deficits after brain tumor resection. *Neurosurgery, 59,* 60–66. doi:10.1227/01.NEU.0000219218.43128.FC

Kris, M.G., Hesketh, P.J., Somerfield, M.R., Feyer, P., Clark-Snow, R., Koeller, J.M., ... Grunberg, S.M. (2006). American Society of Clinical Oncology guideline for antiemetics in oncology: Update 2006. *Journal of Clinical Oncology, 24,* 2932–2947. doi:10.1200/JCO.2006.06.9591

Lewis, D.A., & Smith, R.E. (1983). Steroid-induced psychiatric syndromes. A report of 14 cases and a review of the literature. *Journal of Affective Disorders, 5,* 319–332.

Lipsman, N., Skanda, A., Kimmelman, J., & Bernstein, M. (2007). The attitudes of brain cancer patients and their caregivers towards death and dying: A qualitative study. *BMC Palliative Care, 6,* 7. doi:10.1186/1472-684X-6-7

Litofsky, N.S., Farace, E., Anderson, F., Jr., Meyers, C.A., Huang, W., & Laws, E.R., Jr. (2004). Depression in patients with high-grade glioma: Results of the Glioma Outcomes Project. *Neurosurgery, 54,* 358–366.

Litofsky, N.S., & Resnick, A.G. (2009). The relationships between depression and brain tumors. *Journal of Neuro-Oncology, 94,* 153–161. doi:10.1007/s11060-009-9825-4

Locke, D.E.C., Cerhan, J.H., Wu, W., Malec, J.F., Clark, M.M., Rummans, T.A., & Brown, P.D. (2008). Cognitive rehabilitation and problem-solving to improve quality of life of patients with primary brain tumors: A pilot study. *Journal of Supportive Oncology, 6,* 383–391. Retrieved from http://www.supportiveoncology.net/journal/articles/0608383.pdf

Lukins, M.B., & Manninen, P.H. (2005). Hyperglycemia in patients administered dexamethasone for craniotomy. *Anesthesia and Analgesia, 100,* 1129–1133. doi:10.1213/01. ANE.0000146943.45445.55

Mainio, A., Hakko, H., Niemelä, A., Koivukangas, J., & Räsänen, P. (2005). Depression and functional outcome in patients with brain tumors: A population-based 1-year follow-up study. *Journal of Neurosurgery, 103,* 841–847. doi:10.3171/jns.2005.103.5.0841

Mainio, A., Tuunanen, S., Hakko, H., Niemelä, A., Koivukangas, J., & Räsänen, P. (2006). Decreased quality of life and depression as predictors for shorter survival among patients with low-grade gliomas: A follow-up from 1990 to 2003. *European Archives in Psychiatry and Clinical Neuroscience, 256,* 516–521. doi:10.1007/s00406-006-0674-2

Manninen, P.H., & Tan, T.K. (2002). Postoperative nausea and vomiting after craniotomy for tumor surgery: A comparison between awake craniotomy and general anesthesia. *Journal of Clinical Anesthesia, 14,* 279–283.

Marciniak, C.M., Sliwa, J.A., Heinemann, A.W., & Semik, P.E. (2001). Functional outcomes of persons with brain tumors after inpatient rehabilitation. *Archives of Physical Medicine and Rehabilitation, 82,* 457–463. doi:10.1053/apmr.2001.21862

McCorkle, R., & Quint-Benoliel, J. (1983). Symptom distress, current concerns and mood disturbance after diagnosis of life-threatening disease. *Social Science and Medicine, 17,* 431–438.

McGirt, M.J., Chaichana, K.L., Gathinji, M., Attenello, F., Than, K., Ruiz, A.J., ... Quiñones-Hinojosa, A. (2008). Persistent outpatient hyperglycemia is independently associated with decreased survival after primary resection of malignant brain astrocytomas. *Neurosurgery, 63,* 286–291. doi:10.1227/01. NEU.0000315282.61035.48

McGirt, M.J., Than, K.D., Weingart, J.D., Chaichana, L., Attenello, F.J., Olivi, A., ... Quiñones-Hinojosa, A. (2009). Gliadel (BCNU) wafer plus concomitant temozolomide therapy after primary resection of glioblastoma multiforme. *Journal of Neurosurgery, 110,* 583–588. doi:10.3171/2008.5.17557

Mendoza, T.R., Wang, X.S., Cleeland, C.S., Morrissey, M., Johnson, B.A., Wendt, J.K., & Huber, S.L. (1999). The rapid assessment of fatigue severity in cancer patients: Use of the Brief Fatigue Inventory. *Cancer, 85,* 1186–1196. doi:10.1002/(SICI)1097-0142(19990301)85:5<1186::AID-CNCR24>3.0.CO;2-N

Meyers, C.A., Weitzner, M.A., Valentine, A.D., & Levin, V.A. (1998). Methylphenidate therapy improves cognition, mood, and function of brain tumor patients. *Journal of Clinical Oncology, 16,* 2522–2527.

Mitchell, S.A., Beck, S.L., Hood, L.E., Moore, K., & Tanner, E.R. (2009). ONS PEP resource: Fatigue. In L.H. Eaton & J.M. Tipton (Eds.), *Putting evidence into practice: Improving oncology patient outcomes* (pp. 155–174). Pittsburgh, PA: Oncology Nursing Society.

Morey, C.E., Cilo, M., Berry, J., & Cusick, C. (2003). The effect of Aricept in persons with persistent memory disorder following traumatic brain injury: A pilot study. *Brain Injury, 17,* 809–815. doi:10.1080/0269905031000088586

Mulhern, R.K., Khan, R.B., Kaplan, S., Helton, S., Christensen, R., Bonner, M., ... Reddick, W.E. (2004). Short-term efficacy of methylphenidate: A randomized, double-blind, placebo-controlled trial among survivors of childhood cancer. *Journal of Clinical Oncology, 22,* 4795–4803. doi:10.1200/JCO.2004.04.128

Narayana, A., Kelly, P., Golfinos, J., Parker, E., Johnson, G., Knopp, E., ... Gruber, M.L. (2009). Antiangiogenic therapy using bevacizumab in recurrent high-grade glioma: Impact on local control and patient survival. *Journal of Neurosurgery, 110,* 173–180. doi:10.3171/2008.4.17492

National Cancer Institute Cancer Therapy Evaluation Program. (2006). *Common terminology criteria for adverse events* [v.3.0]. Retrieved from http://ctep.cancer.gov/protocolDevelopment/electronic_applications/docs/ctcaev3.pdf

National Cancer Institute Cancer Therapy Evaluation Program. (2009). *Common terminology criteria for adverse events* [v.4.02]. Retrieved from http://evs.nci.nih.gov/ftp1/CTCAE/CTCAE_4.02_2009-09-15_QuickReference_5x7.pdf

National Comprehensive Cancer Network. (2010). *NCCN Clinical Practice Guidelines in Oncology™: Cancer-related fatigue* [v.1.2010]. Retrieved from http://www.nccn.org/professionals/physician_gls/PDF/fatigue.pdf

Nijboer, C., Tempelaar, R., Triemstra, M., van den Bos, G.A., & Sanderman, R. (2001). The role of social and psychological resources in caregiving of cancer patients. *Cancer, 91,* 1029–1039. doi:10.1002/1097-0142(20010301)91:5<1029::AID-CNCR1094>3.0.CO;2-1

Norden, A.D., Young, G.S., Setayesh, K., Muzikansky, A., Klufas, R., Ross, G.L., ... Wen, P.Y. (2008). Bevacizumab for recurrent malignant gliomas: Efficacy, toxicity, and patterns of recurrence. *Neurology, 70,* 779–787. doi:10.1212/01. wnl.0000304121.57857.38

Olson, J.J., McKenzie, E., Skurski-Martin, M., Zhang, Z., Brat, D., & Phuphanich, S. (2008). Phase I analysis of BCNU-impregnated biodegradable polymer wafers followed by systemic interferon alfa-2b in adults with recurrent glioblastoma multiforme. *Journal of Neuro-Oncology, 90,* 293–299. doi:10.1007/s11060-008-9660-z

Osoba, D., Aaronson, N.K., Muller, M., Sneeuw, K., Hsu, M.-A., Yung, W.K., ... Newlands, E. (1996). The development and psychometric validation of a brain cancer quality-of-life questionnaire for use in combination with general cancer-specific questionnaires. *Quality of Life Research, 5,* 139–150. doi:10.1007/BF00435979

Osoba, D., Brada, M., Prados, M.D., & Yung, W.K. (2000). Effect of disease burden on health-related quality of life in patients with malignant gliomas. *Neuro-Oncology, 2,* 221–228. Retrieved from http://www.ncbi.nlm.nih.gov/pmc/articles/PMC1920595/pdf/11265231.pdf

Pasternak, J.J., McGregor, D.G., & Lanier, W.L. (2004). Effect of single-dose dexamethasone on blood glucose concentration in patients undergoing craniotomy. *Journal of Neurosurgical Anesthesiology, 16,* 122–125.

Patil, C.G., Patil, T.S., Lad, S.P., & Boakye, M. (2008). Complications and outcomes after spinal cord tumor resection in the United States from 1993 to 2002. *Spinal Cord, 46,* 375–379. doi:10.1038/sj.sc.3102155

Pelletier, G., Verhoef, M.J., Khatri, N., & Hagen, N. (2002). Quality of life in brain tumor patients: The relative contributions of depression, fatigue, emotional distress, and existential issues. *Journal of Neuro-Oncology, 57,* 41–49. doi:10.1023/A:1015728825642

Pinquart, M., & Sörensen, S. (2003). Differences between caregivers and noncaregivers in psychological health and physical health: A meta-analysis. *Psychology and Aging, 18,* 250–267. doi:10.1037/0882-7974.18.2.250

Pinquart, M., & Sörensen, S. (2004). Associations of caregiver stressors and uplifts with subjective well-being and depressive mood: A meta-analytic comparison. *Aging and Mental Health, 8,* 438–449.

Prados, M.D., Lamborn, K.R., Chang, S., Burton, E., Butowski, N., Malec, M., ... Kelley, S.K. (2006). Phase 1 study of erlotinib HCl alone and combined with temozolomide in patients with stable or recurrent malignant glioma. *Neuro-Oncology, 8,* 67–78. doi:10.1215/S1522851705000451

Sawaya, R., Hammoud, M., Schoppa, D., Hess, K.R., Wu, S.Z., Shi, W.M., & Wildrick, D.M. (1998). Neurosurgical outcomes in a modern series of 400 craniotomies for treatment of parenchymal tumors. *Neurosurgery, 42,* 1044–1055.

Sherwood, P.R., & Given, B. (2008, April). Measuring oncology nursing sensitive patient outcomes: Evidence-based summary. Retrieved from http://www.ons.org/Research/PEP/media/ons/docs/research/measurement/caregiver-strain.pdf

Sherwood, P.R., Given, B.A., Doorenbos, A.Z., & Given, C.W. (2004). Forgotten voices: Lessons from bereaved caregivers of persons with a brain tumour. *International Journal of Palliative Nursing, 10,* 67–75.

Silvani, A., Gaviani, P., Lamperti, E.A., Eoli, M., Falcone, C., Dimeco, F., ... Salmaggi, A. (2009). Cisplatinum and BCNU chemotherapy in primary glioblastoma patients. *Journal of Neuro-Oncology, 94,* 57–62. doi:10.1007/s11060-009-9800-0

Sinha, S., Bastin, M.E., Wardlaw, J.M., Armitage, P.A., & Whittle, I.R. (2004). Effects of dexamethasone on peritumoural oedematous brain: A DT-MRI study. *Journal of Neurology, Neurosurgery, and Psychiatry, 75,* 1632–1635. doi:10.1136/jnnp.2003.028647

Sloan, A.E., Dansey, R., Zamorano, L., Barger, G., Hamm, C., Diaz, F., ... Wood, G. (2000). Adoptive immunotherapy in patients with recurrent malignant glioma: Preliminary results of using whole-tumor vaccine plus granulocyte-macrophage colony-stimulating factor and adoptive transfer of anti-CD3 activated lymphocytes. *Neurosurgical Focus, 9*(6), e9. doi:10.3171/foc.2000.9.6.10

Sörensen, S., Pinquart, M., & Duberstein, P. (2002). How effective are interventions with caregivers? An updated meta-analysis. *Gerontologist, 42,* 356–372.

Stein, K.D., Jacobsen, P.B., Blanchard, C.M., & Thors, C. (2004). Further validation of the Multidimensional Fatigue Symptom Inventory-Short Form. *Journal of Pain and Symptom Management, 27,* 14–23. doi:10.1016/j.jpainsymman.2003.06.003

Strang, S., Strang, P., & Ternestedt, B.M. (2001). Existential support in brain tumour patients and their spouses. *Supportive Care in Cancer, 9,* 625–633. doi:10.1007/s005200100258

Struik, K., Klein, M., Heimans, J.J., Gielissen, M.F., Bleijenberg, G., Taphoorn, M.J., ... Postma, T.J. (2009). Fatigue in low-grade glioma. *Journal of Neuro-Oncology, 92,* 73–78. doi:10.1007/s11060-008-9738-7

Sturdza, A., Millar, B.A., Bana, N., Laperriere, N., Pond, G., Wong, R.K., & Bezjak, A. (2008). The use and toxicity of steroids in the management of patients with brain metastases. *Supportive Care in Cancer, 16,* 1041–1048. doi:10.1007/s00520-007-0395-8

Tang, P., Roldan, G., Brasher, P.M., Fulton, D., Roa, W., Murtha, A., ... Forsyth, P.A. (2006). A phase II study of carboplatin and chronic high-dose tamoxifen in patients with recurrent malignant glioma. *Journal of Neuro-Oncology, 78,* 311–316. doi:10.1007/s11060-005-9104-y

Taphoorn, M.J., van den Bent, M.J., Mauer, M.E., Coens, C., Delattre, J.Y., Brandes, A.A., ... Bottomley, A. (2007). Health-related quality of life in patients treated for anaplastic oligodendroglioma with adjuvant chemotherapy: Results of a European Organisation for Research and Treatment of Cancer randomized clinical trial. *Journal of Clinical Oncology, 25,* 5723–5730. doi:10.1200/JCO.2007.12.7514

Taylor, M.D., & Bernstein, M. (1999). Awake craniotomy with brain mapping as the routine surgical approach to treating patients with supratentorial intraaxial tumors: A prospective trial of 200 cases. *Journal of Neurosurgery, 90,* 35–41. doi:10.3171/jns.1999.90.1.0035

U.S. Department of Health and Human Services. (1998). *Informal caregiving: Compassion in action.* Retrieved from http://aspe.hhs.gov/daltcp/Reports/carebro2.pdf

Vercoulen, J.H., Swanink, C.M., Fennis, J.F., Galama, J.M., van der Meer, J.W., & Bleijenberg, G. (1994). Dimensional assessment of chronic fatigue syndrome. *Journal of Psychosomatic Research, 38,* 383–392.

Verhoef, M.J., Hagen, N., Pelletier, G., & Forsyth, P. (1999). Alternative therapy use in neurologic diseases: Use in brain tumor patients. *Neurology, 52,* 617–622.

Vitaliano, P.P., Zhang, J., & Scanlan, J.M. (2003). Is caregiving hazardous to one's physical health? A meta-analysis. *Psychological Bulletin, 129,* 946–972. doi:10.1037/0033-2909.129.6.946

Vredenburgh, J.J., Desjardins, A., Herndon, J.E., 2nd, Marcello, J., Reardon, D.A., Quinn, J.A., ... Friedman, H.S. (2007). Bevacizumab plus irinotecan in recurrent glioblastoma multiforme. *Journal of Clinical Oncology, 25,* 4722–4729. doi:10.1200/JCO.2007.12.2440

Wada, K., Yamada, N., Sato, T., Suzuki, H., Miki, M., Lee, Y., ... Kuroda, S. (2001). Corticosteroid-induced psychotic and mood disorders: Diagnosis defined by DSM-IV and clinical pictures. *Psychosomatics, 42,* 461–466. Retrieved from http://psy.psychiatryonline.org/cgi/reprint/42/6/461

Walker, W., Seel, R., Gibellato, M., Lew, H., Cornis-Pop, M., Jena, T., & Silver, T. (2004). The effects of donepezil on traumatic brain injury acute rehabilitation outcomes. *Brain Injury, 18,* 739–750. doi:10.1080/02699050310001646224

Weitzner, M.A., Meyers, C.A., Gelke, C.K., Byrne, K.S., Cella, D.F., & Levin, V.A. (1995). The Functional Assessment of Cancer Therapy (FACT) scale. Development of a brain subscale and revalidation of the general version (FACT-G) in patients with primary brain tumors. *Cancer, 75,* 1151–1161. doi:10.1002/1097-0142(19950301)75:5<1151::AID-CNCR2820750515>3.0.CO;2-Q

Wellisch, D.K., Kaleita, T.A., Freeman, D., Cloughesy, T., & Goldman, J. (2002). Predicting major depression in brain tumor patients. *Psycho-Oncology, 11,* 230–238. doi:10.1002/pon.562

Wen, P.Y., Schiff, D., Kesari, S., Drappatz, J., Gigas, D., & Doherty, L. (2006). Medical management of patients with brain tumors. *Journal of Neuro-Oncology, 80,* 313–332. doi:10.1007/s11060-006-9193-2

Wideheim, A.K., Edvardsson, T., Påhlson, A., & Ahlström, G. (2002). A family's perspective on living with a highly malignant brain tumor. *Cancer Nursing, 25,* 236–244.

Yano, S., Matsuyama, H., Matsuda, K., Matsumoto, H., Yoshihiro, S., & Naito, K. (2004). Accuracy of an array comparative genomic hybridization (CGH) technique in detecting DNA copy number aberrations: Comparison with conventional CGH and loss of heterozygosity analysis in prostate cancer. *Cancer Genetics and Cytogenetics, 150,* 122–127. doi:10.1016/j.cancergencyto.2003.09.004

Yeh, S.A., Ho, J.T., Lui, C.C., Huang, Y.J., Hsiung, C.Y., & Huang, E.Y. (2005). Treatment outcomes and prognostic factors in patients with supratentorial low-grade gliomas. *British Journal of Radiology, 78*(927), 230–235. doi:10.1259/bjr/28534346

Zhang, L., Plotkin, R.C., Wang, G., Sandel, M.E., & Lee, S. (2004). Cholinergic augmentation with donepezil enhances recovery in short-term memory and sustained attention after traumatic brain injury. *Archives of Physical Medicine and Rehabilitation, 85,* 1050–1055. doi:10.1016/j.apmr.2003.10.014.

CHAPTER 12

Evidence-Based Practice: Where We Are Now

Nancy E. Villanueva, PhD, CRNP, BC, CNRN

Introduction

The care of a patient with a tumor of the brain or spinal cord is complex and involves a multidisciplinary approach. The various treatment modalities (surgical, chemotherapy, and radiation) used to treat these tumors were presented in the preceding chapters. This chapter will focus on both nursing and medical practices used to treat these patients and discuss the evidence or lack of evidence supporting these practices. Specific areas will include preoperative site preparation; postoperative management of pain and nausea; and patient instructions concerning bathing, shampooing, and activity level. In addition, the psychosocial issues and effects will be examined. Recommendations for future research to strengthen practice conclude the chapter.

Evidence-Based Practice

Evidence-based practice (EBP) is the conscientious use of current best evidence in making decisions about patient care. Research findings have shown that patients who receive care based on the best and latest evidence experience better outcomes. In addition, research has shown that practitioners who use an evidence-based approach to patient care experience higher levels of satisfaction as compared to practitioners who provide care based on traditional methods (Melnyk & Fineout-Overholt, 2005).

Evidence-based nursing is the foundation for professional nursing practice. Using the best evidence to support nursing practice and generating new knowledge for use in practice are hallmarks of excellence (Mcilvoy & Hinkle, 2008; Schultz, 2009). Using EBP requires practitioners to be flexible and open to ongoing change. This requirement is necessary because a major characteristic of EBP is the continual changes in practice based on the most current and relevant evidence (Porter-O'Grady, 2010).

A triad model has been used to illustrate the components of EBP (Melnyk & Fineout-Overholt, 2005). The three compo-

nents of the triad are listed in Figure 12-1. These components continually interact to provide improved patient outcomes. The categories of best available clinical evidence can be ranked from the strongest to the least strong. It is important that nurses understand what comprises each category. The strongest evidence includes meta-analyses and systematic reviews of current research investigations and randomized trials. The next solid evidence includes well-designed controlled trials without randomization, case-controlled studies, and cohort studies. Lower levels of evidence include systematic reviews of several descriptive or qualitative studies and single quantitative or qualitative studies. The last category, or the least strong, includes opinions of respected authorities and reports of expert consensus panels or committees. Individual clinical expertise includes clinical judgment and skills. It provides insight into whether the evidence, policy standard, or guideline applies to the individual patient and, if so, how does it apply. Nurses depend upon both external evidence and strong clinical expertise. The third component of the triad is the patient's values and expectations. Nurses must be culturally sensitive and respect the patients' and families' values and beliefs when using EBP (Melnyk & Fineout-Overholt, 2005).

The Oncology Nursing Society (ONS) created the ONS Putting Evidence Into Practice (PEP) resources as a means of summarizing current evidence so nurses could incorporate current practice recommendations into their individual practices (Tipton, 2009). ONS initially used the ONS Levels of Evidence (Hadorn, Baker, Hodges, & Hicks, 1996; Ropka & Spencer-Cisek, 2001) and the Evidence Rating System for the Hierarchy of Evidence (Melnyk &

Figure 12-1. Components of Evidence-Based Practice

- Best available external clinical evidence
- Individual clinical expertise
- Patient's values and expectations

Note. Based on information from Melnyk & Fineout-Overholt, 2005.

Fineout-Overholt, 2005) to rate the level of evidence for studies incorporated into the PEP guidelines. Ultimately, the decision was made to identify the weight of evidence for each intervention with the review of the study design and limitations, as opposed to the previously used levels of evidence for each study (Tipton, 2009). See Table 12-1 for additional information about the ONS Weight-of-Evidence Classification Model.

Nurses have the unique opportunity in every practice setting to positively affect their patients and families. Implementing EBP guidelines in everyday practice provides nurses and their patients the confidence that the desired outcomes will be achieved. The ONS symptom-related evidence-based guidelines are applicable for use in the continuum of care for patients with a CNS cancer (see www.ons.org/Research/PEP/Topics). Figure 12-2 lists the PEP guidelines for use in delivering effective symptom management. In addition, the figure highlights those that are observed in patients with CNS cancers in order to provide nurses with additional resources to use throughout this population's continuum of care. Although these guidelines present the intervention research for symptom management, nurses need to carefully consider the impact that tumor location may pose on the frequency, severity, or persistence of particular symptoms (Batchelor & Byrne, 2006; Mukand, Blackinton, Crincoli, Lee, & Santos, 2001). Tumor location and unresolved

cerebral edema can promote symptoms of anxiety, depression, nausea and vomiting, pain (particularly headache), peripheral neuropathy, and bowel inconsistencies of diarrhea or constipation (Armstrong, Cohen, Eriksen, & Hickey, 2004; Batchelor & Byrne, 2006; Fox, Lyon, & Farace, 2007). Most particularly observed in neuro-oncology are persisting symptoms of fatigue, sleep-wake disturbances, and cognitive impairment, which can become increasingly severe with a negative impact on patients' perceived quality of life (Lovely, Miaskowski, & Dodd, 1999). Finally, caregiver strain and burden can be observed through the continuum of care (Farace, Shaffrey, Huang, Litofsky, & Laws, 2002). These EBP guidelines are an invaluable resource for nurses and their patients and families.

Preoperative Site Preparation

Historically, preparing the patient for surgery involved shaving the surgical wound site. For the patient undergoing a craniotomy, the entire head was shaved, and then the procedure changed so that a smaller area was shaved. This practice came under examination because of concerns for surgical site infections (SSIs). It is known that shaving can affect the protective skin flora and cause microtrauma of the area, which can increase the bacterial colonization of the area,

Table 12-1. Oncology Nursing Society Putting Evidence Into Practice Weight-of-Evidence Classification Model	
Classification	**Definition**
Recommended for practice	Interventions for which effectiveness has been demonstrated by strong evidence from rigorously designed studies, meta-analyses, or systematic reviews, and for which expectation of harms is small compared with the benefits
Likely to be effective	Interventions for which effectiveness has been demonstrated by supportive evidence from a single rigorously conducted controlled trial, consistent supportive evidence from well-designed controlled trials using small samples, or guidelines developed from evidence and supported by expert opinion
Benefits balanced with harms	Interventions for which clinicians and patients should weigh the beneficial and harmful effects according to individual circumstances and priorities
Effectiveness not established	Interventions for which insufficient or conflicting data or data of inadequate quality currently exist, with no clear indication of harm
Effectiveness unlikely	Interventions for which lack of effectiveness has been demonstrated by negative evidence from a single rigorously conducted controlled trial, consistent negative evidence from well-designed controlled trials using small samples, or guidelines developed from evidence and supported by expert opinion
Not recommended for practice	Interventions for which ineffectiveness or harmfulness has been demonstrated by strong evidence from rigorously conducted studies, meta-analyses, or systematic reviews, or interventions where the costs, burden, or harms associated with the intervention exceed anticipated benefit
Expert opinion	Low-risk interventions that are (1) consistent with sound clinical practice, (2) suggested by an expert in a peer-reviewed publication (journal or book chapter), and (3) for which limited evidence exists. An expert is an individual who has published articles in a peer-reviewed journal in the domain of interest.

Note. From "PEP Up Your Practice: An Introduction to the Oncology Nursing Society Putting Evidence Into Practice Resources" (p. 6), by B.H. Gobel and J.M. Tipton in L.H. Eaton and J.M. Tipton (Eds.), *Putting Evidence Into Practice: Improving Oncology Patient Outcomes,* 2009, Pittsburgh, PA: Oncology Nursing Society. Copyright 2009 by the Oncology Nursing Society. Reprinted with permission.

Figure 12-2. Oncology Nursing Society Putting Evidence Into Practice Guidelines

Anorexia
Anxiety*
Caregiver strain and burden*
Chemotherapy-induced nausea and vomiting*
Cognitive impairment*
Constipation*
Depression*
Diarrhea*
Dyspnea
Fatigue*
Hot flashes
Lymphedema
Mucositis
Pain*
Peripheral neuropathy*
Prevention of bleeding
Prevention of infection
Radiodermatitis
Skin reactions
Sleep-wake disturbances*

---

* May be more likely to be observed in patients with central nervous system cancers.

Note. Based on information from Oncology Nursing Society, n.d.

---

thus increasing infection risk (Celik & Kara, 2007). A number of individual studies using different methodologies (e.g., prospective, retrospective, randomized, nonrandomized) addressed this question (Celik & Kara, 2007; Miller, Weber, Patel, & Ramey, 2001; Tang & Sgouros, 2001). Most recently, Tanner, Woodings, and Moncaster (2006) conducted a Cochrane Database Systematic Review with the primary objective of determining if routine preoperative hair removal would result in fewer SSIs than not removing hair. Eleven randomized clinical trials were included in the review. The reviewers found no difference in the SSI incidence among patients who had hair removed prior to surgery and those who did not. However, it was recommended that if hair removal was necessary, the preferred method was clipping the hair. Fewer SSIs occurred in patients whose hair had been clipped than those whose hair was shaved.

Postoperative Nausea and Vomiting

Following the administration of anesthesia, postoperative nausea and vomiting (PONV) is the most frequent side effect. For patients who have undergone a craniotomy, vomiting has the potential to cause harm. Physiologic response to vomiting results in an increased arterial blood pressure and intra-abdominal pressure, which has the potential to cause an elevation in intracranial pressure. In the immediate postoperative period, strict blood pressure parameters must be maintained. For those patients who have an intracranial pressure monitoring device, the pressures are closely monitored and interventions

taken for the maintenance of intracranial pressure and cerebral perfusion pressure (Eberhart et al., 2007).

Research into the risk factors associated with PONV began in the 1990s and has provided a body of knowledge of the independent risk factors. The risk factors that have been identified include female gender (from puberty), nonsmoker, PONV history or motion sickness, duration of surgery, type of anesthesia used, and use of postoperative opioids (Gan, 2006). Because these risk factors were identified in studies of patients undergoing general surgery, the question of the applicability of these factors to postcraniotomy patients must be addressed. In addition, in this particular patient population, unique factors are related to PONV. Eberhart et al. (2007) conducted a systematic literature search in various databases (MEDLINE®, Embase®, and Cochrane Library) starting with 1994. Only seven studies were found to meet the inclusion criteria, which were double-blinded, prospective, randomized controlled trials in adult patients, with the primary endpoints of postoperative nausea and/or vomiting. All of the studies focused on the prevention of PONV with the use of 5-HT$_3$ antagonists. The reviewers concluded that no difference existed in the efficacy of these agents in postoperative craniotomy patients compared to the general surgical population.

Neufeld and Newburn-Cook (2007) performed a meta-analysis to assess the efficacy of prophylactic intraoperative administration of 5-HT$_3$ antagonists for PONV in neurosurgical patients. The analysis included seven randomized placebo-controlled trials. Adults who received prophylactic 5-HT$_3$ antagonists exhibited a reduced risk of vomiting at 24 and 48 hours when compared to the placebo group. No significant difference in nausea was reported. These findings did support the use of intraoperative administration of a 5-HT$_3$ antagonist, but the question was raised as to the acceptability of these findings. Although the treatment effect was significant, the rates of postoperative emesis remained high. If the nausea and vomiting were combined and the efficacy of the agent calculated based on the combination, the overall efficacy would be considerably lower.

Nurses caring for this population must be knowledgeable about the known risk factors for PONV and tailor their care accordingly. The American Society of PeriAnesthesia Nurses has established EBP guidelines for the prevention and management of PONV. These recommendations include a simplified risk scoring tool used to predict PONV as a part of the preoperative assessment (Neufeld, Newburn-Cook, & Drummond, 2008). Although this would appear to be an easy task, it is quite the opposite. A number of prognostic models are available, and Gan (2006), in a systematic review, provided no evidence of models or risk scores to effectively predict PONV after craniotomy in adults or children.

Studies in the craniotomy literature for PONV suggest that unique areas of concern for this population are not included in the model. A study by Fabling et al. (1997) identified the site of surgery (infratentorial) as predictive of PONV. This was later contradicted by Irefin et al. (2003), whose study did not support a relationship between craniotomy location and nausea. This concept continues to be debated.

Clearly, this area needs continued research to support EBP. At this time, clinical decision making is based upon the current evidence, knowledge of the risk factors, and expert clinical judgment.

Pain and Craniotomy

Postoperative pain management after a craniotomy presents a major challenge with potential detrimental effects if not effectively controlled. Moderate to severe pain can cause agitation and sympathetic stimulation with increases in blood pressure. These increases may induce or aggravate an already edematous brain with impaired autoregulation. The recognition that poor pain control has been associated with poor outcomes and increases in many postoperative complications demands that pain control after a craniotomy be a priority for the individuals caring for the patient (Durieux & Himmelseher, 2007; Nemergut, Durieux, Missaghi, & Himmelseher, 2007). Reports conflict concerning the severity of pain experienced after a craniotomy with earlier articles reporting a lower incidence of pain. However, more recent studies have identified that pain is a greater problem than previously believed, with up to 80% of patients reporting moderate to severe pain that persisted for several postoperative days (de Gray & Matta, 2005; Kincaid & Lam, 2007; Thibault et al., 2007).

Kincaid and Lam (2007) conducted a prospective study to evaluate the incidence, severity, and treatment of postoperative pain in patients undergoing major intracranial surgery. A total of 187 adult patients were enrolled, with 129 patients undergoing supratentorial surgery and 58 patients having infratentorial surgery. Moderate to severe pain (defined as greater than 4 on scale of 0–10) was reported by 69% of the patients during the first postoperative day. In 48% of the patients, on the second postoperative day, the pain scores were reported as 4 or greater. Patients who underwent infratentorial procedures reported more severe pain at rest as compared to those who had a supratentorial approach. Examination of pain medication use revealed that patients who had an infratentorial approach used more opioids and nonopioids in the first 48 hours than those who had surgery using a supratentorial approach.

Kincaid and Lam's (2007) finding that the craniotomy site influenced the degree of postoperative pain was also found by Thibault et al. (2007). This was a retrospective study designed to assess the intensity of postoperative pain in relation to the location of the craniotomy. A total of 522 charts of patients who had undergone a craniotomy within the year prior to the study were examined. Of these charts, 222 were excluded. The reasons for exclusion were a prolonged

postoperative intubation or impaired state of consciousness, less than two verbal ratings of pain over the study period, postoperative complications requiring a second operation, craniofacial surgery, burr holes, postoperative pain not related to the cranial surgery, simultaneous craniotomies at two different sites, and craniotomy incision over more than one location (e.g., parieto-occipital). The data were categorized according to the location of the craniotomy. Postoperative pain data collected included median verbal rating scale scores for the initial 48 hours, cumulative doses of analgesics, and occurrence of PONV. Analysis of the data revealed a 24% incidence of mild pain, 51.5% for moderate pain and 24.5% for severe pain. A significant ($p < 0.0001$) relationship exists between the severity of pain and the different craniotomy sites, with the frontal craniotomy having the lowest pain scores and least analgesic use. In addition to craniotomy location, other factors (presence of preoperative pain, postoperative steroid use, gender, and age) were entered into a logistic regression model. Craniotomy site was the only independent predictor of postoperative pain. These results support the belief that a higher incidence of severe pain is a result of the degree of muscle manipulation needed in different approaches with higher pain scores reflected in those patients undergoing an occipital or posterior fossa approach, with postoperative muscle spasms playing a factor in postoperative pain. In addition to pain, the incidence of PONV in relation to craniotomy site was evaluated, and no interaction was found.

With the realization that significant degrees of postoperative pain are experienced following a craniotomy, the adequacy of postoperative pain control then becomes the question. No consensus exists regarding pain control in this population (Ortiz-Cardona & Bendo, 2007). Fear of the side effects of analgesic drugs often leads to the undertreatment of postcraniotomy pain. The occurrence of postoperative sedation is a concern often stated because of the need for frequent neurologic examinations, which lead to the avoidance of opioids (e.g., morphine) for control. Studies in the literature support the use of opioids in this patient population. In a study by Sudheer, Logan, Terblanche, Ateleanu, and Hall (2007), the effects of patient-controlled analgesia (PCA) using morphine or tramadol were compared to each other and codeine delivered intramuscularly. Sixty patients were randomized to receive either the PCA or codeine with six patients excluded (four required ventilation and two were not experiencing pain). Physiologic parameters of heart rate, blood pressure, oxygen saturation, respiratory rate, pain rating, Glasgow Coma Score, and arterial blood gas results were recorded at baseline, 30 minutes, and 1, 4, 8, 12, 18, and 24 hours. Analysis revealed that morphine produced significantly better analgesia than tramadol at all the time points ($p < 0.005$) and better analgesia than codeine at 4, 12, and 24 hours. Morphine use was associated with better patient outcomes compared with tramadol or codeine ($p < 0.001$). This study supported previous studies in that the patients having had a frontal approach experienced the least amount of pain as compared to the other approaches. PONV was greater in those patients who received tramadol (50%) as compared to morphine (20%) and codeine (29%).

Nemergut et al. (2007), with the goal of improving the postoperative care of patients undergoing craniotomy, reviewed the evidence on short- and long-term outcomes of analgesic therapy after craniotomy. The MEDLINE database was searched from 1994 to April 2007. Only randomized controlled trials and nonrandomized controlled or cohort trials of adults were included. These criteria yielded 17 articles. Their analysis supported the use of morphine in the early period after craniotomy. Morphine was found to provide better analgesia and more consistent pain reduction than codeine. No serious complications were reported, but none of the studies had sufficient power to detect differences in safety issues with opioids. Non-narcotics (e.g., tramadol) were seen as a useful supplemental opioid-sparing medication.

Showering and Shampooing

"When can I wash my hair?" is a frequent question that patients ask after having a craniotomy. The feeling of matted hair with residual prep solution and dried blood is both unpleasant and visually disturbing to the patient. Although this would seem to be a straightforward question, answers provided by clinicians vary widely. Variations range anywhere from 48 hours to 2 weeks. Studies addressing this question are scarce. Only one study was able to be located after a search of the databases (CINAHL®, PubMed, MEDLINE, Web of Knowledge) from 1995 to the date of the study. In this study (Ireland et al., 2007), the primary goal was to assess the effect of postoperative hair washing on incision infection and health-related quality of life. A cohort of 100 adult patients was randomized to hair washing 72 hours postoperatively or no hair washing until the sutures or clips had been removed. Patients were excluded from the study if they were severely immunocompromised related to recent chemotherapy or radiation, unable to provide consent for the study, had an open wound or ventricular drain, or had an active infection. The sutures or clips were removed 5–10 days postoperatively. Those patients randomized to the hair washing group kept a record of the number of times they shampooed and used a gentle shampoo that was provided to them. The incisions were assessed using the ASEPSIS Scale at the time of suture/clip removal and at 30 days. Analysis was performed and resulted in no significant difference between the groups in the incidence of postoperative wound infection.

Ireland et al. (2007) have provided the first study to address the issue of shampooing after craniotomy. Additional studies are required to provide more evidence for practice. Questions that need to be addressed include issues such as whether the type of closure (dissolvable versus indissoluble sutures) and location of the incision (supra- versus infratentorial) influence the infection rate. "When is the patient permitted to swim?" is often asked during the summer months and year-round in warmer climates. Does the location (pool, freshwater, saltwater) influence the time period? No studies address these questions, and current practice varies and is based upon individual clinical judgment.

For patients who have undergone spinal surgery for removal of a tumor, the question is asked regarding getting the incision wet and taking a shower. As in the case of shampooing after a craniotomy, answers vary and research-based evidence is scarce. After a search of the databases (CINAHL, PubMed, MEDLINE, Web of Knowledge) from 1995 to the present, only one article could be located that addressed this issue. Carragee and Vittum (1996) conducted a prospective study to determine if early bathing after posterior spinal surgery resulted in increased wound problems. (Although Carragee and Vittum use the term *early bathing*, they are actually referring to showering.) Of the 100 consecutive patients who were enrolled, the patients who had a microdiscectomy were permitted to shower after 48 hours. Other spinal surgery patients in the group were instructed to wait five days. Patients were advised not to swim or soak in a spa, Jacuzzi, or hot tub. The results were compared against a historic control of 100 patients who were operated on by the authors the preceding year. These patients were not permitted to shower until the staples had been removed, 10–14 days after surgery. Analysis of the data revealed no statistical difference between the groups.

Although this study provides initial information for showering after spinal surgery, many questions regarding practice need to be addressed. Since this study, advancements have been made in wound closure and techniques. The use of staples, once popular, is now rare. Suture material is now dissolvable and indissoluble. External wound closure may be with a solution such as DermaBond® (Ethicon). When to permit a patient to take a tub bath, sit in a spa or Jacuzzi, or swim either in a pool or a natural setting are questions raised by patients that have no evidence-based answers. These are areas in which studies need to be designed.

Activity Level

Following surgery for a brain or spinal cord tumor, nurses are continually preparing the patient and family/significant other for discharge. An important part of that instruction involves the patient's activity level and permitted and prohibited activities. "What am I allowed to do?" is a frequent question. Typical discharge instructions include statements such as "avoid strenuous activities," "no lifting greater than X pounds," and "rest frequently." Although these are the usual statements, a search of the databases (CINAHL, PubMed, MEDLINE, and Web of Knowledge) from 1995 to the present elicited no studies addressing these questions. Taking a more general approach, the database was again searched for postoperative restrictions for patients undergoing spine surgery (no longer limited to only tumors). Despite the fact that this was a much broader category, only a few studies were obtained and were limited to lumbar microdiscectomy. A study by McGregor, Dicken, and Jamrozik (2006) illustrated the variations in postoperative restrictions that patients receive. In this article, a survey was distributed to members of the British Association of Spinal Surgeons and Society for Back Pain Research. Of the 89 distributed, 63 were returned and 51 were able to be used. The survey asked what time frames were provided to postoperative patients concerning the duration of lifting and driving restrictions and when they may return to work. The results showed a wide variety of recommendations. These study results mirrored an earlier study by Magnusson, Pope, Wilder, Szpalski, and Spratt (1999), which examined surgeons' restrictions on lifting. No evidence was found in the literature to support the restrictions even when they incorporated mechanical factors.

Clearly research is needed that provides guidance with activity restrictions. If practitioners are questioning the rationale behind the restrictions, imagine the confusion the postoperative patient experiences with rather vague instructions such as "avoid strenuous activities and no heavy lifting." This need for better-defined activity restrictions can be seen in a study by Williamson, Bulley, and Coutts (2008). They conducted a qualitative study with individuals following lumbar surgery to investigate what they felt they were able to do after surgery. One of the identified themes was labeled "wish for precise movement boundaries." In this, the participants verbalized their fear of movement, fear of reinjury, and uncertainty regarding altered movement and activity boundaries.

Driving

Patients will ask when they can resume driving. The loss of the ability to drive has numerous implications, which range from minor disruptions of the patient's social and work-related activities to more severe consequences such as loss of independence, impact on income, and social isolation (Bittar & Fabinyi, 2004). After surgery for a tumor resection, the ability to resume driving will need to be individually determined based upon the patient's functional status. For patients who have undergone surgery and remain cognitively intact and have no motor deficits to prohibit them from driving, the question becomes, what is a safe time frame before resuming? No guidelines are available to assist with this decision, and answers vary. Healthcare providers must assess the individual patient and clearly state what restrictions are being placed and the length of the restriction. Patients who are taking medications that can affect level of consciousness

(e.g., narcotics, muscle relaxants) should be instructed not to drive while using those medications. Healthcare providers must also become knowledgeable about the laws of the state in which they practice with regard to driving restrictions after a seizure. Patients must be informed about driving restrictions that apply in their state and the need to adhere to these restrictions. Elliott and Long (2008) examined the perceived risk, resources, and perceptions concerning driving and epilepsy from a patient's perspective. A 46-item questionnaire was completed by 213 individuals with epilepsy. Results of the survey showed that individuals were not completely honest with their seizure frequency, and reports of having had a car accident as a result of a seizure were provided. In this study and in previous studies, noncompliance was related to occupation.

Supportive Care Needs

Studies in the area of supportive care needs of patients with a brain tumor and their caregivers are limited. This is an area in which nursing, in collaboration with other disciplines, has the opportunity to make significant contributions to the literature. Identifying the needs of patients and families allows for the development of interventions that will help to support them as they move along their disease trajectory.

Janda et al. (2008) surveyed patients and caregivers with the goal of assessing the type and magnitude of supportive care needs of patients and caregivers. The patients were provided with a short form of the Supportive Care Needs Survey, and caregivers received the Partners and Caregivers form. A total of 363 letters of invitation were sent, with completed questionnaires returned from 94 households, a response rate of 29.8%. The majority of the patients reported that they had a diagnosis of a malignant tumor and were within five years of diagnosis.

The five highest unmet supportive needs that patients identified were very different from caregivers' top five. For patients, the highest unmet need was for help with the physical side effects of the tumor and treatment. This demonstrates the importance and need for the work being conducted on symptom management (e.g., fatigue, nausea, vomiting) and symptom clusters (Barsevick, 2007; Donovan et al., 2008; Fox et al., 2007). The patients' second-highest unmet need dealt with needing help with the changes experienced in their mental or thinking ability. For the caregivers, this unmet need was expressed as adjusting to changes in the mental and thinking ability of the person with the brain tumor and was their number-one unmet need (Janda et al., 2008). A recommendation made by caregivers was for healthcare professionals in the early stage of the illness to suggest having the patient settle any outstanding affairs, arranging for enduring power of attorney and wills. Completing these tasks very early in the treatment process, preferably before treatment began, allowed the individual the ability to make decisions before any mental or intellectual impairment occurred. Early preparation also removes this burden from the caregiver, who has myriad issues and items that are additional stressors (Janda, Eakin, Bailey, Walker, & Troy, 2006). Adjusting to the changes has been discussed in other articles and described as changes in the family roles for both patients and the caregivers. This can be seen in a statement by a spouse who says, "We have a different relationship. I've lost my partner and I've lost equality, and that is what is hardest for me" (Schmer, Ward-Smith, Latham, & Salacz, 2008, p. 81).

For caregivers, the second highest unmet need was help with managing the difficult aspects in the patients' behavior (Janda et al., 2008). This high ranking should not be surprising to healthcare professionals because behavioral changes (e.g., impulsiveness, decreased safety awareness, short attention span) also present management challenges even with their professional knowledge of why these behaviors occur. Naturally, family caregivers may struggle because they do not have the same experience and coping mechanisms with the behavior as professionals do. This information has been presented and discussed previously in the literature for many years. A qualitative study performed more than a decade ago identified that families have difficulty dealing with the behavior changes because they lacked the skills and knowledge to manage them (Salander, 1996). Clearly, this is an area where healthcare professionals have not met the families' and caregivers' need to understand and cope with the behavioral changes.

Feeling as if they were not the same person as before the brain tumor was the third highest unmet need of patients. For the caregivers, feeling alone in caring for the person with a brain tumor was the third highest need for which they required support (Janda et al., 2008). Having access to information was seen as a way to help caregivers to cope and feel less alone as they cared for patients. Providing caregivers with information and a mechanism by which they could obtain information to their questions as the situation changed was seen as decreasing the feeling of isolation. Written communication and access to technology provides ways for this to be achieved. The Internet and e-mail have opened new avenues for caregivers to find information and support (Catt, Chalmers, & Fallowfield, 2008). Another recommendation was for a designated contact person for the caregiver to communicate with regarding medical and practical questions (Janda et al., 2006). Having a consistent resource helps to establish cohesion and a sense of security for the caregiver. Help with obtaining information on the latest developments in research and treatment of brain tumors was the fourth highest supportive care need of the patients, whereas adjusting to changes in the personality of the person with a brain tumor was fourth for the caregiver (Janda et al., 2008).

An interesting finding in Janda et al.'s 2008 study was that patients identified help with changes in their ability to work as their fifth highest unmet need. But for the caregivers, this unmet need was not in their top five. This was a surprising finding given the economic impact of having a brain tumor. Also, the need for support with financial issues and dealing with government agencies was identified as a need by both patients and caregivers in the Janda et al. 2006 study.

Bradley et al. (2007) conducted a qualitative study to explore the financial impact of a primary malignant brain tumor. A unique feature of this population was that they all were covered by health insurance. Four major themes were identified from the interviews. The first theme involved paying for medication and health care. Despite the fact that they had insurance, they discussed frustrations with failing to meet insurance and other assistance qualifications and dealing with institutional bureaucracy. Another theme was labeled *strategies*, and the participants described the various strategies they used to cope with the cost of care. These strategies included "cashing in," which meant using their savings or other funds or selling off assets to cover the cost of care. Another strategy was trade-offs/choices, where something was not done or was altered for cost containment. An example was forgoing a family vacation and putting off household improvements. Taking out loans, borrowing money, and using credit cards were other measures. A third theme was impact. In this, the participants discussed the cost to family, change in income and change in job, anxiety, and unease. In the cost to the family, the need for others to assume new roles was addressed. Examples of this included a teenager being asked to get a job in order to provide their own spending money and an at-home parent reentering the work force. Where previous articles have discussed the changes in role experienced by the caregiver, these discussions are often in the context of a single caregiver. This article illustrates how caring roles, especially in the context of a family, are complex and overlapping. The concept was explored in an article by Lingler, Sherwood, Crighton, Song, and Happ (2008) in which the traditional model of unidirectional caregiving was discussed and expanded to include the phenomena of multiple caregivers, shifting, and shared caregiver roles.

The studies by Janda et al. in 2006 and 2008 identified the needs of patients with brain tumors. These studies included both tumors that were benign and malignant. The question then becomes: Are there differences in the needs between patients with benign tumors and those with malignant tumors? Schmer et al. (2008) explored caregiving using a phenomenologic methodology for the patient with a malignant brain tumor during the first six months of treatment. During this period, the caregivers identified the psychosocial issues as being overwhelming, whereas the physical demands were low. The need to address and deal with these issues is of paramount importance for the caregiver. Not having dealt with these issues places the caregivers at risk for physical or psychological conditions that may affect their ability to provide necessary caregiving later in the disease process. The time frame for the patient's needs to begin diversifying was identified as between six months to one year after the initial diagnosis. The patient's ability to return to activities of daily living, including work, was the catalyst for the change. For patients who were unable to return to work as long as their functional status remained impaired, the caregiver's focus became establishing a long-term care structure (Janda et al., 2006).

Directions for the Future

In the various sections presented in this chapter, many areas exist where either initial research is needed to provide a beginning for EBP or additional research is required to strengthen the practice. This section will focus on gaps in knowledge and future directions for EBP (see Figure 12-3).

PONV is a frequent side effect following anesthesia and can have deleterious consequences for patients after a craniotomy. Research has identified known risk factors for PONV in the general surgery population. Nurses need to evaluate their patients for these risk factors, thus providing them with a high suspicion that PONV may occur in their patients. Research with a focus on patients undergoing a craniotomy needs to be developed to discover any risk factors specific to this population. In addition, what medications work best for patients undergoing a craniotomy and the best timing of administration (e.g., intraoperative, scheduled versus as-needed) are other areas needing investigation. The studies discussed involved only the use of 5-HT$_3$ antagonists with quite variable results. Studies that look at different antiemetics would contribute to this body of knowledge.

Although the literature concerning pain management after a craniotomy supports the fact that these individuals do have moderate to severe pain and that opioids can be employed safely, additional studies could strengthen this body of

knowledge. Non-narcotics (e.g., tramadol) as a supplemental opioid-sparing medication are increasingly being used and discussed in the literature. Questions regarding the best time and strategy for switching from an opioid to non-opioid, the use of a staggered administration schedule, and scheduled pain medication with medication for breakthrough pain are topics to be considered.

The instructions provided to a patient upon discharge have a significant number of areas that require research-based information. The previous example of when a patient should be permitted to shampoo after surgery and the discovery of only one article that addresses this question confirms this need. Answers to this question vary depending on the preferences of the neurosurgeon and can range from 48 hours to 2 weeks. Additional studies are needed to address this question, which will give healthcare professionals sufficient power to answer the question and help to standardize and change practice. The questions about when a person may go swimming, whether a chlorinated pool or in freshwater or saltwater, need to be answered. An answer based in research with clinical expertise would be useful the next time a patient asks, "We have a trip planned in six weeks. Can I go swimming?"

Similar to patients who had a craniotomy, patients who had spinal surgery need advisement about showering, tub bathing, using a hot tub, and swimming. Do factors such as the type of closure (e.g., sutures, DermaBond adhesive) or presence of a postoperative drain affect the time frame? Currently, no studies have been conducted, and practitioners use their clinical judgment, which results in varied recommendations. Research studies will help practitioners to make better-informed decisions and provide some practice uniformity.

Postoperative activity restrictions, including lifting and driving, is another area where research would help to clarify and support the discharge instructions provided to patients. For the patient who has had a seizure or has a deficit that prohibits driving (e.g., confusion, visual deficit, motor weakness), the inability to resume driving is clear. When to advise neurologically intact patients to resume driving is not clear; again, clinical expertise is used in this situation. Time frames vary and can range anywhere from two to four weeks. Qualitative studies exploring patients' experiences of resuming driving could provide information regarding the readiness for driving and establishing evidence-based guidelines.

Researchers have multiple opportunities to assist with the psychosocial concerns that both patients and caregivers experience. Interventions that have been recommended from previous studies of individuals with CNS disorders that address psychosocial concerns could be integrated into a study. The study's outcome measures would be their efficacy in addressing patients' and caregivers' concerns. Longitudinal studies could assist in the identification of the patients' and caregivers' needs, when these needs change along the illness trajectory, and intervention development that could be implemented to provide appropriate assistance.

Figure 12-3. Areas of Research Deficits Regarding Care of Patients With Central Nervous System Tumors

- Preoperative site preparation
- Postoperative nausea and vomiting
- Postcraniotomy pain management
- Postcraniotomy and post–spinal surgery discharge instructions
- Postoperative activity restrictions
- Postoperative shampooing
- Postoperative showering
- Postoperative lifting
- Postoperative swimming
- Postoperative driving
- Postoperative symptom management
- Long-term activity restrictions
- Identification of acute and long-term supportive care needs for patient and family

Summary

The concept of EBP was explored in the beginning of this chapter. The existing research that supports a number of nursing and medical practices was discussed. Preoperative site preparation, postoperative pain management, PONV, and patient instructions regarding showering, shampooing, activity restrictions, and driving were areas of special focus. Also, the supportive care needs of patients and caregivers were discussed. Directions for the future and recommendations for research to address the indentified gaps in knowledge were presented at the conclusion of the chapter.

References

Armstrong, T.S., Cohen, M.Z., Eriksen, L.R., & Hickey, J.V. (2004). Symptom clusters in oncology patients and implications for symptom research in people with primary brain tumors. *Journal of Nursing Scholarship, 36,* 197–206. doi:10.1111/j.1547-5069.2004.04038.x

Barsevick, A.M. (2007). The elusive concept of the symptom cluster. *Oncology Nursing Forum, 34,* 971–980. doi:10.1188/07.ONF.971-980

Batchelor, T.T., & Byrne, T. (2006). Supportive care of brain tumor patients. *Hematology/Oncology Clinics of North America, 20,* 1337–1361. doi:10.1016/j.hoc.2006.09.013

Bittar, R.G., & Fabinyi, G.C. (2004). Driving guidelines and neurological illness. *Journal of Clinical Neuroscience, 11,* 455. doi:10.1016/j.jocn.2003.11.003

Bradley, S., Sherwood, P.R., Donovan, H.S., Hamilton, R., Rosenzweig, M., Hricik, A., … Bender, C. (2007). I could lose everything: Understanding the cost of a brain tumor. *Journal of Neuro-Oncology, 85,* 329–338. doi:10.1007/s11060-007-9425-0

Carragee, E.J., & Vittum, D.W. (1996). Wound care after posterior spinal surgery: Does early bathing affect the rate of wound complications? *Spine, 21,* 2160–2162.

Catt, S., Chalmers, A., & Fallowfield, L. (2008). Psychosocial and supportive-care needs in high-grade glioma. *Lancet Oncology, 9,* 884–891. doi:10.1016/S1470-2045(08)70230-4

Celik, S.E., & Kara, A. (2007). Does shaving the incision site increase the infection rate after spinal surgery? *Spine, 32,* 1575–1577. doi:10.1097/BRS.0b013e318074c39f

de Gray, L.C., & Matta, B.F. (2005). Acute and chronic pain following craniotomy: A review. *Anaesthesia, 60,* 693–704. doi:10.1111/j.1365-2044.2005.03997.x.

Donovan, H., Sherwood, P., Bender, C., Cohen, S., Crighton, M., Lu, X., & Sereika, S. (2008). A comparison of three methods of symptom cluster identification [Abstract 3079]. *Oncology Nursing Forum, 35,* 552–553. Retrieved from http://ons.metapress.com/content/0285628p518235k4/fulltext.pdf

Durieux, M.E., & Himmelseher, S. (2007). Pain control after craniotomy: Off balance on the tightrope? *Journal of Neurosurgery, 106,* 207–209. doi:10.3171/jns.2007.106.2.207

Eberhart, L.H., Morin, A.M., Kranke, P., Missaghi, N.B., Durieux, M.E., & Himmelseher, S. (2007). Prevention and control of postoperative nausea and vomiting in post-craniotomy patients. *Best Practice and Research Clinical Anaesthesiology, 21,* 575–593.

Elliott, J.O., & Long, L. (2008). Perceived risk, resources, and perceptions concerning driving and epilepsy: A patient perspective. *Epilepsy and Behavior, 13,* 381–386. doi:10.1016/j.yebeh.2008.04.019

Fabling, J.M., Gan, T.J., Guy, J., Borel, C.O., el-Moalem, H.E., & Warner, D.S. (1997). Postoperative nausea and vomiting: A retrospective analysis in patients undergoing elective craniotomy. *Journal of Neurosurgical Anesthesia, 9,* 308–312.

Farace, E., Shaffrey, M., Huang, W., Litofsky, N.S., & Laws, E.R. (2002). Depression as an independent predictor of survival in malignant gliomas: Findings from the Glioma Outcomes Project [Abstract 152]. *Neuro-Oncology, 4,* 349. doi:10.1093/neuonc/4.4.308

Fox, S.W., Lyon, D., & Farace, E. (2007). Symptom clusters in patients with high-grade glioma. *Journal of Nursing Scholarship, 39,* 61–67. doi:10.1111/j.1547-5069.2007.00144.x

Gan, T.J. (2006). Risk factors for postoperative nausea and vomiting. *Anesthesia Analgesia, 102,* 1884–1898.

Hadorn, D.C., Baker, D., Hodges, J.S., & Hicks, N. (1996). Rating the quality of evidence for clinical practice guidelines. *Journal of Clinical Epidemiology, 49,* 749–754.

Irefin, S.A., Schubert, A., Bloomfield, E.L., DeBoer, G.E., Mascha, E.J., & Ebrahim, Z.Y. (2003). The effect of craniotomy location on postoperative pain and nausea. *Journal of Anesthesiology, 17,* 227–231. doi:10.1007/s00540-003-0182-8

Ireland, S., Carlino, K., Gould, L., Frazier, F., Haycock, P., Ilton, S., … Reddy, K. (2007). Shampoo after craniotomy: A pilot study. *Canadian Journal of Neuroscience Nursing, 29,* 14–18.

Janda, M., Eakin, E.G., Bailey, L., Walker, D., & Troy, K. (2006). Supportive care needs of people with brain tumours and their carers. *Supportive Care in Cancer, 14,* 1094–1103. doi:10.1007/s00520-006-0074-1

Janda, M., Stegina, S., Dunn, J., Langbecker, D., Walker, D., & Eakin, E. (2008). Unmet supportive care needs and interest in services among patients with a brain tumour and their carers. *Patient Education and Counseling, 71,* 251–258. doi:10.1016/j.pec.2008.01.020

Kincaid, M.S., & Lam, A.M. (2007). Pain and craniotomy. *Journal of Neurosurgery, 106,* 1136–1137. doi:10.3171/jns.2007.106.6.1136

Lingler, J.H., Sherwood, P.R., Crighton, M.H., Song, M., & Happ, M.B. (2008). Conceptual challenges in the study of caregiver-care recipient relationships. *Nursing Research, 57,* 367–372. doi:10.1097/01.NNR.0000313499.99851.0c

Lovely, M.P., Miaskowski, C., & Dodd, M. (1999). Relationship between fatigue and quality of life in patients with glioblastoma multiforme. *Oncology Nursing Forum, 26,* 921–925.

Magnusson, M.L., Pope, M.H., Wilder, D.G., Szpalski, M., & Spratt, K. (1999). Is there a rational basis for post-surgical lifting restrictions? I. Current understanding. *European Spine, 8,* 170–178.

McGregor, A.H., Dicken, B., & Jamrozik, K. (2006). National audit of postoperative management in spinal surgery. *BioMed Central Musculoskeletal Disorders, 7*(47). doi:10.1186/1471-2474-7-47

Mcilvoy, L., & Hinkle, J.L. (2008). What is evidence-based neuroscience nursing practice? *Journal of Neuroscience Nursing, 40,* 371–372.

Melnyk, B.M., & Fineout-Overholt, E. (2005). *Evidence-based practice in nursing and health care: A guide to best practice.* Philadelphia, PA: Lippincott Williams & Wilkins.

Miller, J.J., Weber, P.C., Patel, S., & Ramey, J. (2001). Intracranial surgery: To shave or not to shave. *Otology and Neurotology, 22,* 908–911.

Mukand, J.A., Blackinton, D.D., Crincoli, M.G., Lee, J.J., & Santos, B.B. (2001). Incidence of neurologic deficits and rehabilitation of patients with brain tumors. *American Journal of Physical Medicine and Rehabilitation, 80,* 346–350.

Nemergut, E.C., Durieux, M.E., Missaghi, N.B., & Himmelseher, S. (2007). Pain management after craniotomy. *Best Practice and Research Clinical Anaesthesiology, 21,* 557–573.

Neufeld, S.M., & Newburn-Cook, C.V. (2007). The efficacy of 5-HT$_3$ receptor antagonists for the prevention of postoperative nausea and vomiting after craniotomy: A meta-analysis. *Journal of Neurosurgical Anesthesiology, 19,* 10–17. doi:10.1097/01.ana.0000211025.41797.fc

Neufeld, S.M., Newburn-Cook, C.V., & Drummond, J.E. (2008). Prognostic models and risk scores: Can we accurately predict postoperative nausea and vomiting in children after craniotomy? *Journal of PeriAnesthesia Nursing, 23,* 300–310.

Oncology Nursing Society. (n.d.). ONS PEP topics. Retrieved from http://www.ons.org/Research/PEP/Topics

Ortiz-Cardona, J., & Bendo, A.A. (2007). Perioperative pain management in the neurosurgical patient. *Anesthesiology Clinics, 25,* 655–674. doi:10.1016/j.anclin.2007.05.003

Porter-O'Grady, T. (2010). A new age for practice: Creating the framework for evidence. In K. Malloch & T. Porter-O'Grady (Eds.), *Introduction to evidence-based practice in nursing and health care* (2nd ed., pp. 1–10). Sudbury, MA: Jones and Bartlett.

Ropka, M.E., & Spencer-Cisek, P. (2001). PRISM: Priority Symptom Management project phase I: Assessment. *Oncology Nursing Forum, 28,* 1585–1594.

Salander, P. (1996). Brain tumour as a threat to life and personality: The spouse's perspective. *Journal of Psychosocial Oncology, 14*(3), 1–18. doi:10.1300/J077v14n03_01

Schmer, C., Ward-Smith, P., Latham, S., & Salacz, M. (2008). When a family member has a malignant brain tumor: The caregiver perspective. *Journal of Neuroscience Nursing, 40,* 78–84.

Schultz, A.A. (2009). Evidence-based practice. *Nursing Clinics of North America, 44,* xv–xvii. doi:10.1016/j.cnur.2008.10.011

Sudheer, P.S., Logan, S.W., Terblanche, C., Ateleanu, B., & Hall, J.E. (2007). Comparison of the analgesic efficacy and respiratory effects of morphine, tramadol and codeine after craniotomy. *Anaesthesia, 62,* 555–560. doi:10.1111/j.1365-2044.2007.05038.x

Tang, K., & Sgouros, S. (2001). The influence of hair shave on the infection rate in neurosurgery: A prospective study. *Pediatric Neurosurgery, 35,* 13–17. doi:10.1159/000050379

Tanner, J., Woodings, D., & Moncaster, K. (2006). Preoperative hair removal to reduce surgical site infection. *Cochrane Database of Systematic Reviews,* 2006, Issue 3. Art. No.: CD004211. doi:10.1002/14651858.CD004122

Thibault, M., Girard, F., Moumdjian, R., Chouinard, P., Boudreault, D., & Ruel, M. (2007). Craniotomy site influences postoperative pain following neurosurgical procedures: A retrospective study. *Canadian Journal of Anesthesia, 54,* 544–548.

Tipton, J.M. (2009). PEP up your practice: An introduction to the Oncology Nursing Society Putting Evidence Into Practice resources. In L.H. Eaton & J.M. Tipton (Eds.), *Putting evidence into practice: Improving oncology patient outcomes* (pp. 1–8). Pittsburgh, PA: Oncology Nursing Society.

Williamson, J., Bulley, C., & Coutts, F. (2008). What do patients feel they can do following lumbar microdiscectomy? A qualitative study. *Disability and Rehabilitation, 30,* 1367–1373. doi:10.1080/09638280701639915

Index

The letter f *after a page number indicates that relevant content appears in a figure; the letter* t, *in a table.*